Outcome Measurement in Psychiatry

A CRITICAL REVIEW

Outcome Measurement in Psychiatry

A CRITICAL REVIEW

Edited by

Waguih William IsHak, M.D.
Tal Burt, M.D.
Lloyd I. Sederer, M.D.

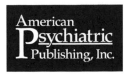

American Psychiatric Publishing, Inc.

Washington, DC
London, England

Copyright © 2002 American Psychiatric Publishing, Inc.
ALL RIGHTS RESERVED

Manufactured in the United States of America on acid-free paper
07   06   05   04   03   02   7   6   5   4   3   2   1
First Edition

American Psychiatric Publishing, Inc.
1400 K Street, N.W.
Washington, DC 20005
www.appi.org

Library of Congress Cataloging-in-Publication Data
Outcome measurement in psychiatry : a critical review / edited by Waguih William IsHak, Tal Burt, Lloyd I. Sederer.
    p. ; cm.
   Includes bibliographical references and index.
   ISBN 0-88048-119-6 (alk. paper)
    1. Outcome assessment (Medical care) 2. Psychiatry. I. IsHak, Waguih William, 1964–
II. Burt, Tal, 1960– III. Sederer, Lloyd I.
   [DNLM: 1. Psychiatry—organization & administration. 2. Outcome Assessment
(Health Care) WM 30 O938 2002]
   RC454.4 .O84 2002
   616.89—dc21

2001060301

British Library Cataloguing in Publication Data
A CIP record is available from the British Library.

To Drs. William, Nawara, Rafik, and Asbasia (one amazing woman) IsHak, for their inspiration, encouragement, and love.
WWI

To my family.
LIS

Contents

PART
I

Understanding Outcomes Assessment

PART
III

Challenges and
Opportunities

Contributors

Asher Aladjem, M.D.
Director, Consultation-Liaison Psychiatry Service, Bellevue Hospital Center; Clinical Assistant Professor, Department of Psychiatry, New York University School of Medicine, New York, New York

Antonio Almoguera-Abad, M.D.
Deputy Director, Forensic Psychiatry Service, Bellevue Hospital Center; Clinical Assistant Professor in Psychiatry, Department of Psychiatry, New York University School of Medicine, New York, New York

Murray Alpert, Ph.D.
Research Professor, Department of Psychiatry, New York University School of Medicine, New York, New York

Drew A. Anderson, Ph.D.
Assistant Professor, Department of Psychology, University at Albany–State University of New York, Albany, New York

Harry Baker, M.D.
Chief, Sleep Disorders Center; Coordinator, Psychiatry and Mental Health Department, Hospital Medica Sur, Mexico City, Mexico

Laura Berman, L.S.C.W., Ph.D.
Assistant Professor of Urology and Psychiatry, Department of Urology, Women's Sexual Health Clinic, University of California at Los Angeles, Los Angeles, California

Jennifer Berman, M.D.
Assistant Professor of Urology, Department of Urology, Women's Sexual Health Clinic, University of California at Los Angeles, Los Angeles, California

Carol A. Bernstein, M.D.
Director, Residency Training in Psychiatry; Associate Professor of Clinical Psychiatry, New York University School of Medicine, New York, New York

Tal Burt, M.D.
Medical Director, Depression/Anxiety Worldwide Team, Pfizer Inc.; Assistant Professor of Clinical Psychiatry, Columbia University College of Physicians and Surgeons, New York, New York

Alisa B. Busch, M.D., M.S.
Assistant Psychiatrist, McLean Hospital; Instructor in Psychiatry, Harvard Medical School, Belmont, Massachusetts

Annmarie Caracansi, M.D.
Fellow in Forensic Psychiatry, New York University School of Medicine, New York, New York

Gary R. Collins, M.D.
Clinical Instructor, Department of Psychiatry, New York University School of Medicine, New York, New York

Paul Crits-Christoph, Ph.D.
Professor of Psychology in Psychiatry and Director, Center for Psychotherapy Research, University of Pennsylvania, Philadelphia, Pennsylvania

Mary Beth Connolly, Ph.D.
Assistant Professor of Psychology in Psychiatry, University of Pennsylvania, Philadelphia, Pennsylvania

Donald Davidoff, Ph.D.
Psychologist in Charge, Special Care Unit, McLean Hospital; Instructor in Psychology (Department of Psychiatry), Harvard Medical School, Belmont, Massachusetts

Barbara Dickey, Ph.D.
Associate Professor, Department of Psychiatry, Harvard Medical School, The Cambridge Hospital, Cambridge, Massachusetts

Susan V. Eisen, Ph.D.
Health Research Scientist, Center for Health Quality, Outcomes, and Economic Research (CHQOER), E. N. Rogers Memorial Veterans Hospital, Bedford, Massachusetts; Research Associate, Health Services Department, Boston University School of Public Health, Boston, Massachusetts

William E. Falk, M.D.
Director, Outpatient Geriatric Psychiatry, Massachusetts General Hospital; Assistant Professor of Psychiatry, Harvard Medical School, Boston, Massachusetts

Peter Fonagy, Ph.D., F.B.A.
Freud Memorial Professor of Psychoanalysis, University College London; Director of Research, The Anna Freud Centre, London, United Kingdom; Coordinating Director, Child and Family Center and Center for Outcomes Research and Effectiveness, Menninger Foundation, Topeka, Kansas

Madeline Gladis, Ph.D.
Assistant Professor of Psychology in Psychiatry, University of Pennsylvania, Philadelphia, Pennsylvania

Shelly F. Greenfield, M.D., M.P.H.
Medical Director, Alcohol and Drug Abuse Ambulatory Treatment Program, McLean Hospital; Assistant Professor of Psychiatry, Harvard Medical School, Belmont, Massachusetts

Richard C. Hermann, M.D., M.S.
Assistant Professor of Psychiatry and Health Policy and Management, Harvard Medical School and Harvard School of Public Health; Director, Center for Quality Assessment and Improvement in Mental Health, Department of Psychiatry, Cambridge Hospital, Cambridge, Massachusetts

Waguih William IsHak, M.D.
Research Assistant Professor of Psychiatry, New York University School of Medicine; Director, Psychiatry Residency Training Program, Cedars-Sinai Medical Center, Los Angeles, California

Craig L. Katz, M.D.
Clinical Instructor, Department of Psychiatry, New York University School of Medicine, New York, New York

Monika E. Kolodziej, Ph.D.
Assistant Psychologist, McLean Hospital; Instructor in Psychology, Department of Psychiatry, Harvard Medical School, Belmont, Massachusetts

Russell F. Lim, M.D.
Assistant Clinical Professor, Department of Psychiatry, University of California, Davis, School of Medicine, Davis, California

Ciara Marley, B.A., M.A.
Medical Student, Boston University School of Medicine, Boston, Massachusetts

Joseph P. Merlino, M.D., M.P.A.
Professor of Psychiatry, New York University School of Medicine; Director, Ambulatory and Community Psychiatry Division, Bellevue Hospital Center, New York, New York

Vivian M. Mougios, M.A.
Doctoral Candidate, Doctoral Program in Clinical Psychology, Long Island University (Brooklyn Campus), Brooklyn, New York

Grayson S. Norquist, M.D., M.S.P.H.
Director, Division of Services and Intervention Research, National Institute of Mental Health, Bethesda, Maryland

John M. Oldham, M.D.
Professor and Chair, Department of Psychiatry, Medical University of South Carolina, Charleston, South Carolina

Lewis A. Opler, M.D., Ph.D.
Director, Research Division, New York State Office of Mental Health; Adjunct Professor of Psychiatry, Columbia University College of Physicians and Surgeons, New York, New York

Anand A. Pandya, M.D.
Associate Unit Chief, Inpatient Teaching Unit, Bellevue Hospital Center; Clinical Instructor, Department of Psychiatry, New York University School of Medicine, New York, New York

Roy H. Perlis, M.D.
Staff Psychiatrist, Department of Psychiatry, Massachusetts General Hospital; Instructor in Psychiatry, Harvard Medical School, Boston, Massachusetts

J. Christopher Perry, M.P.H., M.D.
Professor of Psychiatry, McGill University; Director of Research, Institute of Community and Family Psychiatry, Sir Mortimer B. Davis Jewish General Hospital, Montreal, Quebec, Canada; Lecturer in Psychiatry, Harvard Medical School at The Austen Riggs Center, Stockbridge, Massachusetts

Eric D. Peselow, M.D.
Research Professor of Psychiatry, New York University School of Medicine, New York, New York

Paul Michael Ramirez, Ph.D.
Associate Professor, Doctoral Program in Clinical Psychology, Long Island University (Brooklyn Campus), Brooklyn, New York

Donald L. Round, Ph.D.
Assistant Director, Neuropsychological and Psychodiagnostic Testing Center; Assistant Director, Neuropsychology Fellowship Program, McLean Hospital; Instructor in Psychology, Department of Psychiatry, Harvard Medical School, Belmont, Massachusetts

Natali H. Sanlian, M.Ps.
Research Assistant, Institute of Community and Family Psychiatry, Sir Mortimer B. Davis Jewish General Hospital, Montreal, Quebec, Canada

Manuel Santos, M.D.
Attending Psychiatrist, Consultation-Liaison Service, Bellevue Hospital Center, New York, New York

Melanie Schwarz, M.D.
Attending Psychiatrist, Consultation-Liaison Service, Bellevue Hospital Center; Clinical Instructor, Department of Psychiatry, New York University School of Medicine, New York, New York

Lloyd I. Sederer, M.D.
Director, Division of Clinical Services, American Psychiatric Association, Washington, D.C.; Associate Clinical Professor of Psychiatry, Harvard Medical School, Boston, Massachusetts

Zebulon Taintor, M.D.
Professor of Psychiatry and Vice Chairman, Department of Psychiatry, New York University School of Medicine, New York, New York

Manuel Trujillo, M.D.
Professor of Clinical Psychiatry and Vice Chairman, Department of Psychiatry, New York University School of Medicine; Director, Psychiatry Department, Bellevue Hospital Center, New York, New York

Sumer Verma, M.D.
Director, Geriatric Psychiatry Fellowship Program, McLean Hospital; Lecturer in Psychiatry, Harvard Medical School; Associate Professor of Psychiatry, Boston University School of Medicine, Belmont, Massachusetts

Henry C. Weinstein, M.D.
Clinical Professor of Psychiatry, New York University School of Medicine, New York, New York

Roger D. Weiss, M.D.
Clinical Director, Alcohol and Drug Abuse Program, McLean Hospital; Associate Professor of Psychiatry, Harvard Medical School, Belmont, Massachusetts

Donald A. Williamson, Ph.D.
Chief, Health Psychology, Pennington Biomedical Research Center, Baton Rouge, Louisiana

Mary Christina Zierak, B.A., M.A.
Medical Student, Temple University School of Medicine, Philadelphia, Pennsylvania

Introduction

The price wars in medicine have taken their toll. Fifteen years of for-profit and then not-for-profit corporate medicine, with cost control as the primary demand, have imperiled medicine for the first time in more than 60 years. Nowhere in medicine has the impact been greater than in the field of psychiatry.

But the public is now restive. Not only doctors and hospitals cry concern that patient care is being compromised to the altar of economics. No patient or family is exempt from feeling the hurried, belt-tightened, all too error-prone atmosphere of medicine of this new millennium.

Enter quality. Slowly and steadily the technology of quality has migrated from production and high-technology industries into medicine. Quality can be defined, measured, publicly reported, and compared among sites of service, and the results can be used to improve the care provided. In addition to being protective of the budgets of the government and businesses that chiefly fund the enterprise, medical services must be accountable to the recipients of care. The assessment, reporting, and improvement of patient care offers the public and the medical profession a language and a means of accountability that are needed to help quiet mounting concerns about the current practice of medicine.

Measures of quality link what care was rendered to the results (outcomes) of that care, good and bad. As complex as medical care has become, it need not be opaque to the public eye. What was done, to whom, when, and with what outcome forms the basis of assessing quality. A paucity of reliable, valid, and standardized measures is no longer a barrier to outcomes assessment in medicine in general and psychiatry in particular, although admittedly this remains a young science. Patients, families, clinicians, and purchasers can be scientifically informed about quality and safety, as they have come to expect in so many other vital aspects of their lives.

The assessment of psychiatric care spans a variety of domains, or areas of interest and importance. We can measure whether or not symptoms are improved. We can measure functioning, a domain that includes work and social relations, as well as self-care and daily activities. Related to functioning is quality of life, or the person's experience of how life feels, not just how symptoms and functioning appear. Another important domain is the patient's (or family's) perception of the care he or she received: the humane, interpersonal experience of trust, dignity, and communication that is so vital not only to receiving care, but also to feeling cared for.

The field of outcomes assessment in psychiatry, although young, allows us to assess the actual measures by which care is assessed. Standards are emerging by which we can judge the quality of our measurement instruments. Do these instruments actually measure what they purport to measure (validity)? Do they do so in a reproducible manner (reliability)? Can they be feasibly used in clinical practice without exceeding the already strained margins of clinicians and information systems? Will they generate information that is meaningful to patients and professionals, and will that information be actionable—that is, will it serve as a practical basis for improving care? And finally, will the information gathered allow us to make accurate comparisons of the care provided by different doctors, hospitals, and systems of care? A critical appraisal of measurement instruments needs to judge them by these standards.

We undertook to publish this book because we believed that a critical analysis of outcomes assessment was needed. Our aim was to produce a text—more than an inventory or nosology of measures—that would hold existing instruments to clear standards and thereby provide clinicians and clinical administrators with a reference to guide them in selecting and implementing quality measures in clinical practice.

The text is organized into three parts. Part I has four chapters that offer detailed explanations of many of the fundamental concepts that underlie outcome measurement. The first chapter is a conceptual and policy piece intended to provide a type of "situational analysis" of outcomes assessment and describe the scientific and policy work ahead. The remaining chapters of this part concern the scientific underpinnings of the field as well as clarification and differentiation of important constructs (e.g., process and outcome, efficacy and effectiveness, basic statistics, and quality improvement). Part II is the critical review of a wide variety, albeit a selected set, of instruments. We asked contributors to focus on instruments that had high clinical utility, that preferably were in the public domain or of low cost and burden, and that met many of the standards noted above. The chapters in this section are organized by patient populations to enable readers to home in on measures that more precisely meet the needs of their services; these measures are critically assessed for their scientific integrity and clinical utility. The patient populations are determined by age, diagnoses, and disorders. Within each chapter are included measures that are general mental health instruments as well as those that are specific to a particular disease or disorder. The instruments vary in their respondents (which include patients, families, and clinicians), thereby offering clinicians a choice of whom to sample. The data these instruments generate can be used to assess outcome for individual patients, populations, and programs. Their value is in demonstrating effectiveness; providing comparison among clinicians, service sites and systems; serving as a basis for quality improvement; and meeting a host of accreditation, regulatory, and contractual demands.

Part III reflects many important yet manageable challenges that outcome measurement brings to clinical practice. Five chapters discuss the impediments characteristic to implementing assessment programs; regulatory and accreditation demands; confidentiality and training; and the technology of measurement. These chapters aim to outline challenges and teach solutions based on experience. The final chapter suspends today's limitations and imagines what innovations may come our way in the years to come.

The delivery of psychiatric and substance use services is becoming inextricably bound to outcome measurement. We believe this is warranted to meet the mandate of public accountability, so long as measurement itself does not become a hollow, burdensome, and costly appendage to health care. It is our hope that this text will provide clinicians and clinical leaders with some of the tools needed to meaningfully incorporate quality measurement into clinical practice.

ACKNOWLEDGMENTS

Waguih William IsHak, M.D., would like to aknowledge the priceless mentorship of Benjamin Sadock, M.D., Manuel Trujillo, M.D., and Carol Bernstein, M.D., in addition to the invaluable trust by Norman Sussman, M.D., Robert Cancro, M.D., and Brian Ladds, M.D., at the Department of Psychiatry of NYU School of Medicine.

The editors would like to personally thank Claire Reinburg, Pam Harley, and Martin Lynds, who were instrumental in bringing this volume to light, as well as Jeremy Revell, M.D., for his valuable contribution to graphic designs. We would also like to acknowledge the valuable advice provided by Jean Endicott, Ph.D., in the preliminary phases of this work.

PART
I

Understanding Outcomes Assessment

CHAPTER 1

Role of Outcome Measurement in Psychiatry

Grayson S. Norquist, M.D., M.S.P.H.

The measurement of quality has been important for some time and predates the current concern about how managed care affects quality. The Joint Commission on Accreditation of Healthcare Organizations was established during the middle of the last century to evaluate hospitals. Assessment of the quality of health care expanded as measurement improved and concern arose about the quality of health care in the United States. A number of organizations were formed during the past few years to provide measures of quality and to perform assessments of health care organizations (e.g., National Committee for Quality Assurance, Foundation for Accountability, and various vendors of quality measures). Recent reports by the Institute of Medicine (1999), such as the one on medication errors, have emphasized the importance of measuring quality of care and finding ways to improve it. With the advent of managed care, there has been even greater general interest in ensuring that the quality of care delivered in such systems does not deteriorate.

In the United States, the President's Advisory Commission on Consumer Protection and Quality in the Health Care Industry was established to respond to public concern about health care quality. The commission issued a proposal for a consumer bill of rights that included the right to information and access to appropriate emergency and specialty care. Because the commission decided that the quality of health care provided in the United States was not as good as it could be, it called for the establishment of a national advisory council on quality and a forum in the private sector that would bring various groups together to develop a set of core measures for quality measurement. The Department of Health and Human Services established the Quality Interagency Coordination Task Force to identify opportunities for interagency collaboration to initiate projects that would improve the quality of care in health programs supported by the federal government. In addition, the Institute of Medicine was recently asked to develop recommendations for a national quality report on health care delivery.

As outlined in other chapters of this book, there are various ways to measure quality of care in mental health. Most efforts at assessing the quality of health care are based on a model outlined by Avedis Donabedian. He conceptualized several domains of quality, including structure, process, and outcome (Donabedian 1980, 1996). *Structure* refers to the context in which the care is delivered and includes such things as population, community and provider characteristics, and the type of health care organization. *Process* refers to what happens in the clinician/consumer encounter and includes such aspects as technical and interpersonal excellence. *Outcome* refers to the result of the health care intervention and includes such things as clinical symptoms, functional status, satisfaction, life expectancy, and economic indicators. Although most efforts at measuring quality use some assessment of all three of these aspects, the most popular currently is measurement of outcome.

In addition, many measurement tools have expanded to incorporate other aspects such as access to health care to indicate quality. Other proposed frameworks expand beyond medical care to include a broader look at the health system and aspects other than medical process (e.g., day-to-day living, caregiver support, education). Current efforts are moving from simply measuring structure, process, and outcome and are focusing more on reduction of variation by publicizing evidence-based information and attempting to have providers adhere to guidelines based on this information.

One way of conceptualizing the concerns about quality of health care is to place them into three major areas: 1) underuse of appropriate care, 2) overuse of health services that have greater risk than benefit, and 3) misuse of health services. Access to appropriate care is probably the major issue in the mental health field, although there has been recent concern about the possible misuse of psychotropic medications in children.

Studies of quality of care in mental health have used controlled clinical trials to study the efficacy of an intervention and to link it with a particular outcome; observational studies have also been used to determine what actually happens in clinic encounters. Much of the previous quality work has focused on determining variation in mental health services across sites and determining whether providers within sites adhere to certain treatment guidelines. It is known that there is wide variation in the use of certain psychotropic medications and in the length of hospital stays. However, some of the variation may reflect poor access to services due to inequalities in social services. There is wide undertreatment of depression, and the Schizophrenia Patient Outcomes Research Team showed that treatment practices for schizophrenia often fell short of evidence-based guidelines (Lehman and Steinwachs 1998).

PROMISES AND PITFALLS OF MEASURING QUALITY

Outcomes are the most sought-after measures of quality because they indicate the ultimate impact of the health care delivered to a person. This is what people want to know: If I obtain this intervention, will I get better? The ideal is a single measure that would tell people that if they go to a certain provider they have a better chance of success than if they went to another provider. However, such an ideal does not exist and is not likely ever to exist. It is naïve to assume that a single measure can adequately convey the impact of something as complex as health care. Therefore, research efforts are targeted toward formulating a set of measures that will reflect how a health care intervention and the health system affect a person's health status. Once those measures are identified, it is necessary to find ways of assessing them in populations and health care systems. This is not an easy task. Even more difficult is finding ways to actually improve the quality of health care when there is evidence of a problem.

Because outcome measures are so popular, it is important to consider the potential problems in using them. One concern is how the measure will be used. Is it to help consumers make a choice, or is it to help improve the quality of care being delivered? The answer to this question can affect what measures are used. The problem is that no currently available outcome measure can provide the simple answers that consumers, providers, employers, and policy makers want. Most are very subjective measures without grounding in scientific evidence. In addition, outcomes may be affected by factors outside the control of the medical system, and the relevance of these factors to the particular treatment intervention may not be apparent for years. Many of the available outcome measures were studied on homogeneous populations at limited geographic sites and have not been validated on heterogeneous populations, especially those with comorbid conditions. In addition, some measures are individual based and others are population-based. Although population based measures have the ability to detect potential underuse of services, individual measures are better at focusing on the quality of care given to a person who presents for services. Certain outcomes (e.g., developmental status in children) may change over time (Mangione-Smith and McGlynn 1998). Using an infrequent event for an outcome is problematic, because it may not be possible to detect statistically significant variation. More than 2,000 observations may be needed for a meaningful conclusion to be made. It may be necessary to apply condition-specific measures at the health plan level if sample sizes are constrained at a lower level.

One particularly problematic category of outcome measures is the frequency of adverse events. Measuring such events requires that adjustments be made to account for differences due to severity and case mix. At present there are no reliable ways to do this. Particularly problematic are rare adverse events such as death, because the power to detect statistically significant differences is often lacking. One possible approach is to determine if the adverse event was preventable. A case-control design could be used in such situations, because the sample size needed for comparisons is not large. However, even if adjustments are made for severity and case mix, additional adjustments are still needed for factors outside the health system if the comparisons are to be fair. Therefore, either the measures must be limited to those that cover processes or outcomes under the control of the health system, or adjustments must be made for confounding factors so the actual contribution of the health systems can be determined. Also, good outcomes can occur despite rather than because of the care provided, and bad outcomes can occur despite the best of care.

Clients for outcome measures have similar data requirements, but often their needs conflict and can cause difficulty for providers who must collect the data. A managed care plan may want access, utilization, and cost data, but providers are often interested in specific clinical outcomes and detection of cases. Employers who are making decisions about plans from year to year want immediate results, but meaningful data are not often so readily available. So, the field may be moving toward a system that is concerned only with the quantity of outcome measures rather than ensuring that the mental health care delivered in the system is the best possible.

Process measures are important but are not useful unless they can show a linkage to outcomes (especially functional outcomes). Yet many believe that once a certain process is shown to have a good outcome, then its presence in a health encounter means that good quality of care has occurred. Process measures are particularly helpful because they provide clearer opportunities to determine where one can intervene to improve care. Today process measures come from clinical guidelines. Unfortunately, these guidelines are usually based on studies that are relevant only to very select populations. Also, guidelines are rarely updated and may become irrelevant for current practice.

Structural measures have been used in the past and are still used currently. However, they are of little use unless they can be linked to variations in process and outcomes. Even so, very few have been shown to predict such variation, so their importance has declined in the past several years.

Even with worthwhile quality-of-care measures, there is little evidence that consumers will use the information in a manner that will be helpful to them. For example, most outcome measures used now are not well understood by the average person. Many consumers are not particularly interested in using information for comparative purposes. It is primarily those who are considering changing health plans who would have an interest in such information. Consumers consistently rate cost, choice of providers, and evidence of good doctor-patient relationships as important factors in making a choice about a health plan. Studies show that people value what other people say and what preventive interventions are offered. They are least likely to find reports of adverse events (e.g., number of low–birth-weight infants) helpful. Therefore, consumers may prefer patient ratings and prevention measures (doctor communications, satisfaction, mammogram rates) than more objective, clinically based measures (hospital death rates after heart attack, rates of postsurgery complications) that are not as well understood. General measures of mortality rates seem to mean less than a single unexpected event reported in the press. Therefore, it is important to make sure that what is measured either is important to consumers or is understandable to the public.

CURRENT STATUS AND NEEDS IN THE OUTCOME MEASUREMENT FIELD

Work is needed in several areas. The first is the development of improved measures of quality and the evidence to support them. The second is the area of improved assessment techniques. The third, and probably most important, is the development of interventions to improve the quality of care delivered.

In the measurement area, the most important effort is to be able to link what is done in the patient encounter with the ultimate impact of that intervention (i.e., linking process with outcome). The most important way to do that is to conduct research that shows which interventions work for particular illnesses in specific populations. This is the basis for evidence-based medical practice.

Even with the ability to link process to outcome, there will still be a need for quality measures that are meaningful and reflect the needs of all potential clients of quality data. Such clients include consumers, families, physicians, health systems, employers, payers, policy makers, and researchers. Consumers are interested in indicators of recovery and some sense of empowerment (e.g., Is a clinician willing to listen to my treatment preferences?). In addition, many believe that continuity of care is an important concept that needs to be assessed. Unfortunately, this is not an easy factor to measure and will require qualitative techniques such as ethnographic analyses. In mental health, clinical outcome measures usually focus only on outcomes related to mental illness and do not assess other potential comorbid conditions such as medical illnesses or substance abuse.

Functional outcome measures are important to all users because they measure concepts that are the ultimate goal of any intervention: improved functional status. In addition, because functional measures can be used across a variety of illnesses, they decrease the total number of measures needed in a health system. Yet they will vary depending on who provides the information. Employers are interested not only in measures of function but also in workplace variables (e.g., number of days missed from work). Because relevant workplace variables are hard to measure, employers often fall back on access, utilization, and satisfaction measures. Health plans want to know about clinical indicators, satisfaction, and expenditures (e.g., whether interventions are cost effective). Providers are most interested in clinical status and life expectancy (e.g., whether treatment A works better than treatment B). Policy makers are interested in expenditures and public health (e.g., cost for an incremental increase in public health). Researchers are interested in all outcome domains.

Once meaningful and valid quality measures exist, adequate ways of assessing quality are needed. This requires the availability of various data sources, such as encounter-level data, enrollment data, survey data, and clinical data. Medical records that provide encounter data are helpful for determining the technical aspects of care but are poor at determining interpersonal aspects of care and what happens in the outpatient setting. Surveys of consumers are able to detect clinical symptoms and interpersonal aspects but are poor at technical process. Administrative data are useful for examining the number of visits and the tests that are used but do not provide information about the content of the visit or the results of the tests that are ordered. Therefore, it is necessary to ensure that an appropriate data source is available for the particular aspect of care that is being assessed. For example, information on access to care can be obtained through surveys of consumers, whereas information on use of services is probably best obtained through administrative data systems. Data on clinical outcomes of care can be obtained from medical records, but functional status information is best obtained through consumer surveys.

Many of the factors that affect health are social (e.g., community violence, environmental factors), and their relationship to health is unclear. What interventions are most likely to help these factors and for what should the health system be held accountable? More work in the interface between the social sciences and clinical treatment could help answer this question. If one acts on imperfect information, then one could increase costs, put excellent health plans out of business, disenfranchise groups with special needs, and have an impact on public health.

Methodology is important. Qualitative and quantitative research must be done on quality measures. For example, qualitative techniques such as cognitive testing and readability analyses would be helpful, whereas quantitative techniques such as psychometric testing are essential. Sampling must be such that one can generalize to a population of interest and provide representation of important subgroups. Response rates are important to ensure comparability. A core set of measures helps everyone, but specific measures may be needed for certain illnesses. Once data are ready, the presentation must be such that the amount of information is not overwhelming and provides the detail needed to inform action.

Efforts to improve quality of care have focused on regulation, competition, quality improvement programs, and economic incentives. However, no single one of these approaches works well. Multiple approaches are needed. Regulation can set the norm for what is expected and help to eliminate very poor care. However, there is an opportunity to use regulation to put into place what is known to work. For example, studies show that facilities that do large numbers of a particular intervention (e.g., surgical procedures) have better outcomes than those that do few of the same intervention. With regulation, the number of facilities that are allowed to do these complex interventions could be restricted. In addition, it could be mandated that the same data be collected on all consumers of health services. This would make it possible to produce risk-adjusted data.

Competition can be a powerful tool, but it must be used to actually improve quality. To compete on quality requires that data are valid and useful. If there are a variety of measures of quality, no one hospital will score high on all of them. It is possible that consumers or health plans might segregate themselves to take advantage of the most positive results that relate to them. Thus, it may be better to improve care in general and not focus on showing that one particular clinic is better than another. Given these problems, it is no surprise that competition currently is based on price and not quality.

Efforts to improve the quality of care in the community have primarily been limited to single institutions, although some multisite programs have recently been instituted. However, even those tend to be short-term fixes. Financial incentives can certainly influence the delivery of treatments, but it is still unclear how much of an impact they can have on quality and how best to use them to improve the quality of care delivered. In addition, more basic behavioral research is needed to understand why consumers and providers choose to use or not use particular interventions.

FUTURE DIRECTIONS

More work is clearly needed to improve measures of quality. One particular area that needs development is the evidence base for what interventions to use in mental illnesses and how well they work in various populations. Previous treatment intervention research has utilized restricted populations that cannot be generalized to people seen in most community clinics. In addition, it has not been clear how well these interventions work when not used by highly trained personnel in tertiary treatment centers. Efforts are currently under way to expand treatment intervention research into much broader populations and treatment settings so that results are more relevant to community practice. With results from these new studies there will soon be better evidence on which to base treatment guidelines.

Measures in mental health are either from self-reporting or clinical observation. Without biological measures it is often difficult to have reliable and valid measures for outcome. However, research is being undertaken to look for biological measures in mental illnesses. Work now in progress using new brain imaging technology may one day inform the choice of treatment interventions and indicate changes after treatment that could be used as outcome measures.

Developing a way to assess functional status is a critical part of current research efforts in measurement development. Several studies in the United States and at international sites are now focusing on ways to measure functional status. An important aspect of this research is delineating the contributions of health care and illness to a person's functional status.

To improve the ability to assess quality of care in the community, new methodological research will be needed (Dickey et al. 1998). Research is now incorporating both quantitative and qualitative methods. In addition, researchers have been encouraged to explore the relationship between the mental health field and other disciplines that have had similar issues in quality assessment, such as quality engineering.

Another area of current research is examining the appropriate time to measure an outcome. When has the intervention had enough time to have an effect? Most disorders are chronic, and therefore a number of confounding variables occur during long follow-up periods. Current treatment intervention research is expanding follow-up periods to look for effects at much later times (i.e., several years). Observational studies are being used to study people with illnesses for long periods to determine what variables other than the treatment intervention have an impact on outcomes.

In addition, work is now being devoted to interventions specific to the recovery and maintenance phase of illness.

The need to collect a variety of data to measure all aspects of quality and the impact of health care and the health system on health status can place a burden on providers and consumers. New technological innovations for data collection could be useful in collecting such data and decreasing the burden on respondents. However, the collection of so much personal data raises concerns about protection of confidentiality. Therefore, a compromise will need to be reached to ensure that the data needed are collected but that the individual consumer's confidentiality is protected. Encryption technology and restricting the type of data to only that needed for summary measures may make this compromise easier.

Even with the best evidence for treatments and adequate measures, there is no guarantee that people will use the interventions that are considered to produce the best outcomes. Therefore, work is needed on how to have providers, consumers, and systems change their behavior. In addition, it is necessary to move beyond simply providing information and instead find ways to better educate the public about quality-of-care information and understanding what forms of information are most helpful. Formal continuing medical education programs have minimal effect on what happens in a practice. Information does not change the behavior of consumers, and clinicians do not routinely follow treatment guidelines. Interventions that help people make decisions are needed (e.g., decision support tools). Centrally derived treatment guidelines are less acceptable in the community, where there is no sense of ownership. What may be best is to have a centrally supported site for development of the evidence for guidelines. Local communities could then develop their own guidelines using data from such sites.

The future will see more efforts to develop national and regional reports on health care quality. However, there are no real accepted quality accounting principles, no tradition of public disclosure of health outcomes, no rewards for those whose high quality attracts the worst financial risks, and little evidence that consumers respond to comparative information on quality. It may be necessary to make a choice between measures of health care delivery and measures of health status. If both are needed, then they must be linked. Indicators are most useful if they are nationally representative, actionable, and evidence based and affect a large portion of the population. The challenge for the mental health field is not simply to find better measures of quality of care but to develop interventions that will actually improve the quality of care.

Assessment of quality of care is a part of the future and will likely become even more important in determining resource allocations. Clinicians must become partners in the process of developing measurements and implementation plans. Without such investment, they will lose the opportunity to have a say in a process that will likely have a major impact on the way they practice in the future.

REFERENCES

Dickey B, Hermann RC, Eisen SV: Assessing the quality of psychiatric care: research methods and application in clinical practice. Harv Rev Psychiatry 6:88–96, 1998

Donabedian A: Explorations in Quality Assessment and Monitoring. Vol 1, The Definition of Quality and Approaches to Its Assessment. Ann Arbor, MI, Health Administration Press, 1980

Donabedian A: Evaluating the quality of medical care. Milbank Memorial Fund Quarterly 44:166–206, 1996

Institute of Medicine, Committee on Quality of Health Care in America: To Err Is Human. Washington, DC, National Academy Press, 1999

Lehman AF, Steinwachs DM: Patterns of usual care for schizophrenia: initial results from the schizophrenia PORT client survey. Schizophr Bull 24:1–10, 1998

Mangione-Smith R, McGlynn EA: Assessing the quality of healthcare provided to children. Health Serv Res 33:1059–1090, 1998

SUGGESTED READINGS

Chassin MR: Assessing strategies for quality improvement. Health Aff (Millwood) 16:151–161, 1997

Feldman J: How will mental health outcomes data be used in private systems? New Dir Ment Health Serv 71:103–109, 1996

Hibbard JH, Jewett JJ: Will quality report cards help consumers? Health Aff (Millwood) 16:218–228, 1997

Kassirer JP: The quality of care and the quality of measuring it. N Engl J Med 329:1263–1265, 1993

McGlynn EA, Norquist GS, Wells KB, et al: Quality-of-care research in mental health: responding to the challenge. Inquiry 25:157–170, 1988

Norquist G, Hyman SE: Advances in understanding and treating mental illness: implications for policy. Health Affairs 18:32–47, 1988

Wells KB, Katon W, Rogers B, et al: Use of minor tranquilizers and antidepressant medications by depressed outpatients: results from the Medical Outcomes Study. Am J Psychiatry 151:694–700, 1994a

Wells KB, Norquist G, Benjamin B, et al: Quality of antidepressant medications prescribed at discharge to depressed elderly patients in general medical hospitals before and after prospective payment system. Gen Hosp Psychiatry 16:4–15, 1994b

Outcome Measurement From Research to Clinical Practice

Barbara Dickey, Ph.D.

Measuring the clinical and functional outcomes of mental health treatment is hardly a new idea. Medical practice today rests on centuries of astute observations made by clinical practitioners who sought to alleviate the pain and suffering of their patients. These practitioners learned that trying different treatments led to different results—or, as we would say today, different outcomes. Sometimes these observations were recorded, but when twentieth-century science, with its more systematic methods, shaped the ethos of medicine, the measurement of treatment outcomes became a statistically based discipline. Until recently, the measurement of outcomes has been limited to research. However, among the many changes taking place in health care today, one is the use of outcome measures without research experience.

As the focus of outcome measurement shifts from clinical trials to clinical practice, psychometric standards are being raised. This means that studies that report treatment outcomes can be interpreted with greater confidence than was previously possible. The field of psychometrics has developed reliability and validity standards that ensure that measures are sound and robust. This is important, because the level of measurement "noise" increases as the design of studies shifts away from experimental methods. Measurement noise is the amount of error in a particular measure. It increases as experimental research design gives way to less rigorous data collection protocols. To balance the increase in measurement noise, more psychometrically robust outcome measurements are needed. Fortunately, a number of excellent instruments are available today, although achieving good reliability and validity in outcome instruments is neither quickly done nor cheaply accomplished. In other words, "homegrown" instruments—whether to measure satisfaction or mental health status—do not meet needed psychometric standards.

The purpose of this chapter is to illustrate the range of outcome assessments and to help readers determine what type of assessment best suits their needs. To set the stage, four types of outcome studies that might take place in any health care facility are outlined:

- In some hospital treatment units, medication *efficacy studies* use volunteers from whom consent is sought to randomly assign them to a new experimental treatment or a placebo treatment. The study protocol usually calls for the clinical outcome of each person in the study to be measured.
- Elsewhere in the same facility, patients might be part of an *effectiveness study* examining the quality of their treatment under a certain type of managed care program. These patients are not randomly assigned but give consent to be enrolled in the study and to have their treatment records reviewed and their insurance claims examined. They also give permission to have their treatment outcome assessed.
- All patients admitted for treatment might be given the opportunity on discharge to complete a survey on their perceptions of the care they received. These data can then be used to identify problems so that a *continuous quality improvement* committee can investigate ways to improve those problems.
- Finally, in response to licensing, regulatory, or payer groups, the facility might be required to supply *performance measures* such as rates of seclusion and restraint. These rates might then be used in a report card format to compare the performance of facilities or health networks.

EFFICACY RESEARCH

Measuring outcomes in clinical trials is not the same thing as measuring outcomes in clinical practice. Classic clinical trials, characterized by double-blind experimental research designs, enroll volunteers as subjects if they meet the criteria established by the principal investigator. Subjects are homogeneous and have the same diagnosis and few if any complicating medical problems. The goal of efficacy studies is to test a new treatment (e.g., a new medication) under ideal circumstances. If the treatment does not have the desired effect, then it is very unlikely to work in a less-than-ideal environment. Thus, all new treatments undergo efficacy testing and need to do so for approval by the U.S. Food and Drug Administration. The audience for this type of study generally consists of other investigators, those who sponsor the new treatment, and those who will regulate it.

Careful selection of outcome instruments in efficacy studies means focusing on very specific effects of the new treatment. The well-known Brief Psychiatric Response Scale (BPRS) was designed in 1962 (Overall and Gorham 1962) to test the effects of new antipsychotic medication. These new drugs were developed to directly affect psychotic symptoms and behavior, which became the focus of the BPRS. In clinical trials of antipsychotic drugs, selection of an instrument that measures a global level of functioning would not have been a good choice because of the imprecision of such measures with respect to the particular desired outcomes (see Table 2–1).

EFFECTIVENESS RESEARCH

Once the efficacy of a particular treatment has been established and the treatment has been introduced into practice, a different type of research becomes appropriate. It is well known that medications and other treatments that had a favorable response in clinical trials are often less effective with the general population. This apparent reduction in effect has been repeatedly demonstrated by effectiveness studies. Effectiveness studies assess the outcomes of new treatments under less-than-ideal conditions— conditions that replicate the environment in which most patients are treated. These conditions include busy ambulatory settings such as clinics, outpatient clinics, and emergency rooms. The patients themselves are also not ideal: they may have more than one psychiatric disorder, may have chronic medical conditions, may seek help from multiple providers, or may not follow through with the treatment prescribed.

Compared with efficacy studies, there are several substantial differences in how effectiveness studies are conducted (Brook and Lohr 1985). Researchers relax the enrollment criteria and do not exclude individuals unless participation in the study is medically contraindicated. Furthermore, the analysis is planned in such a way as to include not only subjects

Table 2–1.   Characteristics of outcome research and outcome study activities

Study activities	Design	Target group	Represents	Data sources	Outcomes	Analysis	Audience
Research							
Efficacy	Experimental	Homogeneous, volunteers	Those who comply with treatment	Clinician, patients	Treatment response, side effects	Significance tests, difference	Those who sponsor new treatments
Effectiveness	Observational	Typical patients	Intent to treat	Clinician, patients	Treatment response, side effects	Dropouts in analysis	Clinicians, policy makers, consumers
Clinical practice							
TQM/CQI	Ad hoc	Those receiving treatment	Other patients	MIS, clinicians, patients	Systems performance	Link quality to outcome	Clinical staff, administration
Report cards	Observational	Population treated	Plan members	MIS	Quality of care, morbidity, mortality	Rates	Purchasers of care, consumers, members

Note.   MIS=management information system; TQM/CQI=total quality management/continuous quality improvement.

that get the full treatment, but also those who drop out during the study period (i.e., the design includes those for whom the treatment is intended). The design of the study may not be experimental, but rather observational, which involves observing (and recording) the actual practice of treatment without attempting to intervene in choices that patients make about where they seek treatment or which treatments they receive (Wells et al. 1994).

The outcomes measured in effectiveness studies include effects that are meaningful to patients, policy makers, or consumers who are considering treatment choices. The Medical Outcomes Study (Brook et al. 1986) is a good example of an effectiveness study. In one segment of the study, adults treated for depression were identified, their treatment was recorded, and subjects were followed up with a self-report measure of their outcome. Because this study enrolled thousands of subjects, lengthy, detailed outcome instruments were not a good choice. Both the high cost of collecting the data and the burden on respondents influenced the investigators' decision to use instruments especially suited for a study of the effects of different health plans on medical outcomes. The measurement focused on general physical and mental health status, not specific clinical symptoms or disease-specific outcomes. The advantage to this approach was the capacity to compare physical and mental health status across several disease groups. The study results were useful to policy makers because the results would provide outcomes from treatment in different health care settings (health maintenance organizations, solo practice, group practice).

Data collection in effectiveness studies may be from several sources: patient self-reports and administrative data from insurance companies or health plans, and less frequently from physician assessments. Patients who drop out are usually included in the analysis, because it is important to understand the outcomes of these subjects and why they dropped out.

CONTINUOUS QUALITY IMPROVEMENT

Even effectiveness research does not provide an optimal platform for measuring outcome in everyday clinical practice. The insistent call for improved quality of care and provider accountability has raised outcomes measurement to new importance. However, there is danger in assuming that what is known from studies will meet the challenges of continuous quality improvement (CQI). Although the selection of outcome measures must be guided by criteria that include strong psychometric instrument properties, just as they would in research projects, additional considerations must be incorporated into the decision making. Ideally, measures chosen should be clinically relevant; sensitive to change; tested for cultural sensitivity; and (importantly) minimally burdensome to the patient, to the staff, and to the institution in terms of the cost of collecting and analyzing the data.

CQI activities are not research, at least in the formal sense of the word. CQI was developed to improve quality of care by those who provide the care. It is an in-house activity, and costs must be absorbed within the overhead budget of the institution. Costs are a significant factor at a time when health care organizations are struggling to keep overhead costs to a minimum. Expenditures include not only the fees for using many of the available outcome instruments, but the direct costs of data collection, analysis, and reporting. In addition, there are significant indirect costs when physicians, nurses, or other personnel are asked to collect data in addition to their other duties. Therefore, efficiency of measurement is an important selection criterion. This means reducing the time burden—choosing instruments that can be successfully completed briefly by patients and with minimal staff assistance.

CQI activities differ from research in other ways as well. The patients included in CQI data collection activities generally are not homogeneous. In fact, they may differ widely in socioeconomic background, psychiatric history, comorbidities, and diagnosis. These differences inevitably lead to important questions about selecting the best instruments for specific patients. If an instrument is diagnosis specific, for example, who will make the decision about which instrument for that disorder to use or whether different instruments are needed? Which outcomes will be considered important to measure? There are different perspectives on what constitutes a "good" outcome: Is it independent functioning? Reduced psychological distress? Minimal recurrence of problems? Increased community supports and social integration? There are other questions about instrument selection that also arise. Will the language of the instrument be appropriate and clearly understood? Can patients complete it with minimal assistance? Has it been found to be valid and reliable? Is it cost effective?

Even after the right outcome instruments have been chosen, the task of putting them to use is complicated and demanding. Who within the facility will be responsible for reporting the right information to the right people? Who will carry out the necessary tasks? What concerns will the staff have about CQI activities? Who will alleviate these concerns? Where will the money come from?

Standards of protocol precision that mark research studies are bound to be relaxed. It is hard to follow up on discharged patients, and nursing staff rarely have the same perspective as do researchers on the need for adherence to protocols, even when they enter into CQI projects enthusiastically. Changes in nursing or other staff lead to repeated training sessions for data collectors. Timing of data collection in a pre-post design is often difficult to work out in busy clinical settings.

The audience for CQI reports is internal staff, both clinical and administrative. Some institutions may want to share their CQI successes with regulatory agencies and purchasers of care. The data must be reported in a timely fashion and in understandable formats that support the efforts to improve treatment. This means in ways that clinical staff members without a statistics and measurement background can readily understand. It also means that the data may be fairly fine grained, that is, specific to the situation and detailed at a level that provides sufficient information to inform decisions about systemic solutions.

PERFORMANCE INDICATORS

Performance measurement emphasizes population-level rates for specific treatment processes. It has been chosen by purchasers of care and regulatory agencies to make providers more accountable and to increase market competition among provider groups.

Performance indicators focus on population-level care processes rather than patient-level clinical outcomes. Population-based performance indicators measure processes of care such as the number of patients treated, plan membership, or some similar metric. Because performance indicators are designed to reflect plan-level processes, they are used in report cards to judge the overall quality of the plan. Specific indicators of care are presumed to reflect underlying quality. This approach assumes that better quality of care results in improved clinical outcomes. In addition, instead of collecting outcome data from individual patients, performance indicators are generally derived from administrative data. Although this kind of data collection may be less burdensome, it requires sophisticated technology.

A much wider audience is likely to be interested in performance indicators: accrediting agencies, health network administrators, and purchasers of health plans. Rather than presenting data about small details in the delivery of care, the goal is to provide information on broad categories of processes of care. The categories must be labeled in such a way as to be clearly understood by readers who want to compare performance across multiple health plans or facilities. Performance indicators intended for purchasers of care are also likely to include measures of patient satisfaction with services. Satisfaction is unlikely to be of primary importance in efficacy and effectiveness research. Taken alone, it is usually not the major focus of CQI projects, although it may play a role in any data collection effort related to quality of care. There is notable interest in shifting from global measures of satisfaction to assessing the patient's perception of care, that is, the patient's view of the technical and interpersonal aspects of his or her care.

Report cards have been touted as the means by which consumers will make informed choices. But research on how consumers understand the information provided in report cards has been discouraging (Jewett and Hibbard 1996). Consumers do not understand indicators very well and, in fact, interpret them in unintended ways. This is an area where thoughtful development of this technology needs to occur if report cards and performance indicators are to successfully differentiate poorly performing health plans from ones that are doing better.

CONCLUSION

Outcome measurement has come a long way in the last 50 years. Where once measurement was the province of educational and social psychology, the growth of the pharmaceutical industry has fueled the development of refined and sophisticated outcome instruments, finely tuned to expected symptom improvement. Parallel development efforts have produced more general, nonspecific measures of mental health and mental illness. These measures have encouraged others to study questions linked to health care policies. Understanding why each outcome measure was developed, the population for which it was developed, and its strengths and weaknesses will increase the likelihood that outcome effects, if they exist, will be demonstrated. The chapters in Part II should be a valuable resource in matching specific outcome instruments with specific clinical settings.

REFERENCES

Brook RH, Lohr KN: Efficacy, effectiveness, variations, and quality: boundary crossing research. Med Care 23:710–722, 1985

Brook RH, Chassin MR, Fink A, et al: A method for the detailed assessment of the appropriateness of medical technologies. Int J Technol Assess Health Care 2:53–63, 1986

Jewett JJ, Hibbard JH: Comprehension of quality care indicators: differences among privately insured, publicly insured, and uninsured. Health Care Financing Review 18(1):75–94, 1996

Overall JE, Gorham DR: The Brief Psychiatric Rating Scale. Psychol Rep 10:799–812, 1962

Wells KB, Katon W, Rogers B, et al: Use of minor tranquilizers and antidepressant medications by depressed outpatients: results from the Medical Outcomes Study. Am J Psychiatry 151:694–700, 1994

CHAPTER 3

Linking Outcome Measurement With Process Measurement for Quality Improvement

Richard C. Hermann, M.D., M.S.

Although the principal focus of this book is outcome measurement, another important dimension of quality assessment—process measurement—requires discussion. After decades of debate over process versus outcome measurement, it is now becoming apparent that improving quality of care requires both types of measurement. (Brugha and Lindsay 1996; Hammermeister et al. 1995; Salzer et al. 1997).

Recent changes in health care delivery have accelerated the development of methods for quality assessment. There is growing awareness of the variability in the quality of health care, including underuse, overuse, and

This work was supported by NIMH Grants K08-MH001477 and AHRQ R-01HS10303 to Dr. Hermann.

misuse of certain treatments (Chassin and Galvin 1998; Dickey et al. 1998; Hermann 1996). Cost-containment efforts such as utilization review have stirred concerns about quality and have added urgency to assessment efforts. Market forces in health care have greatly intensified competition among plans and providers. Measures are needed to ensure that plans compete not only on the basis of lower cost, but also on higher quality. Consolidation of providers and hospitals into large networks, combined with information-systems development, has provided new opportunities for addressing quality issues (Hermann et al. 2000c).

The resulting pressure for useful quality assessment methods has revealed the strengths and weaknesses of both outcome and process measurement. Their utility may lie in their complementarity: each is more useful and powerful when linked to the other. This chapter compares characteristics of process and outcome measures, explores this complementarity, and illustrates their combined potential for assessing and improving the quality of mental health care.

DEFINITIONS AND MEASURE CHARACTERISTICS

Drawing from Donabedian's (1980) paradigmatic triad,[1] Eddy (1998) described the roles of process and outcome in population-based quality assessment. In a given population, subgroups of patients are at risk for adverse health states, either by having risk factors for new disorders or by having existing conditions that are subject to recurrence, progression, or exacerbation. Often these conditions can be prevented or lessened through appropriate medical care. Assessing the quality of health care in populations takes one of two basic approaches. One approach is to compare the proportion of patients with an adverse health state (including its severity) before and after treatment; these are *outcome measures*. An alternative approach is to measure the proportion of patients who receive a clinical intervention consistent with evidence-based recommendations; these are *process measures*.

For example, patients with schizophrenia—a chronic relapsing condition—are at risk for acute episodes characterized by psychosis, disorgani-

---

[1] In addition to process and outcome, Donabedian's triad also includes "structure," i.e., the stable characteristics of patients, providers, facilities, and organizations that constitute a health care system. Many concepts discussed in this chapter with regard to process can also be applied to measures of structure, particularly the need to evaluate the significance and validity of such measures.

zation, and decreased functioning. The frequency and severity of relapses can be reduced by the effective use of antipsychotic medications. An outcomes approach to quality measurement would be to assess the severity of psychotic symptoms, level of functioning, or quality of life of a group of patients before and after a pharmacologic intervention. In contrast, a process-based approach would measure aspects of the treatment patients receive or should receive, such as the type of medication and its dose or duration of action (Hermann et al. 2000a).

Case Study: Choosing a Measurement Strategy

BCMHC Inc. is a nonprofit corporation operating five community mental health centers that serve severely mentally ill patients in a New England state. A new Department of Mental Health regulation was issued requiring centers to routinely assess and improve quality of care.

Individuals with schizophrenia constitute the largest proportion of BCMHC's patients. After several years of observation, the organization's chief medical officer had concerns that the quality of care for schizophrenic patients varied among the five centers. He wondered whether some centers were less likely to use state-of-the-art practices to prevent noncompliance and relapse, but he had no data to support his impressions. He resolved to make care for schizophrenia the focus of a quality assessment and improvement initiative. His first question was how to measure the quality of care for schizophrenia in the centers.

Strengths and Limitations of Outcome Measurement

The principal strength of outcome measures can be their clinical relevance. Although clinicians may dispute the best treatment for a given psychiatric disorder, most would agree on desired outcomes such as reduced symptoms, improved functioning, and enhanced quality of life. The importance of these outcomes can serve as a basis for motivating clinicians and other stakeholders to participate in quality improvement work.

Symptoms, functioning, and quality of life can be assessed from both the patient's and the clinician's perspectives. Other views can also be relevant. Employers may be interested in a functional outcome such as missed work days and may use this measure to assess the value of their health plan. A societal perspective might include outcomes within the criminal justice system, such as conviction rates among juveniles. A family perspective could include caregiver burden.

Outcome measurement is efficient, in that it assesses the aggregate impact of all care, whereas process measures provide information about specific interventions. For example, measuring changes in symptoms and functional outcome in a cohort of schizophrenic patients assesses the impact of all treatment modalities: medication, therapy, patient and family education, and case management.

However, outcome measurement has its limitations, which current methodology has yet to surmount. A national system of "outcomes management," as envisioned by Ellwood (1988), remains more tomorrow's technology than today's. Some of the most definitive and routinely tracked outcomes (e.g., death) occur too rarely or too far downstream from treatment to be useful indicators of quality. Although the number of patients with schizophrenia who ultimately commit suicide has been estimated to be as high as 13%, only a small fraction are at risk during any specific point in time (Harkavy-Friedman and Nelson 1997). This limits the utility of suicide incidence as a quality measure in very large populations.

Perhaps the greatest problem in the field is that poor outcomes result from factors other than the treatment provided. Suicide, for example, could be a consequence of a schizophrenic patient's receiving poor care, but it could also occur for reasons unrelated to quality. Outcome measures may be confounded by a patient's clinical characteristics (such as illness severity and comorbid psychiatric, substance-related, and medical conditions) and factors outside the clinical realm, including whether the patient has housing or social support. Case-mix adjustment can provide a statistical means of controlling for nontreatment factors (e.g., characteristics of schizophrenic patients associated with a higher rate of suicide), but methods have not yet been adequately developed for many conditions and measures in mental health (Hermann et al. 2000a). A final problem with outcome measurement is illustrated by the following case example.

Case Study: Implementing Outcomes Measurement

The chief medical officer implemented brief rating scales to measure symptoms and functioning levels among schizophrenic patients at the five centers. After training, clinicians administered the instrument to new patients at the start of treatment and at successive 6-month intervals. The results were collected and analyzed. Adjustments were made for some potentially confounding factors, such as age, gender, substance abuse, and homelessness. The results, illustrated in Figure 3–1, supported the chief medical officer's hypothesis of variation in patient outcome among the centers. Patients at three of the five centers showed comparable degrees of improvement at 6 months. On average, however, patients at clinic C showed greater improvement and those at clinic E showed less. Subsequently, the results were reviewed with the clinical staff at each site. The data interested the clinicians, particularly at clinic E, but did not provide guidance about the reasons patients at clinic E did less well or how to improve care and outcomes.

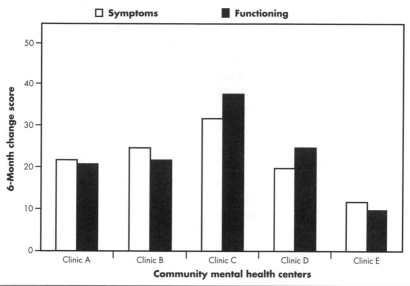

Figure 3-1. Example of measured treatment outcomes of schizophrenia at five community mental health centers. Not shown in this illustrative example, but important for actual use, are data on sample sizes, confidence intervals, and specifications of the case-mix adjustment.

Strengths and Limitations of Process Measurement

Process measurement involves the assessment of the interaction between patients and the health care system, including interpersonal and technical aspects of care. Interpersonal processes, such as the quality of clinician-patient communication and the respect accorded to patients during the delivery of care, are often evaluated by surveying patient satisfaction (Hermann et al. 1998). Technical process measures examine treatment content and are typically expressed as the proportion of patients with a given condition who receive an appropriate treatment.

Process measurement is in many ways the inverse of outcomes measurement. Rather than being rare, as are some significant outcomes, treatment processes are common. In contrast to many outcomes, processes can be evaluated concurrently with the delivery of care. Process measures can help clinicians determine where to focus quality improvement efforts, by identifying processes that show significant variance between actual practice and standards of care.

By relying on previously collected data, such as billing claims or pharmacy records, process measurement can be less costly and burdensome to implement and maintain. However, some process measures also require the collection of new data, for example, from medical records or patient surveys.

Process measures are generally less susceptible to confounding variables—and a need for case-mix adjustment—than are outcome measures. Many processes—such as whether a schizophrenic patient is evaluated for substance abuse during an initial assessment—rely on the clinician's performance rather than a patient's characteristics, and thus are less influenced by differences among patients. However, some treatment processes depend both on provider practice and patient compliance, and thus measurement results may differ based on the characteristics of the population treated by the clinician. For example, one measure of medication treatment is the proportion of patients with schizophrenia who continue taking an adequate dosage of antipsychotic medication throughout a 6-week acute treatment period. Conformance with this measure depends on both the clinician's practice and the patient's agreement and ability to comply. Mediating factors—such as the severity of the patient's thought disorder and the level of social support—may confound results.

The limitations of process measurement lie less with their implementation than with their significance. There has been little study of their validity, which is thought to be highly variable. Although some measures are derived from research-based evidence, others are not and are based on consensus judgments or clinical opinion (Hermann et al. 2000b). The latter measures may represent high-quality practices, but they can also be arbitrary and can reify existing practice rather than promote higher quality. Process measurement may also promote micromanagement by implicitly recommending *how* to achieve desired clinical results, whereas outcome measures enhance accountability but leave decision making to clinicians.

OPPORTUNITIES FOR SYNERGY

Combining process and outcome measures can serve quality improvement more completely than can either alone.

Case Study: Integrating Process and Outcome Measurement

Comparing patient outcomes among the five centers had the desired effect of focusing clinicians on the quality of their care. Initially, clinic E's staff scrutinized the data, convinced that they would show that their patients were sicker than those at other centers, thus explaining the poorer outcomes. Finding no such evidence, they turned to examine their practices.

Over the course of several meetings, clinicians from all five centers discussed their schizophrenia treatment practices. They developed a list of key areas where their practices varied; prioritizing those that they believed may explain differences in outcome. Drawing on the work of Lehman and

Steinwachs (1998) and others, these practices were translated into process measures:

- The proportion of patients with schizophrenia assessed for substance abuse and, if positive, referred for treatment
- The proportion of patients with unremitting psychotic symptoms given a trial of clozapine
- The proportion of patients with poor medication compliance given a trial of depot antipsychotics
- The proportion of patients with multiple hospital admissions enrolled in an assertive community treatment or intensive case management program

These measures were further specified to ensure that the same data sources and measure specifications would be used at each site. At the next 6-month assessment interval, the process measures were implemented in conjunction with the outcome scales.

Developing a Measurement Strategy

With limited resources and a nearly infinite number of measurable processes and outcomes, a necessary step is the development of an assessment strategy. Rather than using measurement to monitor existing practice, clinicians should focus on known or suspected problems (also known as opportunities for improvement). The problem selected for improvement should have a high priority—that is, that it affects patients, has important clinical implications, is under the control of the clinicians and staff, and is meaningful to quality improvement participants.

Although advocating for fewer measures over many, Kaplan and Norton (1992) suggest the use of a "balanced scorecard" of performance measures. This approach can unify an organization around a handful of measures in key domains: processes, outcomes, cost, and patient satisfaction. Adding cost recognizes the need for health care organizations to monitor financial performance and acknowledges that clinical decision making allocates limited health care resources. Adding measures of patient satisfaction reflects a customer-focused perspective that is becoming essential in a competitive environment. Figure 3–2 illustrates an example of a balanced approach by the community mental health centers in the case study, using a compass metaphor developed by Nelson et al. in 1996.

Improvement Methodology

Among the many emerging models for quality improvement in health care, one of the most developed is continuous quality improvement (CQI). Berwick et al. (1990) outlined some of its key principles:

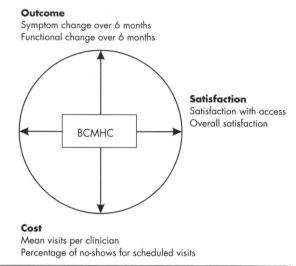

Outcome
Symptom change over 6 months
Functional change over 6 months

Process
Percentage of patients with
  persistent psychosis offered
  clozapine
Percentage of patients with
  multiple hospitalizations
  in ACT

Satisfaction
Satisfaction with access
Overall satisfaction

BCMHC

Cost
Mean visits per clinician
Percentage of no-shows for scheduled visits

Figure 3–2.   Sample elements of a balanced scorecard for the treatment of schizo-phrenia in community mental health centers. Elements are arrayed as balance points on a compass to illustrate differences in direction and utility of varied directions.

1. Quality problems can be viewed as a result of flawed or variable processes.
2. Quality improvement is grounded in statistical analyses of processes and outcomes.
3. Problem selection should focus on that which is meaningful, measurable, and circumscribed.
4. Problem diagnosis should search for root causes of the problem.
5. Improvement interventions should be assessed in terms of measured changes in process and outcome.

Case Study: Using Process and Outcome Measurement in Quality Improvement

After the next measurement cycle, the clinical and administrative staff at clinic E reviewed the results. Their patients' clinical outcomes remained below those of the other centers. Process measurement identified two areas where they also lagged: in the use of depot antipsychotic drugs and assertive community treatment. Clinic E staff developed work groups to address possible deficiencies in these areas. Over the course of several subsequent measurement cycles, they implemented a series of interventions. For example, a monthly chart review was conducted to identify patients with repeated episodes of antipsychotic drug noncompliance followed by relapse. At these patients' next visit, a paper prompt was clipped to the front of these patients' charts recommending that the prescribing clinician consider depot medication. In addition, compliance-enhancing strategies were the subject of several of clinic E's weekly case conferences.

After the interventions, remeasurement of these processes informed them whether the interventions had successfully changed clinical practice. Remeasurement of outcomes determined whether their patients' clinical and functional status had improved.

NEEDS FOR THE FUTURE

For process measurement to become more useful in quality improvement, it will be necessary to improve the meaningfulness, feasibility, and action-ability of these measures.

Validating Process Measures

Validity is a primary consideration in improving the meaningfulness of process measures. A valid measure is one that represents true quality of care. Because there is no gold standard for quality, validity is assessed through indirect means. Face validity can be established by informed judgments of relevant stakeholders (e.g., consumers, clinicians, researchers, and payers). Predictive validity can be determined by establishing a statistical association between conformance with the process measured and subsequent improvement in patient outcome. Linking process measures to clinical outcomes combines their strengths: process measures' ease of use and the evident importance of improved outcomes (Owen et al. 1999).

Statistical analyses of such process-outcome links are few and technically difficult. Large sample sizes are needed, as are accurate measures and multivariate analysis to control for confounding factors. A few preliminary analyses of mental health measures have been conducted. Druss and Rosenheck (1997) studied a Health Plan Employer Data and Information Set (HEDIS) 2.0 measure of ambulatory follow-up after hospitalization for depression, finding the measure to correlate poorly with other proxies for outcome. Melfi et al. (1998) found that adherence to a guideline recommendation for the duration of antidepressant treatment (a HEDIS 3.0 measure) was significantly associated with lower rates of relapse. Owen et al. (1999) determined that patients with schizophrenia who were prescribed lower-than-recommended dosages of oral antipsychotic drugs (a Schizophrenia Patient Outcomes Research Team [PORT] measure) were less likely to respond to treatment than were patients whose dosages were within the recommended range.

Using Core Measure Sets

More than 300 process measures have been proposed by professional groups (e.g., the American Psychiatric Association), managed care organizations, government agencies (including the Center for Mental Health Services), purchasers, accreditation groups (e.g., the National Committee for Quality Assurance's HEDIS initiative), and researchers (particularly RAND's quality-of-care studies and the University of Maryland's Schizophrenia PORT).

Having numerous measures allows for assessment of multiple domains of quality—such as detection of illness, access to care, and appropriateness of treatments—as well as varied patient populations. But the variety of measures also limits the feasibility of their use. Currently, providers must use different measures to meet requirements of each payer, accreditor, and regulatory agency. Even a single measure, such as readmission rates, can have different specifications, requiring reanalysis for each report.

A solution is the development of one or more core sets of measures with established specifications. Core sets could be used by multiple stakeholders and providers, which would reduce the reporting burden, allow for comparisons across sites, and provide a greater pool of data for benchmarking and case-mix adjustment. A number of organizations, including the American College of Mental Health Administration, the Substance Abuse and Mental Health Services Administration, and the National Association of State Mental Health Program Directors, have launched efforts to develop consensus among stakeholders on measures, but to date this has not been achieved.

The U.S. Agency for Health Policy Research has funded the National Inventory of Mental Health Quality Measures, which is cataloguing the properties of existing process measures (e.g., numerator, denominator, rationale, data source, population, sampling, risk adjustment, validity, reliability, scientific basis, norms, and standards) (Hermann and Palmer, in press; Hermann et al. 2000b, in press). This information will allow areas for future measure development and testing to be identified, enable potential users to access measure information, and provide a foundation from which core sets can be developed. The inventory will be disseminated via the Internet by the Center for Quality Assessment and Improvement in Mental Health at Harvard Medical School (http://www.cqaimh.org).

Acting on Measurement Results

Several factors affect a quality measure's "actionability," that is, the capacity of a clinician (or other measure users) to act on a result that may reflect a problem with quality. First, only 20% of proposed measures are in routine use, providing a limited pool of results (Hermann et al. 2000b). Wider use can lead to the identification of norms (average values) and benchmarks (standards reflecting best practices), allowing users to interpret their results—for example, as excellent, average, or inadequate—and if the latter, to set goals for improvement. Ideally, norms and benchmarks should be specific to geographic regions and relevant patient subpopulations. Second, there is a need for a typology among measures by user and purpose. Different measures are needed to drive quality improvement within a hospital than those needed for regulatory oversight by a governmental agency. Still other measures are needed to inform consumers in their selection of clinicians and purchasers in selecting among plans.

CONCLUSION

No single instrument or method will adequately assess the quality of mental health care. A combination of methods—including process and outcomes measurement, satisfaction surveys, and surveillance for errors and adverse events—will be needed to improve care in the increasingly complex health care system. Many measures, scales, and surveys have been developed. The next step is to identify the most promising for further development and rigorous testing, separately and in combination.

REFERENCES

Berwick D, Godfrey A, Roessner J: Curing health care. San Francisco, CA, Jossey-Bass, 1990

Brugha T, Lindsay F: Quality of mental health service care: the forgotten pathway from process to outcome. Soc Psychiatry Psychiatr Epidemiol 31:89–98, 1996

Chassin M, Galvin R: The urgent need to improve health care quality: Institute of Medicine National Roundtable on Health Care Quality. JAMA 280:1000–1005, 1998

Dickey B, Hermann R, Eisen S: Assessing the quality of psychiatric care: research methods and application in clinical practice. Harv Rev Psychiatry 6:88–96, 1998

Donabedian A: Explorations in Quality Assessment and Monitoring: The Definition of Quality and Approaches to Its Assessment. Ann Arbor, MI, Health Administration Press, 1980

Druss B, Rosenheck R: Evaluation of the HEDIS measure of behavioral health care quality. Psychiatr Serv 48:71–75, 1997

Eddy DM: Performance measurement: problems and solutions. Health Aff (Millwood) 17:7–25, 1998

Ellwood PM: Outcomes management. N Engl J Med 12:741–808, 1988

Hammermeister K, Shroyer A, Sethi G, et al: Why it is important to demonstrate linkages between outcomes of care and processes and structures of care. Med Care 33:OS5–OS16, 1995

Harkavy-Friedman J, Nelson E: Assessment and intervention for the suicidal patient with schizophrenia. Psychiatr Q 68:361–375, 1997

Hermann RC: Variation in psychiatric practices: implications for health care policy and financing. Harv Rev Psychiatry 4:98–101, 1996

Hermann RC, Palmer RH: Common ground: a framework for selecting care quality measures for mental health and substance abuse care. Psychiatr Serv (in press)

Hermann R, Ettner S, Dorwart R: The influence of psychiatric disorders on patients' ratings of satisfaction with health care. Med Care 36:720–727, 1998

Hermann R, Finnerty M, Teller T: Measures of treatment quality and guideline adherence for schizophrenia. In Cross-walk of National Schizophrenia Guidelines. Edited by Docherty J, Finnerty M. Clifton Park, NY, RTP, 2000a

Hermann RC, Leff H, Palmer RH, et al: Quality measures for mental health care: results from a national inventory. Med Care Res Rev 57 (suppl 2):136–154, 2000b

Hermann R, Regner J, Erickson P, et al: Developing a quality management system for behavioral healthcare: the Cambridge Health Alliance experience. Harv Rev Psychiatry 8:251–260, 2000c

Hermann RC, Palmer RH, Finnerty M, et al: Process measures fo the assessment and improvement of care for schizophrenia. Schizophr Bull (in press)

Kaplan R, Norton D: The balanced scorecard—measures that drive performance. Harvard Business Review 71–79, 1992

Lehman A, Steinwachs D: Patterns of usual care for schizophrenia: initial results from the Schizophrenia Patient Outcomes Research Team (PORT) client survey. Schizophr Bull 24:11–20, 1998

Melfi C, Chawla A, Croghan T, et al: The effects of adherence to antidepressant treatment guidelines on relapse and recurrence of depression. Arch Gen Psychiatry 55:1128–1132, 1998

Nelson E, Mohr J, Batalden P, et al: Improving health care, Part 1: The clinical value compass. Jt Comm J Qual Improv 22:243–58, 1996

Owen RR, Thrush CR, Kirchner JE: Performance measurement for schizophrenia: adherence to guidelines for antipsychotic dose. Int J Qual Health Care 12:475–482, 2000

Salzer M, Nixon C, Schut L, et al: Validating quality indicators: quality as relationship between structure, process, and outcome. Evaluation Review 21:292–309, 1997

CHAPTER

4

Validity, Reliability, and Other Key Concepts in Outcome Assessment and Services Research

Alisa B. Busch, M.D., M.S.

Consumers, health plans, and payers are concerned with purchasing quality mental health services. This, in addition to the desire of clinicians to provide high-quality care, provides impetus for clinicians to measure what we do, assess and define our effectiveness, and use those assessments to improve care. We are in the midst of an explosion of new treatments in pharmacotherapy and psychotherapy, as well as new ways of delivering services. Although many psychiatric treatments have been tested in rigorous

Supported by a postdoctoral training grant from the National Institute of Mental Health. The author would like to thank Paul Cleary, Ph.D., Arnold Epstein, M.D., Richard Frank, Ph.D., Shelly F. Greenfield, M.D., M.P.H., Sharon-Lise Normand, Ph.D., and Lloyd I. Sederer, M.D., for their helpful advice on outcomes assessment and comments on earlier drafts of this chapter.

clinical trials, we have too often been unable to assess the outcome of treatments as they are used in typical clinical practice where they are applied to real patients in real-life clinical settings. For example, randomized, controlled clinical trials indicate that different classifications of antidepressants, on average, have similar efficacy (Hyman et al. 1995). But these studies look only at very carefully selected patient populations, who are often without comorbid conditions and are more motivated for treatment than is the average patient. It is unclear whether clinical trials would have the same results if they were conducted in usual care settings with patients typically seen in practice.

Assessing the quality of care provided by a program, intervention, or system requires careful consideration to the three main components of care: structure (how the system or program is organized), process (services or treatments that are provided), and outcome (the effect the care has on patient health status and satisfaction) (Donabedian 1966, 1988). Medical and psychiatric journals publish increasing amounts of health services research, including outcome studies. Understanding the relative strengths and weaknesses of studies and how they apply to patients can be a challenge for clinicians. To be able to critically evaluate the results of any study, it is necessary to understand the basic concepts of validity and reliability. This chapter focuses on the validity and reliability of outcome measures. Validity (or accuracy) is the degree to which a result truly represents what is being measured, whereas reliability (or precision) is the reproducibility of the result (Fletcher et al. 1996).

Outcome measures with proven validity and reliability help standardize the measurement of quality and provide a common language to compare outcomes across programs and systems of care. These measures include diagnostic instruments and surveys to assess symptoms and functioning as well as to measure change after an intervention. Outcome measures can also include variables such as homelessness, suicide, workplace performance, and patient and family member satisfaction. Often, several types of measures are combined to provide broader information regarding effectiveness as experienced by patients and family members, as well as clinicians.

Outcome measures must demonstrate more than validity and reliability—they must also be practical. Administering or collecting outcome measures can be costly in terms of money and time for patients, family members, clinicians, and service systems. An outcome measure with excellent validity and reliability is useless if it is too burdensome to be utilized in practice. Outcome assessment involves a balance between maximizing validity, reliability, utility (i.e., clinical relevance), and a measure's potential burden. For example, the Short Form Health Survey (SF-36) was developed to provide good reliability and validity, like the more extensive scales used in the Medical Outcomes Study (MOS), but also to be less burdensome to complete (Ware 1992). The brevity came at the expense of some precision in some of the health subscales (Ware 1996). Despite the efficiency of SF-36, the demand for further brevity prompted the authors to develop an even shorter version (SF-12), but once again at the expense of less precision and measuring fewer aspects of health status than does SF-36 (Ware et al. 1996).

This chapter begins with a review of the main types of validity and reliability, followed by an examination of study power, error, and statistical significance. It concludes with a discussion of study design issues, including bias, that affect the validity and reliability of outcomes studies.

VALIDITY

As noted above, validity reflects the confidence that the results of a measure truly represent the characteristic being evaluated. It is usually a matter of degree rather than an all-or-none attribute; in addition, there are several major types of validity (Table 4–1) (Nunnally and Bernstein 1994).

Table 4–1. Major concepts of validity
Face validity
Construct validity
Content validity
Criterion (predictive) validity
Sensitivity
Specificity
Convergent/divergent validity

Face validity is the degree to which an outcome measure intuitively seems to assess what it is supposed to assess—whether or not it makes clinical sense to measure a particular phenomenon. Face validity is an important starting point. For example, if patient violence were strongly associated with agitation, then an outcome study looking at reduction of patient violence would also need to measure agitation. At times face validity is compromised due to confounding or biases within a measure. A confounder is a characteristic associated with how the patient was selected for treatment (or evaluation) and the outcome. Bias is discussed later in this chapter.

Some example of confounding can be seen by asking whether rehospitalization rate is an appropriate indicator of poor inpatient care. The answer would be yes if poor care were the only predictor of high rehospitalization rates. But clinically it is known that rehospitalization rates may be affected by other factors—such as severity of illness, cognitive limitations, or poor family support. Therefore, despite appropriate care, one group of patients may show a higher rehospitalization rate. Similarly, if one were to compare the patient outcomes at two hospitals without taking into consideration the case mix in the hospitals, the effect of hospital A having sicker patients than does hospital B would not be recognized. Because of this, despite providing the same or better care, hospital A may have a higher rehospitalization rate than does hospital B, which could suggest that hospital B provided higher-quality care. This example illustrates that without case-mix adjustments, rehospitalization rate has poor face validity as an indicator of quality. This is because illness severity confounds the relationship between outcome and patient population.

Face validity can also be compromised if there are other factors, independent of the measure, that affect the outcome. For example, if assessing whether or not patients with schizophrenia who receive appropriate medication and psychotherapy have more stable housing than those without these treatments, a great deal of variation in the outcome can occur from circumstances that are often unrelated to treatment. Examples of other variables that can affect outcome are family supportiveness, neighbor and community supportiveness, severity of illness, patients' cognitive limitations, and financial situation, to name a few. In fact, for severely impaired patients it may be that these other factors play a larger role in housing stability than do pharmacotherapy or psychotherapy.

Construct validity is the presence of a positive correlation between a set of characteristics or variables (e.g., anhedonia, insomnia, low energy) and the main entity that is being measured (e.g., depression). When a patient states that she is experiencing difficulty with low mood, the clinician inquires further about associated symptoms. The clinician is trying to determine the underlying problem (i.e., diagnosis) from which these symptoms emerge so as to guide treatment decisions. In this situation, the diagnosis is really a construct; major depression cannot be directly measured or observed. Instead, the clinician observes a set of clinical signs and symptoms that are believed are related and that have been grouped together and given a name. If the collection of symptoms and signs are an accurate reflection of a specific and real illness (with a particular etiology or pathophysiology), then the diagnosis has construct validity. For example, the current construct of major depression includes difficulties with cognitive and physical function. If these difficulties are true aspects of this disorder, then employees with major depression would be expected to demonstrate impaired workplace performance.

Content validity is the degree to which a measure adequately samples what it is supposed to measure. For an outcome measure to have adequate content validity it must have a sufficient and representative collection of items and be constructed in a way that makes sense. This is usually done by what looks reasonable (Nunnally and Bernstein 1994). For example, in designing SF-36, the authors were careful to incorporate enough questions to address the major domains considered critical in the concept of *health*, such as physical and mental function and well-being, as well as role limitations due to physical or mental distress (Ware 1992).

Criterion (predictive) validity is how well an outcome measure and particular characteristic(s) correlate (Nunnally and Bernstein 1994). Returning to the earlier example of major depression and workplace performance, if depression severity were a good criterion for workplace performance, then one would expect to see changes (either improvement or deterioration) in a person's Hamilton Depression Scale (Ham-D) or Beck Depression Inventory (BDI) scores correlating with workplace performance or absenteeism (Beck and Steer 1993).

Sensitivity and specificity are characteristics of an outcome measure that are also markers of criterion validity. They rely on the assumption that there is a criterion test (i.e., a gold standard) available with which to compare. Sensitivity is the probability that an outcome measure will identify all persons in a sample who have a particular disorder or certain characteristics; it quantifies the proportion of true positives. False negatives decrease sensitivity. Specificity is the probability that an outcome measure will accurately determine who truly does not have the disorder or certain characteristics; it quantifies the proportion of true negatives. False positives decrease specificity. Positive predictive value is the probability that a person truly will have the disorder if the test is positive. Negative predictive value is the probability that a person truly will not have the disorder if the test is negative. Table 4–2 illustrates the relationship between an instrument and its test characteristics.

Table 4–2.   Test characteristics

	Truth (disease present or not)	
	Positive	**Negative**
Test result		
Positive	TP	FP
Negative	FN	TN

Note.   TP=true positive; FP=false positive; FN=false negative; TN=true negative. Sensitivity=TP/(TP+FN); specificity=TN/(FP+TN); positive predictive value=TP/(TP+FP); negative predictive value=TN/(FN+TN).

For example, to learn how a particular treatment benefits patients with borderline personality disorder, it would first be necessary to identify the patients with the disorder. If it is known that 100 people in a particular population of 1,000 people have a borderline personality disorder, then a survey that correctly identifies all 100 of these has a sensitivity of 100%. If there are also no false positives, then the specificity is also 100%. However, if in the same population the survey incorrectly identifies 100 people who do not have the disorder as well as correctly identifying the 100 who do have the disorder, then the sensitivity remains 100% but the specificity decreases to 89%. In this example, the positive predictive value goes from 100% to 50% by the addition of the 100 false-positive test results. False positives occur if a survey indicates a positive result for borderline personality disorder in persons with other disorders that are also marked by impulsiveness and unstable interpersonal relationships (e.g., antisocial personality disorder, histrionic personality disorder, bipolar I or II affective disorder).

No single test has both 100% sensitivity and 100% specificity. In fact, gains in one measure are always at the expense of the other. Although an outcome measure with higher sensitivity will detect a greater number of people in a given population who are true positives, it may also detect a higher rate of false positives, which decreases its specificity. This is because a highly sensitive test will detect persons who have subtler, less severe characteristics or symptoms—which leaves more room for false-positive results. Conversely, when specificity is higher there is more confidence that a negative test represents a true negative. However, because the test is more stringent, there will be more people who actually have the characteristic(s) being sought but who will not be detected (false negatives). For example, to assess the correlation between homelessness and the presence of major depression in a community, it is very important to identify all persons in the study who have major depression. Therefore, a measure with high sensitivity for depression should be selected. The measure would ask questions such as "Have you had any sad or blue thoughts in the past week?" This question would elicit a high "yes" response rate and would therefore increase the sample of test subjects. But people have many reasons for feeling sad, and they are not always related to major depression. As a result, many people in the sample would be false positives for major depression, making this measure high on sensitivity, but with lower specificity.

The cutoff of characteristics chosen in a given survey or test will affect sensitivity and specificity. For example, a BDI score of at least 21 suggests clinical depression (Kendall et al. 1987), but does this mean that a person who scores 19 does not have clinical depression? Not necessarily. Instead, if a lower score were selected as the criterion for the presence of major depression, then the instrument would be more sensitive for detecting major depression at the expense of lower specificity. Persons with a score of 19 may have clinical depression, but they are more likely to be sad for another reason than those with scores over 21.

Convergent or divergent validity is determined by comparing two different tests meant to measure the same thing to ascertain if they are actually measuring the same or different things. If two measures for major depression were convergent, they would be expected to show similar results if administered on the same person. For example, if both the Ham-D and the BDI were administered to a person who was known to be depressed, both tests would be expected to indicate that the person was depressed and to show similar severity of symptoms. Divergent validity describes the ability of a measure to highlight the differences in a population sample (Nunnally and Bernstein 1994). Returning to the example of workplace performance and major depression, deterioration in workplace performance alone does not indicate major depression because there are many other reasons why a person's performance may deteriorate (e.g., a medical condition or an acute stressor). Combining Ham-D scores with workplace performance measures may allow clinicians to distinguish clinically depressed workers from the rest of the population who show impaired performance.

RELIABILITY

Reliability is the extent to which a measurement is consistent when repeated; to have high reliability a measure must be stable over a variety of conditions (Table 4–3) (Nunnally and Bernstein 1994). Consider the earlier clinical example in evaluating someone with a low mood. If several clinicians examine the same patient during the same time period and some of them determine that he has major depression whereas others diagnose an adjustment disorder, then there is a reliability problem: repeated measurements of the same person or problem yielded different results. Reliability can be affected by 1) the properties of the outcome measure itself and how adequately it samples the characteristics it is intended to measure; 2) those who apply the outcome measure (i.e., the raters); and 3) the population being studied. A study must attend to all three. Within each of these three categories, there can also be two types of measurement error: systematic bias and random error (see below) (Nunnally and Bernstein 1994). Reliability is necessary but not sufficient for validity. In other words, a measure cannot be valid if it is not reliable, but it can be reliable even if it is not valid. Using the example above, if all clinicians who examine the patient diagnose major depression and the patient actually is hypothyroid, then there is good reliability in the diagnosis but its validity is poor.

Table 4–3.	Reliability major concepts

Internal consistency (coefficient α/Cronbach's α)
Test/retest reliability
Stability of response over time
Interrater reliability
Generalizability
Systematic error and bias
Random error

Internal consistency (coefficient α or Cronbach's α) is summary score of a measure's overall reliability. By convention, the minimum acceptable score for internal consistency is 0.70 (Nunnally and Bernstein 1994). The Global Assessment of Functioning (GAF) Scale (American Psychiatric Association 2000; Endicott et al. 1976; Luborsky 1962) is an example of a measure with variable reliability, ranging from 0.61 to 0.91. Although the GAF is readily available, easily administered, and understood by many clinicians, its imprecision can limit its usefulness in outcome assessment. In contrast, the Life Skills Profile (LSP) (Parker et al. 1991; Rosen et al. 1989), an instrument developed to measure both function and disability for patients with schizophrenia, has greater precision, with an internal consistency of 0.79 (Parker et al. 1996). The LSP therefore is a more reliable measure of function and disability for patients with schizophrenia than is the GAF. However, its usefulness is limited by the fact that it takes longer to administer than the GAF, is not familiar to many clinicians, and is applicable only to patients with schizophrenia.

Interrater reliability is a property of the rater(s). Interrater reliability describes how consistent and reproducible a score is if more than one rater administers the outcome measure to the same person. For example, if two clinicians administer the Addiction Severity Index (ASI) (McLellan et al. 1992) to the same person, very different scores may occur. Perhaps one clinician is better than another at picking up nonverbal cues from the patient and queries further when answers appear to be disparate from the patient's facial expression or body language. Interrater reliability is important in assessing the effectiveness of particular addiction treatment programs; when different raters perform the before-and-after evaluations with the ASI, the observed effect of the treatment could be exaggerated or minimized from the true effect if the interrater reliability is not good.

Generalizability (external validity) is the extent to which a measure developed for and tested in a particular population yields the same results in a different population. For example, in attempting to determine if a particular program diminishes patient aggression, it would be important to identify which patient populations benefit. What works for an aggressive patient with antisocial personality traits may not work for one who has a head injury or is otherwise cognitively limited. Similarly, an outcome measure tested in an English-speaking population may not be comparable to a population speaking another language, even if translated, because of cultural or dialect differences. The same consideration applies when using a survey measure with known validity and reliability for inpatients that will not necessarily be applicable to outpatients.

Systematic error and bias either can affect all observations equally (error) or can affect certain types of observations differently than others (bias) (Nunnally and Bernstein 1994). An example of systematic error in measuring blood pressure is when the sphygmomanometer is not properly calibrated: the blood pressure will be incorrectly measured in the same way for each person. Systematic bias would occur, for example, if the cuff were too small for obese people: the measurement error would occur only in obese patients. In psychiatric assessment, if one wanted to study the effect of an intervention on psychotic illness, systematic error would occur if the instrument used did not adequately cover the spectrum of psychotic phenomenology and the error was consistent across all subjects. Systematic bias would occur if that same instrument were worded in such a way that people of a particular culture would misinterpret the words and answer erroneously, because all people from that particular culture would show a similarly erroneous score, but others would not.

Random error results from unsystematic ratings (Nunnally and Bernstein 1994). Returning to the sphygmomanometer example, random error will occur if the person measuring blood pressure does not attend to correctly positioning the subject's arm or using the correct arm to measure blood pressure. The error will be random because it will be impossible to predict the direction of the error (i.e., whether the observed result will be higher or lower, or the extent of the error). Similarly, if an interviewer evaluating improvement in psychosis varies the interview questions from person to person, thereby identifying a different psychopathology with each person, then the evaluations will be imprecise: either overreporting or underreporting of symptom changes would occur, but in no predictable manner.

The GAF scale, although commonly used to measure global function in patients, can be unreliable due to both random error and systematic bias. One reason for random error in the GAF is that clinicians have much discretion in the rating, despite having guidelines for determining the severity score. Random error would occur from different clinicians' providing different scores for the same patient because of the clinicians' individual definitions of words like minimal, moderate, and severe. Similarly, even if clinicians agree on the level of symptom severity, random error would occur if they attach different emphasis to symptoms versus functioning when determining a GAF score. What one clinician decides is a 60, another may decide is a 50 or 70. There would be no way to predict the direction or magnitude of the difference. An example of systematic bias is when clinicians overscore or underscore patient GAF scores because of confidentiality concerns or to support insurance approval. This is an example of systematic bias because the direction of error is consistent.

As mentioned at the beginning of this chapter, outcome assessment—including services research—aims to evaluate treatment. Describing outcomes may be useful, but it is also necessary to compare them to determine if there are differences among groups of patients or programs. To determine what constitutes a true difference, rather than a chance difference, one begins by choosing outcome measures with high reliability and validity. However, to detect true differences, additional statistical tools are needed (Table 4–4).

Table 4–4.	Major concepts of power and error

Population sampling concepts
Confidence intervals
P values
False-positive errors
Power
False-negative errors
Statistical significance versus clinical significance

Basic statistical concepts about population sampling are important in understanding how meaningful differences between populations or interventions are determined. Suppose a researcher wanted to measure the number of persons in the United States population who have ever had schizophrenia (i.e., the population rate) and assume that there is an incontrovertible test or evaluation from which to make the diagnosis (i.e., there is excellent validity and reliability to the test). By evaluating the entire United States population, one could determine the true prevalence of schizophrenia. Unfortunately, one cannot realistically evaluate every person in the United States; instead, a representative sample of the population is evaluated and then the expected prevalence of schizophrenia is estimated. Samples, however, show natural variation. Even if a researcher is careful to ensure randomness of a sample to minimize bias, the measured rate of a characteristic will still vary from the true prevalence of that characteristic in the general population. Typically, the variation is smaller when the sample size is larger. For example, if the true prevalence of schizophrenia is 1% in the entire United States population and the researcher samples 100 people, it takes only one additional person with schizophrenia in the sample to double the estimated rate to 2%. Sampling another 100 people may increase or decrease the estimate. As the researcher continues to sample randomly, the laws of probability dictate that he or she will approach the true prevalence. The closer the sample size is to the size of the population, the more reliable is the sample rate. The greater the difference between the sample size and the population size, the more variability there will be in the sample rate.

By chance, calculations may indicate a difference between two groups that does not really exist (i.e., a false-positive result). By convention, the rate of such errors is typically set at a maximum of 5%. Therefore, in 5% of studies that demonstrate a true difference between two groups (not a difference occurring by chance alone), there is really no difference. A statistically significant difference refers to the likelihood that a true difference in rate will be determined, rather than a difference due to chance. If it is known that the true prevalence of schizophrenia in the United States is 1% and one wanted to determine if a particular community with a 1.6% rate has a statistically significant difference, how would that question be answered?

A confidence interval (CI) indicates the frequency that the true result will be located in a range of values. By convention, a 95% CI is a statistical standard. For example, if the 95% CI for the prevalence of schizophrenia in the sample was between 0.5% and 1.5% and the test were repeated 100 times (under the same conditions), then in 95 of those 100 trials the true prevalence of schizophrenia would lie within that confidence interval. In the other five trials, the true prevalence would lie outside it. In the example above of a community schizophrenia rate of 1.6%, because 1.6% falls outside of the 95% CI, 1.6% is statistically different than 1%. Therefore, this community has a higher prevalence of schizophrenia than would be expected by random variation (chance) alone. If instead the rate measured in the community was 1.25%, using the same confidence interval, there is no statistical difference between a rate of 1% and a rate of 1.25%. In other words, the difference of 0.25% occurred by chance.

A *P* value is the probability of obtaining a false-positive result. A *P* value less than 5% (i.e., $P \leq 0.05$) corresponds to a result that was outside of the 95% confidence interval; $P \leq 0.01$ corresponds to a result outside of the 99% confidence interval. By convention, a result has statistical significance if *P* is 0.05 or less.

The power of a study determines if enough data have been gathered to detect a true difference between two groups. Power is affected by four things: 1) the probability of a false-positive result, 2) sample size, 3) variability, and 4) the size of the differences between two groups that one wants to detect (also known as the effect size). Table 4–5 illustrates how these characteristics affect power. By statistical convention, power is usually set at 80%. This means that if there is truly a difference, it will be detectable 80% of the time.

Table 4–5.	Relationship between study characteristics and power

Characteristics that should be minimized to increase power
  Probability of a false-positive result
  Variability
Characteristics that should be maximized to increase power
  Sample size
  Effect size

False-negative errors occur when a difference exists between two groups but it is not detected. Therefore, failing to detect a difference between two groups does not mean there really is no difference between them. The higher the power of the study, the less frequently false-negative errors occur; therefore, false negative-errors are more likely when a study is underpowered. Using the earlier schizophrenia example, suppose a 1.6% prevalence of schizophrenia was observed. A study with lower power may yield a larger confidence interval (for example, between 0.25% and 1.75% rather than 0.5% and 1.5%). If this were the case, then a schizophrenia prevalence rate of 1.6% would not be significantly different than the expected rate of 1%, since 1.6% falls within the larger confidence interval resulting from the lower power of the study.

Differences in a population can be difficult to detect sometimes, even with a large sample of people. There still may be problems with power and error. For example, suppose that a researcher wanted to determine whether hospital A or hospital B is better at decreasing readmission rates for psychiatric patients with dual diagnoses (e.g., major mental illness and substance abuse disorder). The researcher knows of an insurance company that has 100,000 enrollees whom it admits to both hospitals randomly (thereby minimizing selection bias of patients); of these enrollees, about 1% can be expected to be hospitalized for a mental health problem in a given year. Of that 1%, 25% can be expected to have a co-occurring substance abuse problem, for a total of 250 enrollees who will be admitted to either hospital A or hospital B. Because these randomized patient populations are expected to be identical in terms of severity, diagnosis, community support, and other factors, each hospital is expected to have 125 first-time admissions. On the assumption that all patients received appropriate postdischarge care, and hospital A has 38 enrollees (i.e., 30%) readmitted in 1 month whereas hospital B has 50 enrollees (i.e., 40%) readmitted, it would seem that hospital

A is more effective in reducing 1-month readmission rates. But is the sample size large enough to reach this conclusion? The number of enrollees may not be large enough to determine if 30% is significantly different from 40%. The power to detect a difference further diminishes if the researcher attempts to refine the determination of which hospital has lower readmission rates based on severity and type of major mental illness (e.g., schizophrenia, bipolar affective disorder). This is because the number of patients in each category will be smaller than the number of all patients with any illness, and lower patient numbers per category will reduce study power.

To avoid this power problem, it may be tempting to assess readmission rates at the hospital level (i.e., all dually diagnosed patients in hospitals A and B, not just the patients from the same insurance plan). However, this may produce a selection bias that can affect the study results. Selection bias will occur whenever a person is enrolled into a study based on some characteristic (either of the patient, hospital, provider, etc.) that may affect the outcome independent of the treatment received. Because hospitals may have different referral patterns and thereby patients with different illness severity, there could be a selection bias if the study population were all psychiatric patients at hospitals A and B in a given year.

Statistical significance and clinical significance are not the same thing. Statistical significance does not always mean there is clinical significance. When a large database is utilized for a particular study, the opposite of the above example can be observed—that is, adequate power is often easily obtained because there are thousands, or tens of thousands, of observations for a particular variable. Large numbers of patients in a sample allow detection of smaller differences between two groups, which makes it easier to achieve statistical significance even if there is little (or unknown) clinical significance. For example, by preintervention and postintervention assessment, it can be measured whether a particular intervention improves a patient's symptoms as evidenced by a change in score on the Brief Psychiatric Rating Scale (BPRS) (Overall and Gorham 1962). From this evaluation can be calculated an average decline of 2 points in the BPRS score after the intervention. With enough patients evaluated, that 2-point difference may achieve statistical significance. But it may not be clinically meaningful.

IMPORTANT CONSIDERATIONS AFFECTING VALIDITY AND RELIABILITY: DESIGN ISSUES

When evaluating an intervention or program, there are several important considerations to keep in mind that will affect validity and reliability. A full discussion of design issues is beyond the scope of this chapter and is addressed in most standard epidemiological and experimental design texts. Instead, this section focuses on design issues that are of particular significance in quality and outcome assessment (Table 4–6).

Table 4–6.	Major concepts in design issues affecting validity and reliability

The effect of bias
Consideration of overall goal of assessment
Reliability of chart as a data source
Consideration of patient population being studied
Consideration of which level in a system of care is being assessed
Trade-offs and their potential to threaten validity and reliability

Effect of Bias

Bias occurs when the likelihood of participating in an assessment is related to other characteristics that may affect the outcome. These characteristics can either exaggerate or minimize outcome results. For example, when determining if patients are pleased with the care they have received it is important to ensure that either all or a randomly selected sample of patients complete a satisfaction survey. Otherwise, it is very possible that the people who respond to the survey are very different than those who do not (e.g., in terms of illness severity, legal status, or satisfaction), thereby skewing the results. Another example is if an intervention specifically developed for generalized anxiety disorder (GAD) were tested in several patients who were improperly diagnosed as having GAD. The study results would be biased and suggest that the intervention had little effect because it was erroneously (and unknowingly) evaluated in patients without the disorder. This bias essentially reduces the power to detect differences.

Determining Which Measures Will Be Used and How: Effect of the Overall Assessment Goal

In designing a study, it important to know what the goal of the study is—is it to establish a minimum standard to be met, to evaluate a baseline from which to measure further improvement, or to assess practice variation (particularly when the appropriate level of utilization in a given population is unclear)? In a situation in which there is no generally accepted benchmark number or rate, obtaining baseline rates and establishing goals is more tenable. For example, in evaluating the use of seclusion and restraint in a psychiatric unit, one could examine the frequency and duration of their use and compare them to an accepted standard. But how would an accepted standard be selected? Wide variations in rates and duration have been documented among different hospitals (Betemps et al. 1992, 1993; Crenshaw and Francis 1995; Crenshaw et al. 1997; Ray and Rappaport 1995; Way 1986; Way and Banks 1990). Different hospitals may have very different patient populations (in terms of severity or diagnosis). It is therefore difficult to compare these differences and decide on an acceptable standard that maximizes both patient and staff safety and minimizes psychological trauma. Because an accepted minimal standard does not currently exist, one could attempt to decrease the rates of seclusion and restraint (without increasing the violence/assault rate) by also assessing the triggering events. Determining the triggers could lead to interventions that decrease seclusion and restraint. Very different data would be gathered to address the second goal rather than the first. Parenthetically, the importance of including structure and process measures in outcome assessment is exemplified by assessments of use of seclusion and restraint because these interventions may be affected by things such as patient to staff ratio, overcrowding, programming, and utilization of deescalation methods (Brooks et al. 1994; Carpenter et al. 1998; Klinge 1994). Without an understanding of the structure and process of care, accurate comparisons across studies and systems of care are impossible.

Process measures are also useful in outcome assessments if the goal is ensuring that patients receive appropriate treatment, independent of improvement. For treatments with proven patient benefit and outcome, measuring processes of care as a proxy for outcome is particularly helpful if the outcomes are rare or occur considerably after care is delivered. But process measures can only be used if a link between process and outcome has been established. For example, although valproic acid has been shown to be effective in acute and rapid stabilization of mania (Bowden 1994, 1998; Pope et al. 1991), it has not yet been conclusively demonstrated to be effective in prophylaxis of bipolar affective disorder (Bowden 1998). Therefore, one cannot use the appropriate provision (i.e., the right medication, dosage, and duration) of valproic acid as a proxy for long-term improved outcome because there is insufficient data to support that link between process and outcome.

Is the Chart a More or Less Reliable Data Source Than Directly Asking Patients?

Although the question of obtaining information from the chart or from the patient is a consideration for other medical disciplines, psychiatric illnesses in particular can impair patients' insight and judgment. Concerns about the accuracy of patient self-reporting have led to a view that patient self-reports are less reliable than information obtained from the chart. This is not necessarily so, especially for information in the chart that is itself obtained by patient reporting (Cleary 1997). The appropriate data source (i.e., patient survey, chart review, clinician survey, or administrative data) is determined by the goal of the evaluation. The question to be answered and the population being studied inform the choice of which data source is most appropriate. Often, multiple data sources are used. For example, substance abuse research utilizes patient self-reporting, urine tests, and collateral informant reports as complementary outcome measures. There is also some information for which it is very useful to have the patients' perceptions. For example, to determine if patients know the purposes and side effects of their medications it is best to ask them. To improve reliability, it is necessary to ensure that the patient understands the questions being asked.

Patient-level and provider-level information may also be complementary. An outpatient medication sheet may reliably indicate what was prescribed, but a patient survey will help reliably determine whether the medication was taken and whether it was taken as prescribed. The approach chosen should be guided by the study question. If the question is, "Did a patient receive counseling or education about the purposes and side effects of the prescription?" it would not be appropriate to use patient recall alone, because the patient may not remember this information accurately. But if the question is, "Do patients know the purpose and side effects of their medications?" then asking the patient directly would be appropriate.

What Is the Patient Population Being Studied?

There are important differences among patient populations, including demographics (age, gender, ethnicity, educational level), diagnosis, cognitive capacities, and personality traits. Differences between the population to be studied and a reference population (against which the measure was normed or standardized) could make study results uninterpretable. For example, the Client Satisfaction Questionnaire (CSQ) (Attkisson and Greenfield 1994) is a widely used mental health questionnaire to assess patient satisfaction. However, the CSQ was developed for, and tested in, outpatients. Questions pertaining to patients' satisfaction with office procedures, location and accessibility of services, and so on will not be appropriate for inpatients. Unfortunately, removing or altering questions from a measure invalidates its validity and reliability. Consequently, it is better to select an outcome measure tested in a population that most closely mirrors the population one wishes to assess. Similarly, if an outcome measure has been tested and standardized on persons with at least a sixth-grade reading level, then the results for persons with lower reading levels cannot be compared to those of the reference population.

Another consideration in tailoring the choice of an outcome measure to the patient population relates to diagnosis. An outcome measure specific to one diagnosis will generally have more questions specific to that disorder and therefore will detect finer changes than does a broader measure. For example, to assess functional impairment before and after an intervention for patients with uncomplicated major depression, an outcome measure specific to that illness (such as the Ham-D) would be preferable to a general psychopathology outcome measure (such as the BPRS).

At What Level Is a System of Care Being Studied?

The unit of care to be studied (e.g., an inpatient unit; a continuum-of-care service; an outpatient program with psychosocial rehabilitation; or a city-wide, statewide, or federal program) will inform choices of which type of data should be obtained for a particular outcome assessment. All research studies require standardization of the definitions and diagnostic criteria utilized, as well as of methods for obtaining subjects (Regier et al. 1984). It is a more prodigious and costly undertaking to standardize selection or sampling methods and diagnostic and functional criteria over multiple sites of data collection, but it is still important to do so. When assessing an individual unit, because the number of data gatherers (typically clinicians) is usually smaller, it can be feasible to collect more reliable detailed patient information by staff members trained to achieve interrater reliability. Specific definitions of mild, moderate, and severe, which would be reproducible (i.e., reliable) across raters, can more easily be agreed on. Alternatively, when studying large systems of care, readily accessed, less subjective data are more feasible. Examples of system data include demographic information, length of stay, readmission rates, and seclusion/restraint rates. What may be gained in richness of clinical information from a small program may be diminished by the power limitations of the number of subjects available. Larger systems of care allow for the detection of smaller differences than could be observed in small systems, but without the richness of clinical detail.

Different levels of study can be complementary in helping to understand observed outcomes. For example, suicide is a critical psychiatric outcome, but it occurs infrequently. An evaluation of a small program is unlikely to detect significant changes in suicide rate. Although the evaluation of a large program may yield high enough numbers to determine valid and reliable rates of suicide, such an evaluation will likely be unable to determine the reasons those rates were observed. A smaller study could focus more easily than a large study on how a program assesses suicide risk and addresses suicide precautions. Such data could be obtained by chart review (if those data are consistently recorded) or clinician interview.

Tension Between Validity, Reliability, and Assessment Feasibility

Assessment goals must be balanced against cost, time constraints of staff, and administrative burdens. In general, the more burdensome or complicated the measure, the less likely it is that staff members and patients will complete it accurately. Available automated, reliable, and valid data sources can decrease the burden of data collection on clinicians and patients. As mentioned above, there are trade-offs in all studies; what can be validly and reliably accomplished may fall short of expectations. Researchers need to determine how much accuracy and precision can be lost to learn something, even if less refined, about the study question. Assessing patterns of uncommon events such as hospitalization requires greater numbers of subjects and large data sets. These data sets can be expected to have missing or misclassified variables, but those limitations can be accepted if they are minimal. Although it is not ideal, this may be the only feasible way to study a particular issue.

Although researchers can still strive for good validity and reliability, they also need to be realistic about what can be measured. To do so requires understanding the various trade-offs among methods of data collection and measures utilized. For example, scaling back the goals of the evaluation to maximize validity and reliability may allow greater confidence in the results, but a more limited evaluation. For example, if assessing the appropriateness of medication, one might want to know dosage and blood levels—which may not be feasible. If it is not possible to determine the dosage and blood levels, perhaps it could be determined if patients with a diagnosis of major depression received *any* antidepressant medication. This would be useful information and can be reliably obtained. At times, more reliable or valid methods to study a particular intervention are not possible; in those instances, scaling back the confidence in the results may allow at least something to be learned about the intervention being assessed. The decision to scale back the assessment versus accepting lower validity and reliability will depend on the evaluation goals. It will also depend on whether the validity and reliability would be so compromised as to make the study results meaningless.

CONCLUSION

The results of quality assessments will continue to influence the ongoing debates over health care policy. Validity and reliability are the cornerstones of these assessments and they must be considered when designing and interpreting services research and quality improvement studies. The interrelationship among outcome assessment, validity, and reliability depend on more than the measures chosen and their reliability and validity. Careful consideration must also be given to the patient population, study goals, available data sources (and how reliable and valid they are given the population and study goals), and the ability to detect change given the number of study participants available.

Measuring quality and outcomes involves a trade-off between what one would really like to learn and what one *can* learn with as much validity and reliability as possible, given the constraints of cost, time, and burden. These issues are critical in understanding the strengths and limitations of an outcome assessment. They clarify what can and cannot be learned from a given assessment and what its appropriate impact should be on clinical practices and health care policies.

REFERENCES

American Psychiatric Association: Diagnostic and Statistical Manual of Mental Disorders, 4th Edition, Text Revision. Washington, DC, American Psychiatric Association, 2000

Attkisson C, Greenfield T: The Client Satisfaction Questionnaire–8 and the Service Satisfaction Questionnaire–30, in The Use of Psychological Testing for Treatment Planning and Outcome Assessment. Edited by Maruish M. Hillsdale, NJ, Erlbaum, 1994, pp 120–127

Beck A, Steer R: Manual for the Beck Depression Inventory. San Antonio, TX, Psychological Corporation, 1993

Betemps EJ, Buncher CR, Oden M: Length of time spent in seclusion and restraint by patients at 82 VA medical centers. Hospital and Community Psychiatry 43:912–914, 1992

Betemps E, Somoza E, Buncher C: Hospital characteristics, diagnoses, and staff reasons associated with use of seclusion and restraint. Hospital and Community Psychiatry 44:367–371, 1993

Bowden C: Efficacy of divalproex versus lithium and placebo in the treatment of mania. JAMA 271:918–924, 1994

Bowden C: New concepts in mood stabilization: evidence for the effectiveness of valproate and lamotrigine. Neuropsychopharmacology 19:194–199, 1998

Brooks K, Mulaik J, Gilead M, et al: Patient overcrowding in psychiatric hospital units. Adm Policy Ment Health 22:133–144, 1994

Carpenter M, Hannon V, McCleery G, et al: Variations in seclusion and restraint practices by hospital location. Hospital and Community Psychiatry 39:418–423, 1998

Cleary P: Subjective and objective measures of health: Which is better when? Journal of Health Services Research and Policy 2:3–4, 1997

Crenshaw WB, Francis PS: A national survey on seclusion and restraint in state psychiatric hospitals. Psychiatr Serv 46:1026–1031, 1995

Crenshaw WB, Cain KA, Francis PS: An updated national survey on seclusion and restraint. Psychiatr Serv 48:395–397, 1997

Donabedian A: Evaluating the quality of medical care. Milbank Q 44:166–203, 1966

Donabedian A: The quality of care. How can it be assessed? JAMA 260:1743–1748, 1988

Endicott J, Spitzer R, Fleiss J, et al: The Global Assessment Scale: a procedure for measuring overall severity of psychiatric disturbance. Arch Gen Psychiatry 33:766–771, 1976

Fletcher R, Fletcher S, Wagner E: Clinical Epidemiology: The Essentials. Baltimore, MD, Williams & Wilkins, 1996

Hyman S, Arana S, Rosenbaum J: Handbook of Psychiatric Drug Therapy. Boston, MA, Little, Brown, 1995

Kendall P, Hollon S, Beck A, et al: Issues and recommendations regarding the use of the Beck Depression Inventory. Cognitive Therapy Research 11:289–298, 1987

Klinge V: Staff opinions about seclusion and restraint at a state forensic hospital. Hospital and Community Psychiatry 45:138–141, 1994

Luborsky L: Clinicians' judgments of mental health. Arch Gen Psychiatry 7:407–417, 1962

McLellan A, Cacciola J, Kushner H, et al: The fifth edition of the Addiction Severity Index: cautions, additions and normative data. J Subst Abuse 9:461–481, 1992

Nunnally J, Bernstein I: Psychometric Theory. New York, McGraw-Hill, 1994

Overall J, Gorham D: The brief psychiatric rating scale. Psychol Rep 10:799–812, 1962

Parker G, Rosen A, Emdur N, et al: The life skills profile: psychometric properties of a measure assessing function and disability in schizophrenia. Acta Psychiatr Scand 83:145–152, 1991

Parker G, Hadzi-Pavlovic D, Rosen A: Life Skills Profile (LSP), in Outcomes Assessment in Psychiatry. Edited by Sederer L, Dickey B. Baltimore, MD, Williams & Wilkins, 1996, pp 79–81

Pope H, McElroy S, Keck PJ, et al: Valproate in the treatment of acute mania: a placebo controlled study. Arch Gen Psychiatry 48:62–68, 1991

Ray N, Rappaport M: Use of restraint and seclusion in psychiatric settings in New York State. Psychiatr Serv 46:1032–1036, 1995

Regier DA, Myers JK, Kramer M, et al: The NIMH Epidemiologic Catchment Area program. Historical context, major objectives, and study population characteristics. Arch Gen Psychiatry 41:934–941, 1984

Rosen A, Hadzi-Pavlovic D, Parker G: The life skills profile: a measure assessing function and disability in schizophrenia. Schizophr Bull 15:325–337, 1989

Ware JJ: The MOS 36-item short-form health survey (SF-36). Med Care 30:473–483, 1992

Ware JJ: The MOS 36-item short-form health survey (SF-36), in Outcomes Assessment in Clinical Practice. Edited by Sederer L, Dickey B. Baltimore, MD, Williams & Wilkins, 1996, pp 61–69

Ware J, Kosinski M, Keller S: A 12-item short-form health survey: construction of scales and preliminary tests of reliability and validity. Med Care 34:220–233, 1996

Way B: The use of restraint and seclusion in New York State psychiatric centers. Int J Law Psychiatry 8:383–393, 1986

Way BB, Banks SM: Use of seclusion and restraint in public psychiatric hospitals: patient characteristics and facility effects. Hospital and Community Psychiatry 41:75–81, 1990

PART
II

A Critical Review of the Instruments

CHAPTER 5

Outcome Measurement in Children and Adolescents

Peter Fonagy, Ph.D., F.B.A.

THE COMPLEXITY OF OUTCOMES MEASUREMENT

It is hardly self-evident, although it should be, that child mental health outcomes cannot be considered in absolute terms. Even in the arena of high-technology medicine it is now generally agreed that the impact of any intervention must be seen in the context of the totality of that person's life experience, ostensibly qualified as quality-adjusted life years (QLYs). Demographic changes, in particular the rising proportion of older individuals in society, has led to profound questions being asked about the circumstances under which death may be considered a positive rather than a negative outcome. Similarly, when is the preservation of a family unit a positive outcome, or rather for whom is that outcome positive—the child, the parents, the clinician, or the purchaser who would be required to fund alternative care? What if the outcomes diverge: if what is good for the child is less favorable to the family or to the service provider? What monetary value can be placed on symptom reduction? Is it worth more or less than the unity of a family? We should be aware of the adage, "In most instances the most cost-effective intervention is to do nothing."

The assessment of children and adolescents presents special problems. Children, especially those under age 8, are poor at verbalizing their thoughts and feelings. The clinician has to rely on other informants (parents, teachers, pediatricians, and case records). A major problem in the measurement of outcome in children arises from the low level of agreement generally observed among informants about the child's symptoms or adaptation. Even at the level of symptom severity, teachers, mothers, and fathers appear to have little more than 10% of variance concerning the child's internalizing symptoms (Achenbach 1995). It is striking that children's views concerning their own treatment are rarely taken into serious consideration; in fact, very little is known about children's understanding of mental health. It cannot be assumed that parents' perceptions will accurately reflect the child's feelings and needs. It is not surprising that a mother's mental health is a good predictor of her perception of the degree of her child's disability, even when this disability is of a physical nature (Jessop et al. 1988).

There is a danger of imposing ethnically rooted cultural biases on what is designated as "needing treatment" and a "good outcome." For instance, the achievement of selfhood through the separation-individuation process is one of the cornerstones of psychotherapeutic interventions. Yet is Lasch (1978) correct that the emphasis on individual achievement in Western culture is excessive and that an appropriate submission to the goals of the family and community may be a far better indicator of healthy adaptation? Such differences are particularly acute in the area of child development and parenting. Rogler (1989) outlined some of the practical steps that culturally sensitive outcome research requires. In particular, it is important to ensure that interventions are consonant with the subjective culture of the ethnic group to which it is applied and that instruments used are able to integrate cultural and linguistic meanings with the pertinent scientific categories.

A further consideration that complicates the issue of outcomes for childhood interventions is the developmental framework, which has appropriately come to dominate the fields of child psychiatry and psychology. Children's normal development presents a changing backdrop against which current complaints must be assessed. Many of the symptoms of mental disorder are normal in young children (e.g., fearfulness, shyness, difficulties in understanding language), and some may occur at particular developmental phases in the course of development (e.g., outburst of aggression, difficulty in sustaining attention). The clinical significance of problem behaviors change with age, and outcome instruments should (but frequently do not) take account of this.

A clear implication of the developmental approach is that symptoms cannot be considered the sole, or even the most important, criteria of treatment effectiveness. Because psychiatric disorder is not only the result of a complex series of interactions across time of biological, social, and psychological characteristics, but is itself part of a complex transactional causal chain, good outcome might sometimes be an increase rather than a decrease in symptoms.

Finally, the "adult-centrism" of evaluation techniques should be noted. Even diagnostic criteria for childhood disorders are derived from those of adults with only sparse research having been carried out concerning their validity or predictive value. Traditionally, clinicians had little faith in the value of diagnoses for children. However, these views were rapidly reconsidered when reimbursement standards and clinical guidelines became organized according to diagnostic categories. Many instruments available for outcome assessment available for children (like the diagnostic criteria) are translated down from adult versions, and their relevance to childhood problems is assumed rather than demonstrated. This is even more the case for adolescents, for whom there are very few specifically designed measures.

LEVELS OF OUTCOME MEASUREMENT

Five levels of outcome can be conceptually differentiated. They are described below.

Symptomatic or Diagnostic Level

Currently, the most sophisticated level of measurement of child mental health outcomes is the symptomatic or diagnostic level. Both categorical and dimensional checklist-based assessments can be obtained reliably with relative ease, and the computerization of such assessments will overcome many remaining practical problems. Studies comparing structured respondent-based interviews and checklists tend to find that both have reliability and validity, although checklists take far less time to complete. Nevertheless, the agreement between these methods of measurement is only moderate; consequently, the usual advice to researchers is to obtain multiple measurements from different informants. Because the use of multiple measurements inevitably reduces error through aggregation, this approach tends to lead to more robust findings.

The concern that this approach raises is the low level of observed agreement between informants, especially concerning internalizing behaviors. A further problem is that the correlates obtained with data from different informants tend to differ, which causes difficulties in the interpretation of results. There are a number of possible explanations for the poor agreement between two informants, including lack of knowledge of one or both parents. To deal with the disagreement between informants, one could count a symptom as present if it is reported by either of the informants (e.g., parent or child); another method would be the use of structural equation modeling to derive a latent variable. Achenbach (1995) offered a decision-tree approach for making taxonomic assignments from multiple sources of data. This approach, if applied, would enable the researcher to distinguish three reasons for such disagreements: 1) the contextual dependence of the child's problem, 2) comorbidity or multiple syndromes, and 3) distorted perception on the part of some informers. The value of these strategies in outcome research remains to be explored.

A broad range of symptomatic assessments is essential, because about half of individuals in community samples who meet diagnostic criteria for a DSM-IV-TR disorder (American Psychiatric Association 2000) are likely to meet criteria for another disorder as well (Anderson et al. 1987). In clinical samples, the prevalence of comorbidity is likely to be even higher (70%–75%) (Kazdin 1996). Some of this overlap may be the consequence of measurement problems and errors in prevailing psychiatric concepts. Nevertheless, comorbidity may be meaningful in that problems tend to go together. For example, delinquency commonly goes with drug abuse. They go together either because they serve similar functions in relation to development and adaptation (e.g., abuse and delinquency may both be understood in terms of attachment-related considerations) or because one represents a risk factor for the other (e.g., reading retardation may be a risk factor for conduct problems). Without evaluating the full breadth of an individual's symptoms, one will have limited information on the effectiveness of a treatment except for the individual's primary diagnosis.

The assessment of treatment inevitably involves repeated assessments. A recurrent feature in studies that use repeated ratings is that levels of psychopathology on the second rating occasion tend to be systematically lower than those in the first assessment (e.g., Boyle et al. 1997). This underscores the importance of using well-matched control groups as well as supplementing symptom ratings with other assessments. A further limitation of checklist and interview schedule–based measures is the rather obvious one that they can tap only the constructs that are included in them. This is not a problem when the features to be measured are well recognized, but it may well be an issue when exploring the treatment of less well-studied conditions. This argues for the use of investigator-based interviews that elicit descriptions of behavior rather than yes or no answers to structured questions.

A range of structured psychiatric interview schedules are available for the comprehensive assessment of child and adolescent psychiatric morbidity (Hodges 1993). The most impressive of these is the Child and Adolescent Psychopathology Assessment (CAPA) (Angold et al. 1995), which recently has yielded some interesting data from community use (Angold et al. 1999). There are parallel versions for child and parent. Unfortunately, it requires a high level of training (although a clinical qualification is not necessary) and takes several hours to complete, even with a cooperative family. Other than questions concerning symptoms of psychiatric diagnoses, the interview covers the perception of the quality of the child's relationships with the parents and with the siblings, self-care items, and aspects of adaptation, including chores, homework, and school life. It includes separate measurements of symptom intensity and accompanying social incapacity. Although the CAPA can be used to derive both International Classification of Diseases (ICD) (World Health Organization 1992) and DSM diagnoses, the approach is not hierarchical, so it can be adapted for use with any classification system. This is perhaps the most comprehensive interview schedule available, but it is also the lengthiest. The most popular measure is the Schedule for Affective Disorders and Schizophrenia for School-Age Children (K-SADS) (Puig-Antich and Chambers 1978). The interviews are conducted with the parents for younger age groups and take between 30 and 90 minutes, depending on the pervasiveness of the pathology. The K-SADS is a modification of the Schedule for Affective Disorders and Schizophrenia, used in adults. It is suitable for children ages 6–17 years and requires a trained clinician for administration. The first part of the interview is unstructured and permits the elicitation of information concerning the history of the present illness and ongoing episodes. The second part is highly structured and pertains to specific symptoms or behaviors used in the DSM diagnostic scheme. The final part consists of observational items. Its strength is its assessment of change in disorders over time, as it targets the past week, whereas the CAPA targets the past 3 months. There is a considerable body of literature that demonstrates the validity and utility of the instrument. The advent of highly structured assessment tools, such as the National Institute of Mental Health (NIMH) Diagnostic Schedule for Children (DISC), which comes in a spoken version that may be administered through headphones to children and parents and completed online (Shaffer et al. 1996), promises to improve both the accessibility and the validity of diagnostic information. It is highly structured, is focused on DSM criteria, and is suitable for large-scale epidemiological surveys. Even in its original noncomputerized form, it can be administered by trained lay interviewers. There is both a parent and a child version, and it takes at least an hour to complete. It is suitable for children ages 6–17 years.

Questionnaire measures of outcome are readily available. Perhaps the most widely used instrument is the Child Behavior Checklist (CBCL), which exists in various forms for different ages and a range of informants

(Achenbach 1991a, 1991b, 1991c). There are 112 behavior problems listed that are scored in a three-step response scale. The scales include major scales of internalizing and externalizing problems, as well as specific subscales for common problems such as delinquency, attentional problems, and social withdrawal. The scale is normally self-administered and can be completed in about 20–30 minutes. The scale is exceptionally well standardized and validated with well-established clinical cutoff points. There is some concern about the use of this measure as an outcome instrument because it may underreport change (which is not surprising, given the breadth of the measure and the dependence on informants). As always, there are alternatives; for example, the Strengths and Difficulties Questionnaire (Goodman 1997) is highly correlated with the CBCL and may be somewhat more acceptable to parents because of a greater emphasis on prosocial items.

There are questionnaire measures aimed at assessing specific types of problems. For example, a wide range of measures are available for measuring mood disorders, with the Children's Depression Inventory (CDI) (Kovacs 1985) and the Children's Depression Scale (Tisher and Lang 1983) being the most commonly used for depression, and the Children's Manifest Anxiety Scale (CMAS) (Reynolds and Richmond 1984) most commonly used for anxiety. The CDI has 27 items, each consisting of three statements, which the children either read or have read to them. It takes between 10 and 20 minutes to complete and is the best standardized of the self-report depression measures. With adolescents, there is accumulating evidence of the usefulness of the Beck Depression Inventory (BDI) (Beck et al. 1961). The CMAS has 34 items and is suitable for students in grades 1–12. Although it discriminates well between referred and nonreferred groups, it is less sensitive to acute stress. The State-Trait Inventory for Children (Spielberger 1973) is designed to measure response to acute stress, although the independence of the state-trait distinction is controversial.

Behavioral rating scales are often used in the measurement of the effectiveness of parent training interventions for conduct problems (e.g., the Family Interaction Coding Pattern [Patterson 1982] or the Eyberg Child Behavior Inventory [Eyberg and Robinson 1983]). But in this context also, expedience often dictates the use of self-reporting instruments (e.g., the Adolescent Antisocial Self-Report Behavior Checklist [Kulik et al. 1968]). Comprehensive personality assessments are rarely used in outcome investigations but are available (e.g., the Minnesota Multiphasic Personality Inventory–2 [Hathaway and McKinley 1989] or the Millon Adolescent Personality Inventory [Millon et al. 1982]). Self-report questionnaires are in general more appropriate for adolescent patients.

Adaptation Level

The second level of measurement concerns adaptation to the psychosocial environment. Mental health problems impinge on many domains of the child's functioning, yet many treatments are evaluated solely in terms of their impact on core symptoms. Recent meta-analyses demonstrate that such limited evaluations lead to a potentially misleading overestimation of the effect of the treatment, at least in terms of effect size (Weisz et al. 1995). It is known that many treatments leave important areas untouched. For example, stimulants do not benefit the academic performance and peer relations of children with attention-deficit/hyperactivity disorder (ADHD) (Hinshaw 1994). A well-planned study compared cognitive-behavioral therapy (CBT), family therapy, and supportive therapy in adolescents with major depression (Brent et al. 1997). Although the study showed CBT to be effective in reducing depressive symptoms, it did not show parallel gains in social functioning.

At this level, the available measurement options are limited. The most commonly used instrument is the Child's Global Adjustment Scale (CGAS) (see Shaffer et al. 1983). This is a 100-point clinical rating scale, analogous to the Global Assessment of Functioning scale. It is in common use clinically and has been used in some early pharmacotherapy trials. Reliability, however, is a significant problem, and the discriminant validity in relation to symptom severity is poor. There exist a small number of clinician-rated assessments that aim to assess functioning across a number of domains. Perhaps the best-known example is the Child and Adolescent Functioning Assessment Scale (CAFAS) (Hodges 1994), a clinician-rated scale to measure impairment over a 1- to 3-month period. It is suitable for use with children ages 7–17. This measure yields ratings on a four-point scale from severe impairment to no impairment in eight domains (school work, home, behavior toward others, thinking, etc.), yielding five scale scores and a total score. A self-training manual is available to clinicians. The advantage of the CAFAS is that ratings can be based on appropriately tailored clinical interviews. There are two optional scales for rating the young person's caregivers on their ability to provide for the child's material and emotional needs. The measure is a mandated part of publicly funded mental health service delivery in a number of states in the United States.

A new alternative parental interview–based measure, the Hampstead Child Adaptation Measure, was produced by Target and Fonagy (1992). They have identified 14 dimensions of adaptation that may be reliably assessed on the basis of a parental interview. This proved to be superior to simple global measures of functioning such as the CGAS. Unevenness of adaptation may be characteristic of clinical populations, and the presence of prosocial attributes may be particularly important in the comprehensive assessment of outcome. A strength of the approach is the developmental anchoring of adaptation; anchor points are manualized for specific age ranges (2–3 years, 4–5 years, 6–9 years, 10–13 years, and 14–18 years, the latter rated from direct interviews with adolescents) and can thus describe a child in terms of a clinician-rated developmental profile. The amount of psychometric information available on the instrument, however, is limited.

Objective measures of achievement (such as standardized attainment test scores) are often used as a proxy to adaptation measures. For example, one of the few studies of psychodynamic therapy for children used reading attainment as one measure of outcome (Heinicke and Ramsey-Klee 1986). Although such measures are clearly important and have a high level of face validity, they are also strongly correlated with IQ, and school performance may frequently be a function of factors other than the mental health care intervention (e.g., the quality of the school, the teacher, or the parent's support for the child's school work).

Mechanisms Level

The third level concerns mechanisms, the cognitive and emotional capacities that probably underpin both symptoms and adaptation. A cogent case has been argued for grounding outcome research in a theory of both normal and abnormal child development as well as a theory of therapeutic action. This means that outcome measures should be pertinent to the developmental theory within which a treatment is rooted as well as satisfying the practical concerns of patients, families, clinicians, and funders. A good example of the value of this approach was provided by a randomized, double-blind, placebo-controlled trial of methylphenidate (Tannock et al. 1995). In this study, two capacities ostensibly underlying ADHD were explored: response inhibition and response reengagement. The researchers administered three doses of the drug and found different dose-response functions for these two capacities. Whereas response reengagement had a linear relationship to dose, response inhibition was optimal in lower or middle doses. This finding argues against a typical clinical practice of determining the response to a stimulant from a single measure, such as a parent's report of child behavior.

Measurement is quite sophisticated in this area, and the literature is rapidly expanding (Sparrow et al. 2000). The domains most commonly assessed are attention, which is frequently measured using the freedom from distractibility factor of the Wechsler scales (digit span and arithmetic); perceptual functions such as recognition, discrimination, and patterning; memory, which can be assessed using standard IQ tests or specific memory tests such as the Wide Range Assessment of Memory and Learning; and executive functioning, that is, the integration of information from the external world, its transformation into symbols, and its combination with memories and internal states (most commonly assessed using the Wisconsin Card Sorting Test or the Tower Test).

Capacities that are important in the developmental outcome of psychological disorders include dimensions such as affect regulation, understanding of emotions, self-representation, understanding of mental states in self and others, forming emotional bonds, and making moral judgments and attributional biases. This level of measurement may be particularly important with younger children, in whom self-reporting data are the hardest to obtain. An excellent example is offered by Harter's (1990) work on self-esteem, because self-esteem is considered in many theories to be a critical determinant of mood disorder (e.g., Beck 1967). This comprehensive Self Perception Profile measures the child's perception of his or her competency within specific and global domains of self-esteem (Harter 1990). The measure covers scholastic, social, and athletic competence, physical appearance and behavior, and overall self-perception. A social support scale is available to cover the perceived regard the child receives from parents, classmates, teachers, and close friends. There are both parent and teacher versions as well as a child version, and it takes about 10 minutes to complete. The psychometric properties of this self-reporting instrument are reported to be good.

As biological approaches to mental health treatments develop, the reality of physiological measures of treatment outcome come ever closer. There are several studies that have demonstrated that the outcome of psychosocial interventions may be assessed by brain imaging techniques (e.g., Schwartz et al. 1996). In the behavioral health field, physiological measures of outcome for psychosocial interventions, such as growth or blood glucose levels in the treatment of poorly controlled diabetes (Fonagy and Moran 1990), have been available for some time. These measures, where they are already available and validated, are to be preferred, as they are less reactive with the treatment intervention than are self-reporting or parent-reporting measures of outcome.

It should be noted that although both symptoms and adaptation may be directly assessed from informants' reports or observations of behavior, capacities such as understanding of affect must be inferred from the child's performance on specially designed tasks. This creates measurement problems and challenges; for example, researchers are required to distinguish between competence and actual performance. What the child is capable of and what he or she tends to do are often rather different. The theoretical background of the clinician may determine the dimensions identified as being critical to specific interventions. An adequate demonstration of effectiveness must include measuring change in capacities (or mental processes) that the clinician believes may underpin or place the child at risk of developing symptoms or maladaptation. Surprisingly, outcome studies measuring change at this level frequently fail to demonstrate that symptomatic change was associated with modifications of underlying mechanisms. For example, CBT is sometimes successful without demonstrable changes in cognitive structures (Jacobson et al. 1996).[1]

Treatment studies provide an invaluable opportunity to explore causal mechanisms. Outcome gains should correlate and be a function of changes in the postulated mediating mechanisms. Treatment studies, particularly those with random allocation, offer an opportunity to experimentally manipulate key variables of potential causal significance. Even within-group comparisons can yield important information concerning the relationship between the success of the therapy and the extent of change in key mediating variables. The collection of information at the level of mechanism provides an important bridge between research on the causes of disorders and studies of treatment efficacy.

Transactional Level

The fourth level concerns transactional aspects of development. Child mental health professionals and developmentalists have traditionally been concerned with the contextual influences on the child's adaptation and generally see progression and mutual accommodation between the individual and changing environments. Because developmental psychopathology posits transactional interactions between the mental state and behavioral predispositions of the child and the reactions of the environment to him or her over time, it seems essential that evaluators should assess the quality of these transactions. Research on conduct disorder during the past 10 years has indicated how risk factors such as temperament and parents' personal and interpersonal problems (e.g., maternal depression) may interact to cause increased noncompliance. The caregiver's failure to cope with the

-----

[1] This is of more than passing significance in the evaluation of outcomes. Klein (1996) argues that if the Food and Drug Administration (FDA) were responsible for the evaluation of psychotherapy then "no current psychotherapy would be approvable" (p. 84) since the FDA requires that the efficacy of *active ingredients* of any medication be demonstrated. As long as outcome studies cannot show that the changes observed are explicable on the basis of the hypothesized mechanisms of action, a key link in the chain of evidence will be absent.

oppositional behavior of the child may be further aggravated by the absence of social support and the high level of psychosocial stress associated with the environment in which the family lives. Thus the contextual influences that may have transactional relations with the child's problem include the parents, family relations, characteristics of the community, the child's school, and more general cultural factors (Rutter and Smith 1995). Effective treatments address these risk factors, which must be evaluated alongside the child's characteristics.

A good example of the pertinence of the transactional dimension for outcome studies comes from family-based treatments of schizophrenia. High levels of expressed emotion (parents' hostility, criticism, and overinvolvement) predict onset of schizophrenia in adolescence as well as relapse after discharge. A number of well-conducted outcome studies (e.g., Tarrier et al. 1988) have demonstrated that intervention programs addressing expressed emotion reduce the likelihood of relapse in individuals taking medication.

Many effective interventions are directly aimed at bringing about change at the level of transactional processes. For example, parent training and social skills development programs for conduct problems of the kind described by Patterson and others (e.g., Patterson et al. 1992) are effective in improving child management skills, increasing prosocial behaviors, and reducing behavioral problems in middle childhood.

Adequate global measures of family functioning are now available. The Global Family Environment Scale (Rey et al. 1997) is a single 100-point rating scale that permits the easy assessment of family functioning. Although reliabilities reported for the scale are promising, too little data exist on this measure to encourage undue optimism. A better-established measure is the Parenting Stress Index (Abidin 1997), a questionnaire measure of the parents' attitudes to the problem child. It has 101 items rated on a five-point scale, with a brief checklist of life events over the last 12 months. It has two domains, the first corresponding to problematic characteristics of the child, which make it difficult for parents to fulfill their parenting role, and the second in which dysfunction of the parent-child system may be related to dimensions of the parents' functioning. There is also a total score, with a clinical cutoff. Importantly, an extremely low total score is interpreted as being dysfunctional or being associated with defensiveness or a lack of investment in the child. Each of the main domains has subscales associated with specific sources of difficulty, such as child adaptability, child demandingness, parent depression, and parent sense of incompetence.

It has been well demonstrated that approaches that bring about symptomatic improvement in the child also tend to reduce the extent to which parents report hostile and often aggressive feelings in the context of the parent-child relationship. This is of particular significance, because these attitudes are known to aggravate the child's condition, particularly in the case of oppositional and conduct problems. Another group of measures aim to assess the quality of the family system as a whole. There are many laboratory-based measures that aim to provide a view of family process (Grotevant and Carlson 1989). They are mostly difficult to set up; involve relatively complex scripts, such as mock family discussions; and have face, rather than empirical, validity. A frequently used self-reporting instrument for the measurement of family functioning is the Family Functioning Assessment (Olson 1994). This brief instrument, which provides the investigator with the family members' perception of family functioning, can be considered only a proxy for this domain, because it is confounded by the biases of the informant concerning the family process.

Such measures, moreover, carry severe limitations in that considerable evidence now suggests that environmental effects are best considered in terms of the effect on individual children rather than as a family influence. Also, global measures are further limited in that family variables that affect one sort of outcome may not be the same as those influencing others. It should also be borne in mind that what appears, from correlational studies, to be an environmental effect may be mediated at least partially by genetics or by gene-environment interactions (Rutter et al. 1997).

A further key dimension in the transactional level of analysis is peer relationships. Like relationships with parents, peer relationships can affect the course and outcome of treatment as well as be an important possible source of the child's difficulties. The measurement of the quality of peer relationships is possible from parental reports. The Index of Friendship Interview (Goodyer and Altham 1989), for example, aims to assess peer relationships in children above age 11. An alternative, more direct method, is the sociometric analysis of peer nominations within a class. The popularity of children within a class can be assessed by asking each of the class members to rate all the children in the class (Williams and Gilmour 1994). For example, the number of times a specific child is rated as "best friend" might be a good indication of the child's ability to make relationships. Reducing levels of aggression may be indexed by an increase in popularity.

Service Utilization Level

The final level of outcome concerns the level of service utilization. A number of interventions make strong assumptions concerning a reduction in posttreatment service utilization. For example, home-based preventive interventions implemented in early childhood may have the power to reduce childhood maltreatment and thus lessen the pressure on child welfare services. A number of studies offer evidence that maltreatment can be prevented, although not all studies demonstrate significant benefit. Mac-Millan et al. (1994) reviewed this literature and concluded that "extended home visitation can prevent child physical abuse and neglect among families with one or more of the risk-markers of single parenthood, teenage parents status and poverty" (p. 854).

Most children currently in mental health facilities have multiple service needs. Service utilization data therefore need to be comprehensive and longitudinal and need to show frequency, intensity, and duration of receipt across a wide range of services. Many instruments have been developed to collect service utilization data. An instrument developed specifically for mental health economic evaluations with a variant in the child and adolescent mental health field is the Client Service Receipt Inventory (Beecham 1995). A structured interview is used to elicit information concerning service use, to which an econometric analysis may be applied. In the United Kingdom, there is now an annual publication, *Unit Costs of Health and Social Care* (Netten and Dennett 1996). In the United States, a survey-based initiative is planned for a major multisite 5-year study of needs, service use, outcomes, and costs for children and adolescents with mental health problems. This survey will yield critical information concerning cost per service unit, total annual direct treatment costs, models of service organization and their respective costs, and the influence of insurance coverage.

Service level outcome may also be conceptualized at the level of general service provision and the quality of integration of various services. Thus an important outcome of intensive case management may be the better integration and greater accessibility of services relevant to child mental health.

Notwithstanding the self-evident usefulness of economic data, there is a remarkable scarcity of useful economic evaluations of child and adolescent mental health interventions (Knapp 1997). Obviously, until relatively recently researchers have been relatively uninterested in the health economist's perspective. However, as Yates (1994) pointed out, "the costs of clinical efforts are not mundane, unimportant, irrelevant, or too predictable to be of interest" (p. 729).

A further aspect of service utilization is satisfaction with service use. A wide range of user satisfaction measures are available (Vibbert and Youngs 1995). In general, however, these measures fail to distinguish variations in quality among interventions. Most interventions are rated by users as quite satisfactory.

CONCLUSION

The multiple-level outcome system described in this chapter has many features in common with the model advanced recently by Hoagwood et al.

(1996), Symptoms, Functioning, Consumer Perspectives, Environments, and Systems (SFCES). However, whereas Hoagwood and colleagues consider consumer satisfaction as a separate dimension of outcome, they combine adaptational and cognitive and emotional capacities into the single domain of functioning. Both systems emphasize that outcomes should be considered across a range of domains and underscore ways in which the measurement of child mental health outcomes is both more complex and yet less well developed than the assessment of adult functioning. Sophisticated evaluations of outcome are essential in addressing the issue of the appropriateness of a particular treatment for a particular individual. It is likely that particular profiles of scores on the five dimensions specified at baseline might predict the differential efficacy of the treatment for patient groups.

The approach outlined in this chapter prompts the question of why there are no measurement approaches that assess more than one of these levels simultaneously. Clearly this would have both practical and psychometric advantages. I know of only one such approach for children and adolescents. Workers at the Menninger Clinic in Kansas are developing a computerized medical record that will yield as a by-product outcome measurement at least at the symptomatic, adaptational, transactional, and service utilization levels (Clifford 1999). This instrument makes use of operationalized clinical judgments on a five-point scale. Separate versions are available for the age groups 3–5, 6–10, 11–13, and 14–18 (Barber et al. 1999). The ratings are based on ordinary clinical assessments by members of a multidisciplinary team, including psychiatrists, nurses, and social workers. There is also a parent self-reporting form. An advantage of such an approach is that information concerning outcome may be collected in the course of routine clinical evaluation in a standardized and reliable way.

REFERENCES

Abidin RR: Parenting Stress Index: a measure of the parent-child system, in Evaluating Stress: A Book of Resources. Edited by Zalaquett CP, Wood RJ. Lanham, MD, Scarecrow Press, 1997, pp 277–291

Achenbach TM: Manual for the Child Behavior Checklist/4–8 and 1991 Profile. Burlington, University of Vermont, Department of Psychiatry, 1991a

Achenbach TM: Manual for the Teacher Report Form and Profile. Burlington, VT, University of Vermont, Department of Psychiatry, 1991b

Achenbach TM: Manual for the Youth Self-Report and 1991 Profile. Burlington, VT, University of Vermont, Department of Psychiatry, 1991c

Achenbach TM: Diagnosis, assessment, and comorbidity in psychosocial treatment research. J Abnorm Child Psychol 23:45–64, 1995

American Psychiatric Association: Diagnostic and Statistical Manual of Mental Disorders, 4th Edition, Text Revision. Washington, DC, American Psychiatric Association, 2000

Anderson JC, Williams S, McGee R, et al: DSM-III disorders in preadolescent children: prevalence in a large sample from the general population. Arch Gen Psychiatry 44:69–76, 1987

Angold A, Prendergast M, Cox A, et al: The child and adolescent psychopathology assessment (CAPA). Psychol Med 25:739–753, 1995

Angold A, Costello EJ, Farmer EM, et al: Impaired, but undiagnosed. J Am Acad Child Adolesc Psychiatry 38:129–137, 1999

Barber CC, Target M, Fonagy P: Child and Adolescent FACE. Topeka, KS, Menninger Clinic, 1999

Beck AT: Depression: Causes and Treatment. Philadelphia, University of Pennsylvania Press, 1967

Beck AT, Ward C, Mendelson M, et al: An inventory for measuring depression. Arch Gen Psychiatry 4:561–571, 1961

Beecham JK: Collecting and estimating costs, in The Economic Evaluation of Mental Health Care. Edited by Knapp MRJ. Brookfield, VT, Ashgate, 1995, pp 157–174

Boyle MH, Offord DR, Racine YA, et al: Adequacy of interviews vs checklists for classifying childhood psychiatric disorder based on parent reports. Arch Gen Psychiatry 54:793–799, 1997

Brent DA, Holder D, Kolko D, et al: A clinical psychotherapy trial for adolescent depression comparing cognitive, family and supportive therapy. Arch Gen Psychiatry 54:877–885, 1997

Clifford PI: The FACE Recording and Measurement System: a scientific approach to person-based information. Bull Menninger Clin 63:305–331, 1999

Eyberg SM, Robinson EA: Conduct problem behavior: standardization of a behavioral rating scale with adolescents. J Clin Child Psychol 12:347–354, 1983

Fonagy P, Moran GS: Studies on the efficacy of child psychoanalysis. J Consult Clin Psychol 58:684–695, 1990

Goodman R: The strengths and difficulties questionnaire: a research note. J Child Psychol Psychiatry 38:581–586, 1997

Goodyer W, Altham PM: Recent friendship in anxious and depressed school age children. Psychol Med 19:165–174, 1989

Grotevant HD, Carlson CI: Family assessment: a guide to methods and measures. New York, Guilford, 1989

Harter S: Issues in the assessment of the self-concept of children and adolescents, in Through the Eyes of the Child: Obtaining Self-Reports From Children and Adolescents. Edited by La Greca AM. Boston, MA, Allyn and Bacon, 1990, pp 292–325

Hathaway SR, McKinley JC: Minnesota Multiphasic Personality Inventory–II. Minneapolis, MN, University of Minnesota, 1989

Heinicke CM, Ramsey-Klee DM: Outcome of child psychotherapy as a function of frequency of sessions. Journal of the American Academy of Child Psychiatry 25:247–253, 1986

Hinshaw SP: Attention deficits and hyperactivity in children. Thousand Oaks, CA, Sage, 1994

Hoagwood K, Jensen PS, Petti T, et al: Outcomes of mental health care for children and adolescents: I. A comprehensive conceptual model. Journal of the American Academy of Child and Adolescent Psychiatry 35:1055–1063, 1996

Hodges K: Structured interviews for assessing children. J Child Psychol Psychiatry 34:49–67, 1993

Hodges K: The Child and Adolescent Functional Assessment Scale. Ypsilanti, MI, Eastern Michigan University Department of Psychiatry, 1994

Jacobson NS, Dobson KS, Truax PA, et al: A component analysis of cognitive-behavioral treatment for depression. J Consult Clin Psychol 64:295–304, 1996

Jessop DJ, Reissman CK, Stein RE: Chronic childhood illness and maternal mental health. Journal of Developmental Behavioral Pediatrics 9:147–156, 1988

Kazdin A: Combined and multimodal treatments in child and adolescent psychotherapy: issues, challenges and research directions. Clinical Psychology: Science and Practice 3(1):69–100, 1996

Knapp MR: Economic evaluations and interventions for children and adolescents with mental health problems. J Child Psychol Psychiatry 38(1):3–25, 1997

Kovacs M: The Children's Depression Inventory (CDI). Psychopharmacology Bulletin 21:995–998, 1985

Kulik JA, Stein KB, Sarbin TR: Dimensions and patterns of adolescent behavior. J Consult Clin Psychol 48:1134–1144, 1968

Lasch C: The Culture of Narcissism: American Life in an Age of Diminishing Expectations. New York, Norton, 1978

MacMillan HL, MacMillan JH, Offord DR, et al: Primary prevention of child physical abuse and neglect: a critical review. Part I. J Child Psychol Psychiatry 35:835–856, 1994

Millon T, Green CJ, Meagher RB: Millon Adolescent Personality Inventory. Minneapolis, MN, National Computer Systems, 1982

Netten A, Dennett JH: Unit Costs of Health and Social Care 1996. Canterbury, University of Kent Personal Social Services Research Unit, 1996

Olson DH: Curvilinearity survives: the world is not flat. Fam Process 33:471–478, 1994

Patterson G: Coercive Family Processes. Eugene, OR, Castalia, 1982

Patterson GR, Reid JB, Dishion TJ: Antisocial Boys. Eugene, OR, Castalia, 1992

Puig-Antich J, Chambers WJ: Schedule for Affective Disorders and Schizophrenia for School-Age Children (Present Episode Version) (K-SADS-P). Unpublished manuscript, 1978

Rey JM, Singh M, Hung S, et al: A global scale to measure the quality of the family environment. Arch Gen Psychiatry 54:817–822, 1997

Reynolds CR, Richmond BO: Revised Children's Manifest Anxiety Scale. Los Angeles, CA, Western Psychological Services, 1984

Rogler LH: The meaning of culturally sensitive research in mental health. Am J Psychiatry 146:296–303, 1989

Rutter M, Smith DJ (eds): Psychosocial Disorders in Young People. Time Trends and Their Causes. Chichester, UK, Wiley, 1995

Rutter M, Dunn J, Plomin R, et al: Integrating nature and nurture: implications of person-environment correlations and interactions for developmental psychology. Dev Psychopathol 9:335–364, 1997

Schwartz JM, Stoessel PW, Baxter LRJ, et al: Systematic changes in cerebral glucose metabolic rate after successful behavior modification treatment of obsessive-compulsive disorder. Arch Gen Psychiatry 53:109–113, 1996

Shaffer D, Gould MS, Brasic J, et al: A children's global assessment scale (CGAS). Arch Gen Psychiatry 40:1228–1231, 1983

Shaffer D, Fisher P, Duclan M, et al: The NIMH Diagnostic Interview Schedule for Children Version 2.3 (DISC 2.3): description, acceptability, prevalence rates, and performances in the MECA study. J Am Acad Child Adolesc Psychiatry 35:865–877, 1996

Sparrow SS, Carter AS, Cicchetti DV: Comprehensive psychological and psycho-educational assessment of children and adolescents: a developmental approach. Boston, MA, Allyn and Bacon, 2000

Spielberger CD: Manual for the State Trait Anxiety Inventory for Children. Palo Alto, CA, Consulting Psychologists Press, 1973

Tannock R, Schachar R, Logan G: Methylphenidate and cognitive flexibility: dissociated dose effects in hyperactive children. J Abnorm Child Psychol 23:235–266, 1995

Target M, Fonagy P: Raters' Manual for the Hampstead Child Adaptation Measure (HCAM). London, Hampsted Clinic, 1992

Tarrier N, Barrowclough CC, Bamrah JS, et al: The community management of schizophrenia: a controlled trial of a behavioral intervention with families to reduce relapse. Br J Psychiatry 153:532–542, 1988

Tisher M, Lang M: The Children's Depression Scale: review and further developments, in Affective Disorders in Childhood and Adolescence: An Update. Edited by Cantwell DP, Garlson GA. New York, Spectrum, 1983, pp 181–202

Vibbert S, Youngs MT: The 1996 Behavioral Outcomes and Guidelines Sourcebook. New York, Faulkner & Gray's Healthcare Information Center, 1995

Weisz JR, Weiss B, Han SS, et al: Effects of psychotherapy with children and adolescents revisited: a meta-analysis of treatment outcome studies. Psychol Bull 117:450–468, 1995

Williams BT, Gilmour JD: Annotation: sociometry and peer relationships. J Child Psychol Psychiatry 35:997–1013, 1994

World Health Organization: International Statistical Classification of Diseases and Related Health Problems, 10th Revision. Geneva, World Health Organization, 1992

Yates BT: Toward the incorporation of costs, cost-effectiveness analysis and cost-benefit analysis into clinical research. J Consult Clin Psychol 62:729–736, 1994

Outcome Measurement in Geriatric Psychiatry

Roy H. Perlis, M.D.
Donald Davidoff, Ph.D.
William E. Falk, M.D.
Donald L. Round, Ph.D.
Sumer Verma, M.D.
Lloyd I. Sederer, M.D.

POPULATION CHARACTERISTICS AND PERTINENT PARAMETERS

An estimated 420 million people worldwide are age 65 and older. More than any other any other age group, these older individuals are more likely to have cognitive and functional disability. In addition, depression and other psychiatric diagnoses may present in unique ways. As psychiatrists are called on to care for these patients, they will need accurate measures of outcome to estimate the impact of their interventions and allocate resources efficiently. For many patients, these results are essential in deciding what supports will be needed and when institutionalization may be required. It is particularly important that clinical information be encapsulated in a concise and standardized manner to facilitate communication among clinicians.

For the clinical psychiatrist, one useful framework for assessing geriatric psychiatric outcome applies four basic axes. The first is cognition, which captures age-associated memory impairment as well as dementia. The second is mood, with a particular focus on depression. The third axis, behavior, may be related to deficits in the first two domains but merits independent consideration because it has important implications for prognosis and treatment. Finally, assessment of overall function assists in planning interventions and monitoring their success.

This chapter includes descriptions of the various domains in which outcomes may be assessed in geriatric psychiatry. For each domain, instruments are identified that may be particularly useful to individual clinicians and service systems, and the strengths and limitations of these tools are described. At the conclusion of the chapter, some directions in which future assessments may evolve are offered.

COGNITIVE ASSESSMENT

With increasing age, people typically experience some loss of sensory acuity, strength, speed, and flexibility or adaptability to new or changing circumstances. Fluid intellectual capacity—the ability to recognize a novel problem, conceptualize relevant factors, and initiate an appropriate response—reaches a peak in early adulthood and subsequently decreases slowly. However, older people do not normally lose their capacity for learning and logical reasoning. Similarly, crystallized intelligence—intellectual or practical knowledge about the world—does not normally show a decrement over the life span. When these sorts of decline do occur, characterization of deficits is important in making an accurate diagnosis.

Currently about 4 million Americans suffer from irreversible dementia. Its prevalence strongly increases with age: at age 65 about 1 in 10 people meet the criteria, compared with nearly 1 in 2 by age 85. Differentiating among dementia, delirium, and depression in a patient can be a particularly difficult task, and the three frequently coexist. Dementia is characterized by diminished functioning in multiple cognitive domains occurring in clear consciousness in a formerly nondemented individual; thus, the presence of amnesia or aphasia does not in and of itself qualify a person as having dementia. In addition to impairment in memory there must be a disturbance of at least one other cortical function (abstract thought, judgment, personality, voluntary movement, or sensory comprehension) such that the individual can no longer carry out normal daily activities. As such, instruments must assess multiple areas of cognitive function.

The brief cognitive assessment tools presented here are suitable for both initial clinical screening and serial reassessment. Although familiarity with the procedure may result in some improvement in test scores, test-retest practice effects among normal elderly persons tend to be clinically inconsequential. On the other hand, statistically significant changes in scores may not constitute clinically meaningful changes in function. Score changes over time should be at least one standard deviation in magnitude using appropriate norms to be considered relevant for clinicians. Specific norms for the elderly are absolutely necessary: extrapolation from data on younger persons is not appropriate. Clinicians should be sensitive to the contribution of mood disorders to cognitive impairment and should utilize a psychiatric interview or depression/anxiety screening instrument, as they deem appropriate.

Although for most of those with a dementing illness the prognosis is for an irreversible downward course, it is impossible to predict the progression of illness for any individual patient. General statements as to whether an individual is doing somewhat better, the same, or worse are often all that can be authoritatively made. An appropriate neuropsychological test battery may provide a more accurate sense of functioning over time.

Of note, accurate assessment of an elderly patient requires that attention be paid to a patient's auditory and visual acuity. Keeping an amplifier-type hearing aid and a pair of magnifying reading glasses on hand is a good idea. Equally important in conducting a useful cognitive examination is cooperation. An elderly person may have little enthusiasm for undergoing a fatiguing and potentially embarrassing set of tests. Taking the time to explain the need for such tests, to establish some rapport, and to pace the testing for best performance is usually worth the effort in increased motivation to succeed and more valid results.

Instruments for Cognitive Assessment

Mini-Mental State Exam

The Mini-Mental State Exam (MMSE) (Folstein et al. 1975) is a well-established screening tool for helping to determine the presence or absence of a cognitive disorder and to distinguish between neurologic and psychiatric illness in the elderly. It includes questions posed by an examiner to assess orientation to time and place, attention/concentration, language, constructional ability, and immediate and delayed recall. There are 11 numbered sections, with scores ranging from 1 to 5 and a resulting total score ranging from 1 to 30. The serial seven subtraction task can be replaced by spelling "world" backward if the patient is uncooperative or unable to perform serial sevens; the correct score for this latter task is the number of letters in correct order (e.g., D L O R W=3 points). The test is easily administered in 5–10 minutes by mental health clinicians without special training.

Care must be paid to the socioeconomic status of those assessed, given the positive correlation between greater educational level and higher scores; some reviewers suggest that the MMSE is inappropriate for individuals who are not fluent in English or who have less than an eighth-grade education. A version in Spanish is also available.

Although more complete data for interpretation are available, age- and education-controlled cutoff scores at about the 16th percentile are shown in Table 6–1.

Table 6–1. Cutoff scores (16th percentile) for the Mini-Mental State Exam

	Age 65–79		Age 80–90	
Years of education	0–8	9+	0–8	9+
Score	22	25	21	25

Scores below the 16th percentile are not necessarily conclusive evidence of a cognitive disorder; however, the 16th percentile is high enough for utility in the clinical setting in identifying possible problem cases for further evaluation and monitoring. Although the use of these cutoff scores will result in more false positives and fewer false negatives, this is acceptable in a screening instrument; a more stringent 5th percentile cutoff point would yield fewer false positives, but also fewer opportunities for earlier interventions. When the test is used for monitoring patients serially, scores may simply be compared with those obtained earlier in treatment.

Clock Drawing Test

The Clock Drawing Test (CDT) is an easily administered test requiring no material other than a blank, unlined sheet of paper and a pen or pencil. It complements the verbally loaded content of most dementia scales, requiring an integration of visuospatial, constructional, and higher-order cognitive abilities such as decoding of language. Paper and pencil are given to the patient with the following instructions: "Please draw the face of a clock. Make it large enough so you can place all the numbers on it, and set the time to 10 after 11." Instructions may be repeated or rephrased but not otherwise changed. Note that the wording requires the person to translate the wording "10 after 11" into an appropriate format, a task that is sensitive to impairment in language and abstract reasoning. Generating a precise score may be unnecessary, but one suggested 10-point scoring system (Spreen and Strauss 1998) is as follows:

10 Normal drawing with numbers and hands in correct position and clear differentiation between the length of the hour and minute hands
 9 Slight errors in hand placement or one missing number
 8 Placement of hands off by one number or appreciable gaps in placement of numbers on the face
 7 Hand placement significantly off (more than one number) or very inappropriate spacing of numbers
 6 Inappropriate use of clock hands (digital display or circling of numbers), crowding of numbers at one end of the clock face, or reversal of numbers
 5 Inappropriate arrangement of numbers (perseveration, dots instead of numbers, etc.); hands may be present but do not point at a number
 4 Numbers missing, written outside clock face, or in wrong order; clock face not represented by a complete circle; hands not clear or outside of clock face
 3 Numbers and face not connected/integrated; hands not recognizable
 2 Some response to drawing instructions but only vague resemblance to a clock; inappropriate arrangement of numbers
 1 No attempt, or irrelevant, uninterpretable figure

   Scores between 7 and 10 are considered normal in elderly persons (over 65), 6 is borderline (13% of unimpaired individuals, 88% of patients with Alzheimer's disease), and a score of 5 or less signals defective performance. This test has been shown to discriminate unimpaired elderly persons (mean age, 76) from individuals with Alzheimer's disease, vascular dementia, or depression. It does not differentiate between types of dementia and can be affected by visuospatial, motoric, and frontal syndromes. Therefore, it should be used only as a screening tool or to suggest other hypotheses for examination. In combination with the MMSE, it may also be useful for serial measurements.

Trail Making Test

The Trail Making Test (Heun et al. 1998) assesses speed and accuracy in attention, sequencing, mental flexibility, visual searching, and motor function. A stopwatch or a watch with a second hand or digital timer is necessary. There are two parts to the test, which is preceded by a short practice section. The entire test takes about 10 minutes to administer. For part A the patient is presented with a single sheet of paper on which are printed circles numbered from 1 to 25 in a random pattern; for part B the patient is given a similar sheet on which the randomly scattered circles contain either a single letter (A–L) or a number (1–13). For both parts, patients are instructed to connect the points in the appropriate order (numbers sequentially in part A, and alternating numbers and letters sequentially in part B).

Part A is a fairly simple test of speed of sequencing (i.e., following a well-known numerical series) and is subject to practice effects with repeated administration. Part B requires, in addition to speed and simple sequencing, that patients alternate between two series while maintaining a visual search that ignores or tunes out visual distractions, a frontally loaded activity. The Trail Making Test is sensitive to brain damage, alcoholism, mild dementia resulting from either Alzheimer's or cerebrovascular disease, and substance abuse; benzodiazepines can also have a deleterious effect on performance. There are no conclusive data supporting its use as a determinant of the site of brain injury, nor can it reliably differentiate between types of dementia. Performance on the Trail Making Test is relatively unaffected by the influence of aphasia, but it is affected by depression, as are all tasks that rely heavily on psychomotor speed.

Scores on this test are also highly associated with IQ and educational level, especially on part B. Although more complete data for interpretation (which incorporate time to complete the task as well as number of errors) are available, simple age-controlled cutoff times in seconds at approximately the 5th percentile (two standard deviations below the mean) are as shown in Table 6–2.

Table 6–2. Cutoff scores (5th percentile) for the Trail Making Test

Age	Part A	Part B
60–69	59	158
70–74	71	250
75–79	83	219
80–85	112	310

Three Words–Three Shapes Test

The Three Words–Three Shapes (3W-3S) Test was developed by Marsel Mesulam (1985) as a semiformalized memory test that could be given as part of a neurology examination. It consists of five forms: a stimulus sheet with three design-word pairs, an alternate version of the form for retesting, multiple-choice recognition sheets for each of the stimulus forms, and a scoring sheet. Patients are instructed to first copy the designs and words directly underneath the shape-word pairs (using photocopies of the stimulus sheet). The exemplar and the reproductions are removed from sight, and the patients are then asked to reproduce onto a blank unlined sheet of paper as much of what they have just copied as they can. This provides a measure of incidental recall, which is the ability to remember information without having been specifically instructed to do so (i.e., the way we take in most everyday information). If criterion is achieved—at least five of the six items reproduced correctly—then recall is assessed at 5-, 15-, and 30-minute delays (see below). If fewer than five items are produced correctly, then the stimulus sheet is presented for 30 seconds and the patient is asked to study the words and shapes and to try to remember them. The sheet is then removed and the patient is asked to reproduce the six items. This study-recall cycle is continued until either criterion has been achieved or five study-recall periods have taken place, after which 5-, 15-, and 30-minute delayed recall is assessed. If fewer than six items are produced in the final (30-minute) recall, then the appropriate multiple-choice recognition form is presented and the patient is asked to circle the words and shapes that he or she copied. There are no published norms for the test, but the clinician is referred to Chapter 2 of *Principles of Behavioral Neurology* (Mesulam 1985) for interpretation of results.

The 3W-3S Test is a useful screen of fine motor control and graphic output, cumulative learning over repeated trials, and memory storage and recall over time. A positive learning curve should be observed with repeated trials, with retention of what was recalled on the previous trial in addition to new material focused on and learned. In a true amnestic condition (such as that caused by Alzheimer's disease), there will be significant loss of material over time (i.e., more than 20% of registered/encoded material), and recall will not be significantly improved in a recognition format. The presence of intrusions, perseverations, or false-positive identifications tends to rule out pseudodementia of depression in favor of a true dementing condition. The 3W-3S Test would be useful in cases where there is a need to discriminate between problems of attention and those of memory registration, storage, and retrieval.

7 Minute Screen

The 7 Minute Screen (7MS) (Solomon et al. 1998) was recently developed to help identify patients with Alzheimer's disease. It consists of four brief tests (Enhanced Cued Recall, Temporal Orientation, Verbal Fluency, and Clock Drawing) that have been shown to reliably distinguish between patients who probably have Alzheimer's disease and healthy control subjects. Because the 7MS was developed specifically for the busy clinician, administration is brief, and scoring and interpretation of results are quite straightforward.

A stopwatch or a watch with a second hand is required. The training videotape is widely available, and the administration manual is written in a clear, step-by-step manner and is easily followed. Results are entered into a calculator (provided with the materials), which uses a logistic regression model to process the raw data and to designate one of three categories ("hi," "lo," or "re"). A score in the high category is consistent with a high probability of dementia characteristic of Alzheimer's disease. It is suggested that a patient who scores in this range undergo a full diagnostic evaluation, with the caveat that it is inappropriate to diagnose Alzheimer's disease based solely on 7MS results. A score in the low category is consistent with a low probability of dementia characteristic of Alzheimer's disease. However, if there is other information suggesting memory and cognitive problems, then further evaluation might be advisable. A score in the rescreen category indicates insufficient data for any judgment; either rescreening in 6–9 months or a diagnostic evaluation may be advisable depending on the patient's background and history.

The 7MS was designed to overcome the limitations of other easily administered assessment instruments. For example, its developers cite studies criticizing the MMSE as being too limited in its assessment of memory because it uses only three items without cueing, has an inadequate delay period, and has an unacceptably high rate of false negatives with more highly educated patients. According to its developers, the 7MS is highly sensitive in detecting Alzheimer's disease; has a low degree of false-positive bias (i.e., is specific); has good test-retest (over 1- to 2-month periods) and interrater reliability; is unaffected by age, sex, or education; and can differentiate reliably among very mild, mild, and moderate Alzheimer's disease. Of the four components, the most sensitive and specific is the Enhanced Cued Recall component: according to the authors, a cutoff point of 15 of 16 items correct accurately classified 59 of 60 Alzheimer's disease patients and 54 of 60 control subjects. However, the authors caution against selective use of just this test as a screening tool for Alzheimer's disease, because a diagnosis of Alzheimer's disease requires more than simple memory impairment (i.e., cognitive deficits in two or more areas) and the 7MS as a whole has significantly greater sensitivity and specificity.

The 7MS appears to constitute a good response to the need for a quick, reliable instrument that can help to identify incipient or actual dementia requiring further workup. Of the various instruments reviewed, the 7MS has the best psychometric properties for a screening procedure for the detection of possible dementia secondary to Alzheimer's disease. Limitations of the 7MS include a current lack of data supporting its utility in detecting dementia with causes other than from Alzheimer's disease, in differentiating Alzheimer's disease from other causes of dementia, and in discriminating between Alzheimer's disease and depression. In addition, its value in assessing outcome remains to be documented: it currently lacks the normative data (i.e., group means and standard deviations) that are necessary for monitoring changes over time and in response to interventions.

MOOD ASSESSMENT

Depression in the geriatric population is quite commonly misdiagnosed or overlooked altogether in the clinical setting. The coexistence of cognitive decline, medical comorbidity, and mood changes can result in a confusing clinical picture. Depressed patients may be particularly prone to somatization, prompting expensive medical workups in lieu of treatment. Moreover, they may present with subsyndromal or partially remitted depressive symptoms.

Some 30 scales purport to assess depression in some form, although they may focus on different symptomatologies. The degree to which somatic symptoms such as anorexia, sleep disturbance, and anergia are assessed is important to keep in mind, because the prevalence of these symptoms in the geriatric population is significant. Other scales assess the personality traits that may predispose to major depressive disorder. Three scales that may be particularly useful in measuring outcome in geriatric depression are reviewed below.

Instruments for Mood Assessment

Hamilton Rating Scale for Depression

Depending on the version used, the Hamilton Rating Scale for Depression (Ham-D) is a 17- or 21-item observer-rated scale for depression, administered by a physician or trained rater (Hamilton 1960). Based on a study of symptoms exhibited by depressed patients in hospitals, the scale was introduced in 1960 for the clinical assessments of depressive symptoms. It is a well-accepted, well-validated scale that is used extensively in clinical research as an outcome measure for treatment strategies. Most studies utilize the 17-item version.

The Ham-D heavily weights the somatic symptoms of depression and relies on the interviewing and clinical skills of the rater. Additional information obtained from others who are familiar with the patient can be used in arriving at a final rating. The interview, which can be administered in approximately 40 minutes, is focused on the patient's state in the immediately preceding few weeks. Each item is scored using a fine (5-point) or a coarse (3-point) scale.

The major value of this instrument lies in its extensive use in research studies. It is reliable and valid and can be particularly useful in assessing change in depression severity over time. The authors of the scale were actually quite specific in instructing users that the scale was not to be used as a diagnostic instrument, although it has often been so applied.

Although it is most useful in assessing major depressive disorders, the Ham-D can be used to assess the severity of affective symptoms in patients with schizophrenia or bipolar disorder. In these situations, it is best to pair this scale with another that is more specific to the other disorder.

The Ham-D has two primary limitations. First, it requires a skilled clinician to administer and interpret the test. Perhaps more significantly, it is heavily weighted to the somatic symptoms of depression. Although this weighting may appropriately identify depression in younger persons, it is less likely to be sensitive in older persons who may have much greater somatic distress consequent to medical illness. For more information, the reader is referred to Chapter 10 in this volume.

Geriatric Depression Scale

The Geriatric Depression Scale (GDS) (Yesavage 1982–1983) is designed to be self-administered, but it can be easily administered by any interviewer in 5–10 minutes. It is available in both a 30-item long form and a 15-item short form, with each question answered with "yes" or "no." Unlike other depression indices, it avoids somatic symptoms, which may be misleading in the geriatric population.

The GDS long form has been compared with a specialist clinical interview, and using a cutoff score of 11 points, it was found to have excellent sensitivity (84%) and specificity (95%) for depression. Both the long and short forms of the GDS are highly correlated and have similarly high sensitivity rates. The GDS has also been validated in cognitively impaired elderly populations: it was found to be a valid measure of mild to moderate depressive disorder in patients with mild to moderate dementia. In fact, the GDS is as accurate a screening test for depression in dementia as it is in cognitively intact subjects. However, given that the reporting of symptoms becomes less reliable with progression of the cognitive loss, the results should be interpreted with some caution in patients with more advanced dementia.

By focusing on the functional and mood symptoms of depression rather than potentially misleading somatic features, the GDS is a useful instrument for assessing the presence of a mood disorder in older patients. Because it is one of the most widely used basic screening instruments to identify depression in older patients, scores may be readily compared with published data. The yes-no response format encourages responses that denote presence or absence rather than more difficult quantification or multiple-choice answers.

Beck Depression Inventory

The Beck Depression Inventory (BDI) may be administered by a clinician, but it is most frequently used as a self-rating instrument (Beck et al. 1961). It is an inventory of 21 multiple-choice questions organized around the symptoms of depression. The respondent is required to rate each instrument on a four-point scale that describes increasing severity; the complete BDI can typically be completed in 5–10 minutes. There are established cut-off scores for nondepression (0–9), mild to moderate depression (10–18), moderate to severe depression (19–29), and severe depression (30–73). A shorter version of the BDI incorporating 13 of the 21 items has also been developed. Both versions have shown good reliability and validity with older adults.

The BDI includes two subscales: items 1–14 constitute the psychological item portion and items 15–21 are the somatic item portion. Older adults tend to score higher on the somatic item portion, and this has led some researchers to suggest that for older persons the psychological item portion alone should be used. The psychological subscale has demonstrated better overall ability to identify depression in the older adult.

The advantages of the BDI are its wide use, relative ease of administration, and brevity. However, its multiple-choice format may be difficult for older persons to follow, particularly individuals with some degree of cognitive impairment. Older persons, particularly depressed respondents, seem to find the GDS easier to complete than the BDI. For more information, the reader is referred to Chapter 10 in this volume.

BEHAVIOR ASSESSMENT

In patients with dementia, behavioral disturbances are quite common; up to 70% of patients will display agitation at some point. Other troublesome activities include wandering, pacing, aggression, shouting, and oppositional behavior. These symptoms contribute significantly to caregiver distress and increased health care costs, and they often lead to institutionalization. On the other hand, many of them respond to a combination of pharmacotherapy and behavioral interventions, making their recognition particularly important.

Several parameters of behavior can be measured. Some scales seek to quantify the severity of particular behaviors. Others sacrifice depth for comprehensiveness, measuring multiple common behavioral problems. A completely different approach seeks to measure the impact of a patient's behavior on his or her primary caregiver, expressed as caregiver burden or strain. All of these measures may be used to study an individual patient over time.

Several scales for the assessment of behavior problems in dementia are often applied in a research setting. These include the noncognitive portion of the Alzheimer's Disease Assessment Scale (ADAS; Rosen et al. 1984), which has 10 items rating such symptoms as depression and delusions, and the behavior rating scale of the Consortium to Establish a Registry for Alzheimer's Disease (CERAD; Morris et al. 1989). Two research-based tools that are potentially useful in the clinical setting, the Neuropsychiatric Inventory and the Behavioral Pathology in Alzheimer's Disease rating scale, are described in more detail below. A third tool, the Scale for Dementia Behavior Disturbance, includes a variety of typical behaviors such as making unwarranted accusations or screaming for no reason, but it is currently less widely used.

A plethora of instruments also attempt to assess the impact of patients' illness, including their behavior on caregivers (Vitaliano et al. 1991b). These tools provide a very different, but equally useful, sort of information, as it is often the primary caregiver who will ultimately decide when a greater level of care is needed. In general, burden may be assessed along multiple dimensions, among them physical, economic, social, and psychological. Measures may focus on caregivers' interpretation of a patient's illness (subjective burden) or on more quantifiable measures (objective burden). The Burden Interview and the Screen for Caregiver Burden are reviewed in more detail below. Of note, the Neuropsychiatric Inventory may also be coadministered with a caregiver distress scale.

Instruments for Behavior Assessment

Neuropsychiatric Inventory

The Neuropsychiatric Inventory (NPI) (Table 6–3) is conducted via a structured interview with a caregiver (Cummings et al. 1994). It includes a total of 12 sections; each begins with a single screening question followed by 7 or 8 subquestions. Symptoms are rated for frequency and severity, with an additional measure for caregiver distress (Table 6–4).

As a means of assessing outcome, the NPI offers several advantages over other instruments. First, it is quite comprehensive and includes items not specifically associated with Alzheimer's disease such as euphoria or frontal disinhibition. At the same time, it has been well studied, with defined psychometric properties and multiple versions available. Because

Table 6–3. Neuropsychiatric Inventory

Author/reference	Cummings et al. 1994
Versions/languages	English, Italian, Spanish
Means of administration	Structured interview with caregiver
Target group	Dementia
Number of items	12 sections, each with 1 screening question, 7–8 subquestions, rating scores for frequency, severity, degree of caregiver distress
Scoring	Domain score=frequency×severity Total score=sum of domain scores
Psychometric properties	Content validity: established via expert panel Concurrent validity with BEHAVE-AD, Ham-D behavior subtest ($P<0.05$) Interrater reliability, 93.6%–100% Test-retest reliability: frequency correlation=0.79; severity correlation=0.86 ($P<0.0001$ for both)
Strengths	Comprehensive Includes items associated with dementia other than Alzheimer's disease (e.g., euphoria, disinhibition seen in frontal dementias)
Contraindications/ limitations	Length of interview
Period of time assessed	Variable (1 month is standard)
Training requirements	Videotape, instructional module available
Source	Dr. Jeffrey L. Cummings, Reed Neurological Research Center, UCLA School of Medicine, 710 Westwood Plaza, Los Angeles, CA 90095-1769

the NPI quantifies specific symptoms, it facilitates a symptom-based approach to treatment in which interventions can be easily monitored. The availability of a separate measure for degree of caregiver distress allows an understanding of the impact of each symptom on the caregiver.

However, this amount of detail may also limit the usefulness of the NPI. It must be administered by a trained interviewer, and the amount of time required may preclude its use in routine office visits. Nonetheless, the amount of information obtained may justify the additional effort required.

Behavioral Pathology in Alzheimer's Disease Rating Scale

The Behavioral Pathology in Alzheimer's Disease Rating Scale (BEHAVE-AD) (Table 6–5) has been widely used in studies of Alzheimer's disease (Reisberg et al. 1987). It utilizes ratings by trained interviewers based on information that may be obtained from caregivers such as spouses or by direct observation. The scale includes seven categories, including paranoid/delusional ideas, hallucinations, activity disturbance, aggression, sleep dis-

Table 6–4.   Neuropsychiatric Inventory Caregiver Distress Scale
               (NPI-D)

Author/reference	Kaufer et al. 1998
Versions/languages	English
Number of items	12 domains (see NPI): delusions, hallucinations, dysphoria/depression, agitation/aggression, anxiety, apathy/indifference, euphoria/elation, irritability/lability, disinhibition, and aberrant motor function
Scoring	6-point scale for each domain
Means of administration	Caregiver survey
Target group	Alzheimer's disease
Contraindications/limitations	Measures caregiver distress *relative to neuropsychiatric symptoms only;* does not assess burden in other domains (physical, economic, social). Focused on symptoms most common in Alzheimer's disease.
Validity/reliability	Validity: robust correlation with Relatives' Stress Scale (a measure of general caregiver stress), $r=0.60$, $P<0.001$ Test-retest reliability: $r=0.92$, $P<0.001$ Interrater reliability: $r=0.96$, $P<0.001$
Strengths	Comprehensive, easily administered as part of NPI, allows correlation with particular symptom domains
Period of time assessed	4 weeks (may be altered easily)
Training requirements	Videotape, instructional module available
Source	Dr. Jeffrey L. Cummings, Reed Neurological Research Center, UCLA School of Medicine, 710 Westwood Plaza, Los Angeles, CA 90095-1769

turbance, affective symptoms, and anxiety/phobia. These are incorporated into 25 items, each with a 4-point rating scale.

Advantages of the BEHAVE-AD include its widespread use and defined psychometric parameters, particularly its good interrater reliability (Patterson et al. 1990). Moreover, it has been shown to be clinically useful, because it correlates well with Alzheimer's disease stage (as measured by global indices) and is sensitive to the effect of neuroleptic medications on behavior.

A primary limitation is its focus on Alzheimer's disease, which may limit its sensitivity in other forms of dementia. In addition, although it does include multiple behavioral measures, it is less comprehensive overall than the NPI.

Burden Interview

The Burden Interview, developed by Zarit and Zarit (1987), utilizes self-reporting by the caregiver of experiences in such domains as finances, health, social life, and interpersonal relations. Items in the interview, derived from

Table 6–5. Behavioral Pathology in Alzheimer's Disease Rating Scale (BEHAVE-AD)

Author/reference	Reisberg et al. 1987
Versions/languages	English
	Modified clinician interview version:
	E-BEHAVE-AD (Auer 1996)
Means of administration	Interview of caregiver
Target group	Alzheimer's disease
Number of items	7 categories with 25 characteristic symptoms
Scoring	Each symptom scored 0–3; total score 0–75
Psychometric properties	Excellent validity, reliability
Contraindications/limitations	Correlation with E-BEHAVE-AD only fair (0.51)
Strengths	Assesses broad range of behavioral pathology
	May be useful in distinguishing among dementia types
Period of time assessed	Specified by interviewer
Training requirements	Minimal
Cost	Free
Source	B. Reisberg, MD, Aging and Dementia Research Program, Department of Psychiatry, New York University Medical Center, 550 First Avenue, New York, NY 10016

the researchers' clinical experience, attempt to capture the caregiver's affective response to a given situation, although the scoring is based on how frequently an experience occurs. A sample question is "Do you feel angry when you are around your relative?" Each of the 22 items is scored on a 5-point scale ranging from never to nearly always. The scale can be administered independently or in conjunction with a 30-item Memory and Behavior Problems Checklist by the same authors.

Reliability and validity of the Burden Interview have been established. However, scores do not correspond to severity of dementia, which is not surprising in light of the nonlinear trajectory of burden described previously.

This scale is useful primarily for its brevity, broad scope, and applicability to all demented patients. One limitation is the lack of distinct indices for objective and subjective burden. Another is the inclusion of fewer questions assessing disruption of social or family situations than is done in some other instruments.

Screen for Caregiver Burden

The Screen for Caregiver Burden (Table 6–6) (Vitaliano et al. 1991a) is also administered by interviewing the caregiver. It includes 25 items generated from a list of upsetting experiences identified by caregivers of

Table 6–6.	Screen for Caregiver Burden
Author/reference	Vitaliano et al. 1991a
Versions/languages	English
Number of items	25
Scoring	Objective burden: number of events
	Subjective burden: distress score (1–4)
Means of administration	Caregiver interview
Target group	Spouses of patients with Alzheimer's disease
Contraindications/ limitations	No subscale scores; content limited to spouses, focused on Alzheimer's disease
Validity/reliability	Test-retest: 0.70 ($P>0.001$), 0.64 ($P>0.001$)
Strengths	Brief screen
Period of time assessed	Duration of illness
Training requirements	Minimal
Source	Dr. Peter P. Vitaliano, Dept. of Psychiatry and Behavioral Sciences, RP-10, Seattle, WA 98195

patients with Alzheimer's disease. Typical items include "My spouse doesn't cooperate with the rest of our family"; "I have to do too many jobs/chores that my spouse used to perform"; and "I worry that my spouse will leave the house and get lost." Scoring explicitly differentiates between objective burden (quantifying the number of behaviors or experiences present) and subjective burden (the amount of distress generated by a particular behavior, rated on a 4-point scale).

Investigation of the psychometric properties of this scale has shown it to have good reliability and validity. It is also sensitive to changes in burden over time, enabling its use as an outcome measure. The major strength of this instrument is its brevity and ease of administration; it is designed to be applied as a quick screen rather than a comprehensive measure. Its primary limitation is its focus on behaviors associated with Alzheimer's disease, although it may be adapted to assess other dementias.

FUNCTIONAL ASSESSMENT

Compared with other groups, older patients may have significant functional limitations, particularly if they have neuropsychiatric illness such as dementia or depression. In fact, a decline in function may be one of the initial indications of either medical or psychiatric illness. A significant portion of the health care resources used by the geriatric population goes for assisting these patients and providing appropriate, safe living situations for them. Targeting these interventions and determining the optimum setting for care are particularly important applications for outcome measures.

Function can be assessed on several levels, including basic self-care (often referred to as basic activities of daily living) and ability to function in the community (or instrumental activities of daily living). Patients who cannot perform most basic activities of daily living often require more than 12 hours a day of assisted care. The degree of support required to achieve a certain level of functioning is yet another level on which function can be assessed; although it is simpler to follow than other aspects, this measure provides less useful information about a particular patient. The caregiver burden scales addressed above also reflect patient functioning (via the impact of loss of function) to some extent.

These parameters can be assessed by caregiver or patient reporting, by direct observation, or by physical testing. Although many instruments exist, two are notable for both their longevity and their simplicity of use and are described in more detail.

Instruments for Functional Assessment

Katz Activities of Daily Living Scale

The Katz Activities of Daily Living (ADL) Scale, described in 1970, assesses basic elements of personal hygiene and self-maintenance (Katz et al. 1970). It is administered by an interviewer, generally to a patient's caregiver. Particular questions assess bathing, dressing, toileting, transferring, continence, and feeding. Multiple scoring systems exist, although the 2- and 3-point scales are the most widely used. A related scale, the Physical Self-Maintenance Scale (PSMS), uses a 5-point observer-rated system (Lawton 1988). Of note, some newer modifications of the ADL scale include other basic activities of daily living such as walking and grooming.

A major advantage of the Katz scale is its ease of use and speed of administration; the complete scale can be completed in 2–4 minutes. It provides useful, concise information about a patient's needs and abilities. As the most commonly applied activities of daily living scale, it has been validated in a wide range of settings, so patients can easily be compared with study populations.

Several disadvantages are also worth noting. The ADL scale was originally described as hierarchical, in that patients were expected to lose functions in a specific order (bathing first, then dressing, toileting, transferring, continence, and feeding) dictated by the underlying neurobiology. This has proved not to be the case; the order in which skills are lost is highly variable. Moreover, the scale has been shown to be sensitive only in the later stages of dementia, so other measures must be employed in patients with more mild illness, such as tracking the ability to perform a particular hobby or type of work. Lastly, most authors agree that continence should not be classified as an activity of daily living. Urinary incontinence is quite prevalent in the geriatric population, particularly among women, and often reflects medical illness such as urinary tract infection.

Lawton Instrumental Activities of Daily Living Scale

The Lawton Instrumental Activities of Daily Living scale assesses more complex activities necessary to function independently in the community (Lawton et al. 1982). These skills include using the telephone, traveling beyond walking distance, shopping for groceries, preparing meals, doing housework or handiwork, doing laundry, taking medication, and managing finances. Several forms are available, including a self-rated (3-point) scale and observer-rated (3- to 5-point) scales.

The strengths and weakness of this scale are similar to those of the Katz scale. It may be administered quickly, provides specific information about areas in which patients need assistance, and allows comparison with a multitude of study populations. On the other hand, it too is nonhierarchical, which limits its predictive value. Certain items may not be applicable to all patients or may reflect traditional gender roles, as many patients have never been responsible for doing laundry or housework.

ONGOING ISSUES IN OUTCOME MEASUREMENT

The geriatric population presents unique challenges in psychiatric outcomes assessment. To begin with, the patients themselves may be difficult to characterize. Many have complex medical comorbidity, which can confound assessment tools or interventions. Others are unable or unwilling to participate in the assessment process because of sensory or cognitive limitations. Moreover, the definition of outcome itself may be difficult, as the requirements for daily function in an 80-year-old retiree may be very different from those of a 35-year-old physician. Close coordination with the primary care provider and other treatment providers helps to overcome some of these limitations; balance and gait assessment and vision and hearing testing are often critical.

In cognitive assessment, time constraints remain a major concern. None of the clinician-administered instruments are designed to replace formal neuropsychological testing, which can require several hours to administer but remains the gold standard for assessing an individual's cognitive strengths and weakness. With repeated testing, neuropsychological testing also provides the most complete information regarding cognitive changes over time. Briefer tests, which still capture a broad range of cognitive data, will be quite helpful for future clinicians.

The major difficulty in mood assessment remains the vast difference in presentation between younger and older patients. Future scales will need to be sensitive to these differences, particularly the confounding effects of somatic symptoms. It may also be useful to include measures of function in addition to the psychological and somatic items that are in the current instruments. Instruments will have to be able to discriminate between the relative contributions of depression and dementia to the functional decline of older persons.

A number of factors complicate the development and interpretation of behavioral instruments, particularly burden scales. Burden tends to follow a nonlinear trajectory in dementia, with certain periods being associated with particularly acute strain. One such time is initial diagnosis; another is onset of incontinence. Thus scores during one period cannot necessarily be used to predict scores during another. In addition, these instruments necessarily reflect aspects of the caregiver as well as of the patient: caregivers differ in their ability to tolerate patient needs. Lastly, most tools overlook the positive aspects of care giving, and in so doing may fail to present a complete picture of the patient-caregiver relationship. As these instruments continue to evolve, investigators will need to find the optimum balance between depth and breadth to make them clinically useful. At the same time, relating symptoms and their impact on caregivers will be essential; the NPI Caregiver Distress index represents a useful first step in this regard.

Future refinements in functional assessment instruments should reflect several needs. The *basic* versus *instrumental* distinction may be overly simplistic; some investigators have suggested that the Katz and Lawton scales actually reflect three scales: basic self-care, intermediate self-care, and complex self-management. More biologically oriented scales with better predictive value for individual patients would be particularly helpful. Newer scales may also substitute gender-nonspecific items. Finally, scales that focus on certain critical tasks will provide a useful adjunct to more general scales. Already, a number of instruments exist that assess such skills as driving a car or managing medications independently.

REFERENCES

Auer SR, Monteiro IM, Reisberg B: The Empirical Behavior Pathology in Alzheimer's Disease (E-BEHAVE-AD) Rating Scale. Int Psychogeriatr 8:247–266, 1996

Beck AT, Ward CH, Mendelson M, et al: An inventory for measuring depression. Arch Gen Psychiatry 4:561–571, 1961

Cummings JL, Mega M, Gray K, et al: The Neuropsychiatric Inventory: comprehensive assessment of psychopathology in dementia. Neurology 44:2308–2314, 1994

Folstein MF, Folstein SE, McHugh PR: "Mini-mental state." A practical method for grading the cognitive state of patients for the clinician. J Psychiatr Res 12(3):189–198, 1975

Hamilton M: A rating scale for depression. J Neurol Neurosurg Psychiatry 23:56–62, 1960

Heun R, Papassotiropoulos A, Jennssen F: The validity of psychometric instruments for detection of dementia in the elderly general population. Int J Geriatr Psychiatry 3(6):368–380, 1998

Katz S, Downs TD, Cash HR, et al: Progress in the development of the index of ADL. Gerontologist 10:20–30, 1970

Kaufer DI, Cummings JL, Christine D, et al: Assessing the impact of neuropsychiatric symptoms in Alzheimer's disease: the Neuropsychiatric Inventory Caregiver Distress Scale. J Am Geriatr Soc 46:210–215, 1998

Lawton MP: Physical Self-Maintenance Scale (PSMS). Psychopharmacology Bulletin 24(4):793–794, 1988

Lawton MP, Moss M, Fulcomer M, et al: A research and service-oriented multilevel assessment instrument. J Gerontol 37(1):91–99, 1982

Mesulam M: Principles of Behavioral Neurology. Philadelphia, PA, FA Davis, 1985

Morris JC, Heyman A, Mohs RC, et al: The Consortium to Establish a Registry for Alzhiemer's Disease (CERAD); Part I: Clincial and Neuropsychological Assessment of Alzheimer's Disease. Neurology 39:1159–1165, 1989

Patterson MB, Schnell AH, Martin RJ, et al: Assessment of behavioral and affective symptoms in Alzheimer's disease. J Geriatr Psychiatry Neurol 3:21–30, 1990

Reisberg B, Borenstein J, Salob SP, et al: Behavioral symptoms in Alzheimer's disease: phenomenology and treatment. J Clin Psychiatry 48(suppl):9–15, 1987

Rosen WG, Mohs RC, Davis KL: A new rating scale for Alzheimer's disease. Am J Psychiatry 141:1356–1364, 1984

Solomon PR, Hirschoff A, Kelly B, et al: A 7 minute neurocognitive screening battery highly sensitive to Alzheimer's disease. Arch Neurol 55(3):349–355, 1998

Spreen O, Strauss E: A Compendium of Neuropsychological Tests: Administration, Norms, and Commentary, 2nd Edition. New York, Oxford University Press, 1998

Vitaliano PP, Russo J, Young HM, et al: The screen for caregiver burden. Gerontologist 37:76–83, 1991a

Vitaliano PP, Young HM, Russo J: Burden: a review of measures used among caregivers of individuals with dementia. Gerontologist 31:67–75, 1991b

Yesavage JA, Brink TL, Rose TL, et al: Development and validation of a geriatric depression scale: a preliminary report. J Psychiatr Res 17:37–49, 1982–1983

Zarit SH, Zarit JM: The Memory and Behavior Problems Checklist–1987R and the Burden Interview (Technical Report). University Park, PA, Pennsylvania State University, 1987

CHAPTER 7

Outcome Measurement in Forensic Psychiatry

Henry C. Weinstein, M.D.

Annmarie Caracansi, M.D.

Gary R. Collins, M.D.

Craig L. Katz, M.D.

Anand A. Pandya, M.D.

The practice of forensic psychiatry is defined by the fact that it relates to people who are involved with the legal process. In this regard, forensic psychiatrists carry out two separate and distinct functions: evaluations for legal purposes and the treatment of patients incarcerated in jails, prisons, and special forensic psychiatric hospitals. In its definition of the subspecialty of forensic psychiatry, the Accreditation Council for Graduate Medical Education (1996) (the accrediting body for fellowships in forensic psychiatry) explicitly identifies these two separate functions.

In its *Ethics Guidelines for the Practice of Forensic Psychiatry*, the American Academy of Psychiatry and the Law (1991) defines forensic psychiatry as "a subspecialty of psychiatry in which scientific and clinical expertise is applied to legal issues in legal contexts." In this chapter, we distinguish between the two functions by referring to the evaluation role as *forensic psychiatry* and the treatment role as *correctional psychiatry*.

The importance of this distinction cannot be overstated. Not only are the professional responsibilities that govern these roles—that is, the ethical principles that guide the psychiatrist in each situation—dramatically different, but the desired outcomes are necessarily quite different in one role than in the other (American Academy of Psychiatry and the Law 1991; Appelbaum 1997; Stone 1984; Strasburger et al. 1997). Briefly, whereas the *treatment* responsibilities of the correctional psychiatrist may, overall, be governed by the usual principles of benefit to the patient and to "do no harm," the *evaluation* responsibilities of the forensic psychiatrist to the legal system are governed by the principles of the search for the truth and the administration of justice.

Considering this important distinction, what should be the measure of outcome in the practice of forensic psychiatry? In this chapter we separate the two functions and discuss the particular instruments suitable to these functions: first the outcome measurements for forensic psychiatric evaluations and then the outcome measurements of treatment in correctional psychiatry. We then note, as an aspect of "outcome" in forensic psychiatry, the special and often unique problems and social concerns with criminal recidivism and its clinical analogs, risk assessment, and the prediction of dangerous behavior. Finally, we suggest some possible future directions for the measurement of outcome in this unique area of psychiatric practice.

OUTCOME MEASUREMENTS OF EVALUATIONS IN FORENSIC PSYCHIATRY

Forensic psychiatrists routinely evaluate the competency and criminal responsibility of criminal defendants. These psychiatrists must determine whether defendants possess a range of capacities necessary at the successive stages in the legal process, including competence to waive Miranda rights, to confess, to stand trial, to plead guilty, to waive representation by counsel, to testify, to waive a jury trial, to waive appeals, and to be executed. Likewise, they must determine whether the defendant has any psychiatric disorder that could preclude criminal intent or knowledge and therefore be invoked as exculpatory evidence (Miller 1994). The extent to which psychiatric illness plays a role in criminal behavior may lead to acquittal of defendants as not guilty by reason of insanity (NGRI) or, at the least, to a mitigating of the charges against them. Sections to follow focus specifically on competence to stand trial (CST) and NGRI for two reasons. First, these two matters exemplify the theoretical and practical difficulties inherent in assessing the outcome of criminal evaluations made by psychiatrists. Second, although they are few and far between, published attempts by forensic psychiatrists to assess the outcomes of their criminal evaluations invariably focus on CST and NGRI.

Forensic psychiatrists also perform evaluations in the arena of civil law. Here, their work broadly encompasses such matters as psychiatric disability, personal injury, capacity to make a will, guardianship, decisions regarding death and dying, informed consent, and refusal of medical treatment. On the surface, psychiatric consultations within many of these domains appear amenable to outcome assessment. For example, when a forensic psychiatrist examines a psychiatric patient who has received disability compensation for his or her illness, one desirable effect might be that if the patient's current psychiatric treatment is deemed inappropriate, he or she can seek better therapy. In practice, however, there is little or no available literature on outcomes in most civil aspects of forensic psychiatry.

Outcome Measurements of Evaluations in Criminal Cases

Competency to Stand Trial

In evaluating a defendant's CAT, the forensic psychiatrist seeks to answer a legal question. The questions to be answered in evaluating an accused criminal's competency (or "fitness") to stand trial in most states are generally based on the U.S. Supreme Court's decision in *Dusky v. United States:* (1960) first, does the defendant have a "rational as well as factual understanding of the proceedings against him?"; and second, does he have "sufficient present ability to consult with his attorney with a reasonable degree of rational understanding?" (Grisso 1988, p. 4). As when focusing on other competencies or criminal responsibility, forensic psychiatrists are asked to address these two issues with the defendant, rather than to treat or necessarily benefit the defendant.

This situation suggests to some that for the forensic psychiatrist, as pointed out above, the physician's traditional duties of benefit to the patient and "do no harm" lose their primacy, giving way instead to the legal goals of the search for the truth and the administration of justice. Therefore, the ambiguity of the forensic psychiatrist's role begets not only ethical problems but also considerable confusion over issues of outcome assessment. If outcome studies in medicine traditionally focus on assessing improvements in patients' suffering and functioning, what standards can the forensic psychiatrist apply when assessing evaluations that have a legal rather than a clinical goal? Although the field of outcomes assessment may be new to traditional medicine, it seems conceptually foreign to psychiatric evaluations of criminal defendants.

What would be the desired outcome in evaluations for CST? The ideal would be a valid assessment—in other words, does the defendant truly meet the criteria spelled out in the Supreme Court's *Dusky* decision? But what makes a CST determination true and hence valid? Several authors, either implicitly or explicitly, have taken the approach that reliability lends validity to CST outcomes. In other words, if forensic psychiatrists are able to reliably reach the same conclusions about specific cases, then the individual consultants must be offering accurate and valid CST assessments. Blashfield et al. (1994) exemplify an interesting example of this approach. They asked members of the American Academy of Psychiatry and the Law to assess CST in specially computer-generated case histories. In the one case that was regarded by the study's authors as the clearest example of lack of competence, 25% of the experts still found the case's defendant competent.

Another study by Rosenfeld and Ritchie (1998) revealed that forensic clinicians working in pairs at one New York City forensic psychiatry clinic reached the same CST determination for defendants 99.5% of the time. On the other hand, a 1980 Canadian investigation bemoaned the "striking" differences in the frequencies of CST and other determinations in forensic clinics across Canada (Menzies et al. 1980). Such variation would indeed be troubling if it said more about the differences in technique among psychiatrists than about actual differences in the defendants.

The study by Menzies et al. (1980) raised the issue of bias in CST evaluations and suggests another criterion for evaluating the outcome of CST determinations: conceptual consistency. Extraneous factors that affected the outcome of a CST evaluation would lessen its validity. In this regard, the study noted that factors such as "psychiatric ideology" and "systemic context," rather than the "pathology" and "criminality" of the examinee, created enormous disparities in CST outcomes across Canada. Blashfield et al. (1994) similarly attributed the unexpected declarations of competence for one of their seemingly incompetent patients to an expressed tendency of the study's participants to declare defendants competent unless there was compelling evidence to the contrary. Personal biases like these may distort the eventual CST outcome by introducing subjective factors into the ostensibly objective domain of CST. However, several more recent studies have allayed such concerns in finding that clinical factors alone, rather than demographic variables such as age and race, influence CST decisions (Cooper and Grisso 1997; Robertson et al. 1997).

However, if the courts may be considered "consumers" of forensic psychiatry evaluations in the same way that patients are consumers of more traditional psychiatric services, then other possibilities for outcome assessment arise. In particular, we can ask, have CST evaluations served the purpose of the courts to which they are addressed? Some investigators have actually asked judges this very question, with generally favorable responses (Owens et al. 1985). The frequency with which the judicial disposition of cases match those suggested by CST evaluations offers another potential standard for quality assessment and outcome measurement. For example, one study found that 85% of eventual court decisions agreed with the findings of CST evaluations (Menzies et al. 1982). It remains for further consideration whether such agreement represents an acceptable outcome standard or a hopelessly circular one wherein the CST evaluation informs the very court decision by which it is then judged.

Grisso (1988) focused on the quality of the various mental health agencies and criminal justice systems in which CST evaluations are conducted. He pointed out that all of the following require monitoring as factors relevant to the quality of CST evaluations: clear and adequate communication between the criminal justice system and the psychiatrist so that the latter has access to all information relevant to the evaluation of a defendant (i.e., reasons for raising the question of CST); cost-efficiency of the evaluation itself; and continuing education for forensic psychiatrists despite inadequate budgets.

Amid the complexities inherent in the study of outcome in CST evaluations, several structured instruments for assessing CST offer the possibility of some clarity. The Competency Screening Test (CSTest) and the Georgia Court Competency Test (GCCT) have been evaluated, and both appear to accurately predict the clinical competency decisions of examiners (Nicholson et al. 1988, 1998). The CSTest consists of 22 items, each of which describes a hypothetical legal situation for which the defendant must give an appropriate response in a fill-in-the-blank fashion. Although it was initially designed for the defendant to give written responses, it has also been used with oral responses. Each item is scored from 0 to 2, with higher scores reflecting greater competency. A cutoff score of at least 22 out of the maximum possible 44 on all questions is considered to be consistent with competency. Although the CSTest is a quick and simple tool with demonstrated predictive validity, the basis of its predictive power remains uncertain. Factor analysis has not revealed how any of its 22 items bear on its predictive validity, thereby handicapping its utility in assessing the many specific functional abilities that collectively inhere in CST.

On the orally administered GCCT, the defendant must answer 17 questions about courtroom procedure, knowledge of the charge, possible penalties, and the ability to communicate with an attorney. Scoring ranges vary for each question, with higher scores reflecting higher competency. The maximum possible score on the questions is 50. The subject's total score is doubled, and a doubled score greater than 70 reflects competency.

Like the CSTest, the GCCT is a rapid and clear instrument with demonstrated predictive validity. Unlike the CSTest, however, the GCCT has the added virtue that its items do predict the overall score and assessment of competency. In particular, items relevant to the defendant's specific legal knowledge were highly correlated with the CST decision.

The MacArthur Competence Assessment Tool–Criminal Adjudication (MacCAT-CA) provides a more recent attempt to assess CST in a structured fashion (Hoge et al. 1999). The MacCAT-CA consists of 22 items divided into three sections: understanding, reasoning, and appreciation. Administration of the interview is estimated to take between 25 and 55 minutes. For the first two sections, a clinical vignette is read to the examinee and questions are posed based on this vignette. The final section then examines the extent to which the subject is able to apply understanding and reasoning to his or her own legal situation. All 22 items are graded from 0 to 2 by the examiner. These individual scores are summed into subtotals for the three domains of understanding, reasoning, and appreciation that reflect whether the individual has minimal/no, mild, or clinically significant impairment within that domain. Unlike the CSTest and the GCCT, the MacCAT-CA thus yields scores on three capacities relevant to CST but no overall score for CST.

The norms for interpreting the MacCAT-CA were developed by comparing 729 defendants after they were divided into three categories: competent without any known mental illness; competent with treated mental illness; and incompetent and hospitalized for restoration of their fitness. The MacCAT-CA was also found to have high interrater reliability, internal consistency, validity, and classification utility. Its authors caution that the MacCAT-CA was devised as a "tool" rather than a "test" of CST that should be employed only in the context of a complete clinical evaluation of a defendant. They also caution that relevance accorded to the various items of the Mac-CAT-CA will likely vary with different courts.

Criminal Responsibility

In light of the preceding survey, it should come as no surprise that the forensic determination of NGRI lacks a clear gold standard by which it may be judged (Janofsky et al. 1989). Nevertheless, the scant literature on outcome in NGRI suggests three potential standards by which to assess the quality of NGRI assessments.

First, as with CST, the reliable rendering of NGRI assessments may indicate the validity of decisions and the quality of individual psychiatrists' work. Thus, a study such as the one by Steadman in 1980, which found considerable discrepancies across New York State in rates of NGRI acquittals, may be interpreted as suggesting that NGRI assessments in the state at the time were of dubious quality. Likewise, agreement between the defense and prosecution in a given case of NGRI would seem like a valuable indicator of the quality of the NGRI assessments. Reliability would avoid the battles of the experts that can take place in the course of a trial. Indeed, Janofsky et al. (1989, 1996) observed that among the respective cohorts in their two studies, few if any of the cases in which criminal responsibility became an issue led to trials where NGRI was disputed by the two sides (Janofsky et al. 1996). In most cases, the sides either agreed to NGRI before going to trial or the defense dropped its NGRI plea before the trial.

Second, and again like the case of CST, agreement between the psychiatrist's conclusion of NGRI and the court's ultimate decision in a given case may define a high-quality outcome. Thus, the finding by Janofsky et al. (1989) of a high correlation between the psychiatric determination of NGRI and court decisions in Baltimore City during a 1-year period may represent an assessment of favorable outcomes in forensic psychiatry.

Third, outcomes may be assessed with respect to their impact on public safety. Several studies have tracked NGRI acquittees over time. One such study found that NGRI acquittees who were eventually released into the community had a high rate of rehospitalization, an outcome that was deemed desirable by reviewers (Packer 1998). This initially counterintuitive conclusion makes sense when rehospitalization is contrasted with reentry into the criminal justice system. One may then ask whether NGRI acquittees who eventually abscond from their forensic units and commit further crimes reflect a poor outcome not only for the responsible facility but also for the initial NGRI evaluation (Nicholson et al. 1991). That is, the NGRI verdict might not have adequately served the public safety in these cases because these acquittees could have been more securely incarcerated in a prison had they instead been found guilty.

The Rogers Criminal Responsibility Assessment Scales (R-CRAS) (Rogers 1984) provide what is perhaps the best-known instrument for assessing criminal responsibility. As such, it offers one tool with which to assess outcome in NGRI evaluations. The R-CRAS consists of 30 different variables (questions) relevant to NGRI that are to be clinically assessed and ranked in terms of the degree to which they characterize the examinee. For example, in item 1 the examiner is asked to rate the reliability of the examinee on a scale of 0 (no information) to 5 (definite malingering). The examiner, who must be a board-eligible or board-certified psychiatrist or have a Ph.D. in clinical or counseling psychology, completes all of the 30 variables immediately after having thoroughly reviewed all available records and then interviewed the examinee. In part 2 the evaluator is asked to translate these variables into decision models, which consist of the various psycholegal criteria (or summary scales) for NGRI—either the American Law

Institute (ALI) or the older McNaughten criteria, depending on which are to be used. For example, in item A1 under the ALI decision model, the examiner is asked to give an opinion regarding the presence of malingering; this opinion is keyed to variables 1 and 2 from the first part. Once all six of these summary scales under the ALI decision tree are completed, these are in turn translated into a composite opinion on the issue of NGRI according to this standard.

The R-CRAS has primarily been tested for reliability and validity for the ALI standard only (the ALI standard is, in fact, the most commonly used standard for NGRI in the United States and differs from the historical standard of McNaughten). As such, the summary scales of part 2 appear to have both internal consistency (α coefficient ranging from 0.28 to 0.8) and reliability (κ ranging from 0.48 to 1.00). The scales also appear to have adequate construct validity. Limitations of the R-CRAS include the need for adequate training in forensics for the examiner, its limited validation in individuals with organic impairment, and the absence of reliability and validity studies using the McNaughten criteria (which are still used in a substantial number of states).

After a defendant is deemed NGRI, retention in a secure psychiatric hospital, rather than incarceration in a prison, follows. That retention then continues only so long as the insanity acquittee is considered dangerously mentally ill. The forensic psychiatrist is therefore periodically called on to assess the dangerousness of the acquittee to evaluate the continued need for his or her retention within the forensic psychiatric system. Therefore, instruments that predict dangerousness in a reliable and valid manner offer one highly desirable route for improving the outcome of NGRI evaluations. One such instrument is the HCR-2 (in which HCR stands for history, clinical assessment, and risk management).

The HCR-2 (Webster et al. 1997) assesses risk for violence by rating 20 different items divided among the three general categories of the patient's history, clinical assessment of the patient, and risk management issues. In fact, it serves not so much as an instrument per se but more as a guide for the major areas that the forensic psychiatrist must consider in assessing the violence risk of individuals such as insanity acquittees. Each of the 20 items, which include such broadly determined risk factors as the presence of mental illness and the presence of a personality disorder, are scored from 0 to 2, with 2 indicating that there is a high likelihood that a given risk factor is present. A conclusion is reached for each individual risk factor based on all data available to the examiner, including prior records, a clinical interview, and psychological testing. Thus, the examiner must have considerable forensic and clinical expertise to be able to use the HCR-2. The scores for the 20 items may be tabulated into subtotals for the history items, clinical items, and risk items as well as an overall total. The HCR-2 ultimately leads the examiner to judge whether the individual poses a low, moderate, or high risk for future violence but does not specify how the various subtotals and total score beget this conclusion. Clinical judgment remains central in the application of this instrument. Its authors thus caution that the current version of the HCR-2 does not yet represent a standardized scale but rather a guide for highlighting the general principles in violence risk prediction.

Outcome Measurements of Evaluations in Civil Cases

Competency to Refuse Medical Treatment

Competency to refuse medical treatment stands out as one civil forensic area where outcomes have at least begun to be explored. Two retrospective studies of consultations by hospital-based consultation-liaison psychiatrists on patients who refused various aspects of their proposed medical care examined the eventual outcome of the study cases (Katz et al. 1995; Umapathy et al. 1999). Both found that, after the competency determination, many (up to 43% in one study) of the patients eventually accepted the disputed treatment or a modification thereof, regardless of whether they were deemed competent or incompetent. The authors thus concluded that the psychiatric consultation facilitated treatment delivery. Validation of this promising conclusion will obviously require future controlled studies. Moreover, it should be kept in mind that the consultant psychiatrists in cases of treatment refusal often engage in both evaluation and treatment of the patient, making it difficult to assess the outcomes of their evaluations alone. This differs from the criminal examples of CST and NGRI, in which the forensic evaluations of defendants are readily distinguished from the treatment that ensues after a defendant has been deemed not competent to stand trial or NGRI, and in which the evaluations and the eventual treatments are often performed by different psychiatrists. One study addressed the question of whether there was any effect on the outcome of electroconvulsive therapy if the depressed patients under study gave informed consent (Wheeldon et al. 1999). The researchers found that consenting and nonconsenting patients had equal rates of response to the treatment.

The MacArthur Competence Assessment Tool for Treatment (Mac-CAT-T) (Grisso and Appelbaum 1998) provides a semistructured interview with which to assess a given patient's abilities in four general areas considered crucial to competence to consent to treatment: understanding, appreciation, reasoning, and expressing a choice. Alternatives to treatment constitute a fifth category that may be considered as well. The MacCAT-T guides the examiner through disclosures of the various details of the patient's disorder, treatment options, risks/benefits, and alternative treatments. Patients are intermittently asked to express their understanding of this information and its relevance for them, and the interviewer rates each answer on a scale of 0 to 2, where 2 indicates that the patient is believed to meet full criteria on a given item. These are then summed to reach individual summary ratings for each category of understanding, appreciation, reasoning, expressing a choice, and, where applicable, alternative treatments. These scores reflect the patient's relative strengths in the different categories, but no total score to reflect overall competency is used. In this way, the MacCAT-T serves as a semistructured supplement to a standard clinical/forensic examination and helps to highlight particular areas of strength or weakness in the patient. In testing, the MacCAT-T has yielded very high interclinician reliability for its various items (ranging from 0.82 to 0.98) and its categories (ranging from 0.87 to 0.99) (Grisso and Appelbaum 1999).

Involuntary or Civil Commitment

Assessing the outcome of a decision to place a patient in a psychiatric hospital against his or her will poses numerous challenges. To start, who is the consumer of this service—the state, the public, the patient, or some combination thereof? From the patient's perspective, being civilly committed may have a number of consequences, not all of which are desirable. Liberty is sacrificed for safety, suggesting that the benefits of one outcome may override the ill effects of another. Lastly, as with consultation-liaison psychiatry, it is difficult to evaluate the outcome of a civil commitment evaluation apart from the psychiatric treatment that ensues in its wake. Nonetheless, researchers have at least begun to broach the issue of outcome in civil commitment. In a manner similar to studies of outcome in CST, one group has observed that the disposition of commitment hearings usually follows the recommendation of physicians, attorneys, and witnesses rather than being influenced by demographic factors such as age, race, and gender (Miller et al. 1983). Civil commitment and compulsory treatment for substance abusers, in particular, has received some attention, with research suggesting that long-term relapse rates are lower following such treatment (Leukefeld and Tims 1990). More recently, Olson et al. (1997) developed the Commitment Response Form as a reliable tool to measure the outcome of involuntary treatment of dually diagnosed alcoholics.

    In the related area of informed consent in clinical research trials, one group has reviewed the existing literature to determine the effect of various consent techniques on outcome measures of subject anxiety, subject understanding, and consent rate (Edwards et al. 1998). They found that giving more information to people enhances their knowledge of the research, which in turn reduces their anxiety. However, the more information that is imparted, the less likely are people to consent to participate. Interestingly, then, in this instance several outcome measures are potentially at odds with one another. Researchers and the public alike might hope that better information would lead to more ready availability of research subjects.

Finally, because malingering is a significant concern in forensic evaluations, it should be noted that special instruments have been developed to assess it. One of these instruments, the Structured Interview of Reported Symptoms (SIRS), has been used extensively since its development in 1985. It consists of a 172-item structured interview. It is estimated by its authors to take about 30–40 minutes (Rogers et al. 1992).

The response to each question is scored as X (no information), 0 (not present), 1 (qualified yes), or 2 (definite yes). The SIRS generates eight subscores that assess whether the individual has endorsed rare symptoms, uncommon symptom combinations, improbable or absurd symptoms, blatant symptoms, subtle symptoms, a higher number of symptoms than is generally found in genuine patients, severity of symptoms, and discrepancy between reported and observed symptoms.

The SIRS is not designed to give a definitive answer to whether or not an individual is malingering. Rather, it is designed to suggest further investigation of feigning if any subscore crosses a threshold to the "definite" range, if three or more subscales have scores in the "probable feigning" range, or if the total SIRS score exceeds a certain threshold.

The SIRS has demonstrated high interrater reliability (Rogers et al. 1992), and it has been validated as a reliable discriminator in both clinical and nonclinical populations (Rogers 1997). In one study, the SIRS was shown to discriminate effectively between inpatients and simulators who were coached (Rogers et al. 1991). In this study, it demonstrated 100% positive predictive value and 100% negative predictive value for the uncoached population and a 96.7% positive predictive value and 84.6% negative predictive power for the coached population.

The SIRS has been validated in English but not in other languages. In addition, the wording and sentence complexity of some items on the SIRS may become problematic for individuals with very low levels of education. The SIRS has also not been validated on a population with severe head trauma. Because it is not uncommon in correctional settings to see individuals who do not speak English, individuals with low levels of education, and individuals with a history of head trauma, these limitations are important considerations and suggest future directions for research on this instrument.

OUTCOME MEASUREMENTS OF TREATMENT IN CORRECTIONAL PSYCHIATRY

This section describes the outcome measurement of psychiatric patients in correctional and forensic facilities. It is worthwhile to note that this group of patients—unique in that it is defined by its involvement with the criminal justice system—is quite substantial: of the almost 2 million people incarcerated in the Unites States' jails and prisons, more than 280,000 have been classified as "mentally ill offenders" (U.S. Bureau of Justice Statistics 1999; Lamb and Weinberger 1998). To these must be added patients who are on probation or parole and those being held in special forensic psychiatric facilities.

The correctional psychiatric population includes many subpopulations, each of which may require special types of treatment considerations (American Psychiatric Association 2000) and therefore special measurement of the outcome of treatments. These include patients with co-occurring mental illness and substance abuse disorders, women in correctional facilities, youths in adult facilities, geriatric patients, and those with mental retardation or developmental disabilities. Treatment selection—and therefore the outcome measurements of treatment—must take into consideration each subset of this population and its specific concerns. Moreover, because psychiatric treatment of correctional patients ranges from substance abuse treatment to behavioral strategies, anyone undertaking assessment of treatment must be prepared to measure a variety of treatment modalities.

Although few instruments exist that are specifically designed for measuring outcomes in correctional psychiatry, various outcome assessment tools used in general psychiatry may be employed, such as the Hamilton Rating Scale for Depression, the Beck Depression Inventory, or the SIRS. These tools are discussed in other sections of this book. The use of standardized measures in outcome evaluation maximizes reliability and sensitivity.

In general, the goals of effective treatment from the patient's perspective are relief from primary symptoms and restoration of unimpaired or improved functional status; however, forensic psychiatry must also take into account societal goals, such as safety.

Suggested criteria for treatment effectiveness, including societal as well as individual concerns, are reduction of primary symptoms, improved health and personal and social functioning, the cost of care, and the reduction of public health and safety concerns.

Relief of primary symptoms and improved functioning can be measured by the same criteria used by the U.S. Food and Drug Administration in controlled clinical trials (Sederer and Dickey 1996; U.S. Food and Drug

Administration 1980). Reduction of primary symptoms can be measured by independent evaluators. Effectiveness of substance abuse treatment can be assessed by urinalysis, Breathalyzer measurement, and self-reporting.

Threats to public safety include criminal acts committed by the mentally ill with or without the influence of substances. Crimes committed under the influence of drugs and alcohol can be measured by confidential self-reports, interviews, and questionnaires. Objective measures of treatment outcome include review of public arrest and conviction measures, but these measures typically underestimate the extent of the criminal and dangerous activities actually engaged in.

Three types of classification and analysis are needed to assess treatment outcomes: first, a risk/adjustment scheme to systematically identify the differences in severity of mental illness, (such as comorbidity); second, a treatment definition scheme to describe the nature, duration, and intensity of treatment intervention including the context and setting in which the treatment is delivered; and third, measured outcome variables to address a range of outcomes, including social functioning.

Specific instruments that may be applied to the correctional population include the Addiction Severity Index (ASI) and the Treatment Services Review (TSR). The ASI is designed to evaluate the nature and severity of the problems presented by substance abusers at the start of treatment and after discharge. The TSR is designed as a companion to the ASI to characterize the functions of a treatment program. (See Chapter 12 in this volume for a review of both scales.)

The ASI may not be an appropriate measure for the criminal population, because it depends on disclosure by the patient in a setting in which help is sought and trust in the provider exists. There is reason to suspect denial, conclusion, or misrepresentation among those in criminal populations and those with chronic psychiatric disabilities (Sederer and Dickey 1996). One recently developed instrument is discussed here as an example. The Correctional Program Assessment Inventory (CPAI), developed by Gendreau and Andrews (1996) at the University of New Brunswick, is a structured assessment of the rehabilitative potential of correctional programs with high-risk patients both in community and in institutional settings. Although it is a helpful, comprehensive instrument, it does not provide an assessment of the treatment of the mentally ill in a correctional setting. (This test is further discussed below with regard to its relevance to the study of recidivism.) Briefly, the CPAI assesses the strengths and weaknesses of programs in the following areas: program implementation, client preservice assessment, program characteristics, staff characteristics and practices, evaluation, and other. The CPAI provides a percentage score of program quality.

The Carlson Psychological Survey (CPS) (Carlson 1999) assesses behavior or substance abuse problems in offender populations. This assessment tool, which may be used with adults and adolescents, evaluates the effectiveness of intervention programs. The CPS has a five-category response format consisting of a 50-item questionnaire, which takes about 15 minutes to complete. It may be used for research or evaluation of intervention programs. There are four scale scores and one validity check. The CPS includes chemical abuse, thought disturbance, antisocial tendencies, self-deprecation, and validity. This tool has been assessed with regard to correlations with the Minnesota Multiphasic Personality Inventory.

There is a growing body of evidence that treating the mentally ill in the correctional setting favorably changes outcome. Metzner (1998) has detailed the significance of treatment for the mentally ill in the correctional setting. Evidence shows that inmates with schizophrenia have more trouble functioning in a prison environment than do nonschizophrenic inmates, and consequently they have more prison infractions and spend more time in lockdown and in prison.

In another study (Metzner 1998), inmates in the New York State prison system who received psychiatric care (which included milieu therapy, individual and group therapy, psychotropic medications, recreational therapy, task and skills training, educational instruction, vocational instruction, and crisis intervention) were shown to have reductions in rules infractions, suicide attempts, correctional discipline, the use of crisis care, seclusion, and hospitalization. The American Psychiatric Association practice guidelines for treatment of patients with schizophrenia in a correctional setting include medication and psychosocial and rehabilitative programs. They warn against placing patients with schizophrenia in lockdown for behaviors resulting from their illness, because such intervention not only will not ameliorate the behavior but might make it worse (Metzner 1998).

The end point for the assessment of treatment needs to be explicit before the appropriate measure can be applied. If the goal of treatment is restoration of competency, then measures that assess competency will measure treatment outcome. If the goal of treatment is that the forensic patient no longer commits crimes, then recidivism measures (discussed in the next section) must be applied. If the goal of treatment is amelioration of psychiatric signs or symptoms, then a host of other measures may be applied— both subjective evaluations, in which a patient assesses the degree of symptoms, and objective measures, in which an evaluator rates psychiatric signs and symptoms. Another measure of treatment may be rehospitalization rates or lengths of stay as indicators of treatment outcome. These measures would include hospitalization in a psychiatric unit within a correctional facility or hospitalization of forensic patients from the community.

In summary, the importance of effective treatment for the mentally ill correctional patient should be obvious, because treatment for the sick and safety in the community are shared societal goals. Important work has begun on defining measures and designing outcome assessment instruments. This section should have demonstrated not only the uniqueness and the complexity of this task but also the significant need for it.

OUTCOME MEASUREMENTS IN RECIDIVISM

Society seeks to protect its citizens; therefore, it seeks to prevent criminal behavior. Forensic psychiatric evaluations are invoked to predict criminal behavior. Correctional psychiatric treatment may be invoked to prevent future criminal behavior.

Thus, from the perspective of society, it is highly desirable that forensic psychiatric evaluation and correctional psychiatric treatment predict and prevent future criminal behavior. In criminology, *recidivism* is defined as repeated criminal offense (with the recidivist frequently labeled as a "habitual offender") (Hanson and Bussiere 1998). The corollary in psychiatry relates to the prediction of "dangerousness," which many now prefer to discuss in terms of "risk assessment."

Although prediction of dangerousness is an evaluation frequently requested of forensic psychiatrists (Luettgen 1998), it is fraught with legal, ethical, and societal complications. Even determining the most appropriate tools or measurements to facilitate this task requires scholarly endeavor. Perhaps the most simplistic tool of assessment of dangerousness risk occurs by way of corroborating the treatment failures, or repeated criminal offenses—that is, recidivism.

However, the determination of individual deterrents to recidivism is an important and extremely challenging function of criminal law. For example, in the landmark case, *Barefoot v. Estelle*, a psychiatrist testified that he was "100% sure" that a person with the characteristics of the defendant would be violent in the future. After this testimony, the jury subsequently decided against the defendant and sentenced him to death. The American Psychiatric Association responded in brief by casting doubt on the psychiatrist's ability to predict danger. Although years have passed since this monumental case, many of the questions it raised remain largely unanswered.

Despite the tremendous implications and pressures associated with attaining valid and reliable measures for risk management, there are few measurement tools in place to predict recidivism and dangerousness (Hanson and Bussiere 1998; Kaplan and Sadock 1998; Leong 1994; Rogers 1994; Sederer and Dickey 1996). Studies indicate that up to 22% of male inmates and 80% of female inmates have major mental illnesses (Kaplan and Sadock

1998). Most of these inmates are not incarcerated for life, and the rate of recidivism, or rearrest, of mentally disturbed offenders exceeds that of non–mentally ill offenders (McCarthy 1993). Therefore, the need for measures to assess the risk of recidivism—which is most simply measured by future incarceration for repeated offense—is clearly important for the forensic mental health practitioner and society at large.

However, studies measuring specific psychiatric traits and the likelihood of future crime have produced mixed results. Two frequently used measures in predicting recidivism are the Weinberger Adjustment Inventory (WAI) (Weinberger 1989) and the Hare Psychopathy Checklist (PCL) (Hare 1991, 1993, 1999). Both measures attempt to analyze past crime paths in an effort to assess the likelihood of future arrest for repeat offenses. Using a number of categorical assessments of criminal behavior, both have been shown to measure above predictions based on criminological or demographic factors. Several previous studies have established the ability of the WAI to assess and discriminate among samplings of juvenile delinquents. The WAI was used to assess nearly 200 rehabilitative programs, and congruent and predictive validity was found in samples of juvenile delinquents.

In addition, the PCL measures callousness and narcissism in an individual as a means to measure that individual's risk of recidivism. The assessment is based on a series of clinical interviews and has been validated in forensic psychiatric populations. The PCL distinguishes psychopathy as a subset of DSM-IV-TR diagnosis of antisocial personality disorder (American Psychiatric Association 2000). Psychopathy, the more refined concept, is intended to identify especially dangerous offenders. Most prison populations show a 50%–75% incidence of antisocial personality disorder and a 15%–25% rate of psychopathy.

Despite the existence of these highly accepted risk management tools, their ability to predict an inmate's future dangerousness if released back into general society remains controversial.

One category of inmates about whom there is great concern in society at present is sexual offenders. There are no universally accepted measures for the prediction of recidivism among sex offenders (Travin 1994). The most common kind of measurement remains the self-report, which includes a detailed sexual interview and varying combinations of scales, questionnaires, and inventories. The major disadvantage of this kind of measure is that reports are dependent on the truthfulness of the offender's personal account (Steiner 1999). The reliability of such accounts can be affected by an offender's motivations—particularly the anticipation of a more favorable outcome if the reporting of active pathologic symptoms is minimized.

Physiologic measurements of penile erections serve as the most specific physiologic indexes available to assess male sexual arousal (Kaplan and Sadock 1998). These measures have serious limitations, the major problem being that deviant sexual arousal in the laboratory is not necessarily generalizable to actual abnormal sexual behavior. Measuring penile erection responses to various stimuli, Abel et al. in 1978 introduced a "rape index" as a predictive measure for recidivistic rape. These results have not been replicated. Also noteworthy is the fact that the objective risk scales designed for general (nonsexual) recidivism (described earlier) do not similarly predict sexual recidivism. Thus, the tremendous hope initially suggested by this rape index scale was not realized.

The recently developed Sexual Violence Risk–20 (SVR-20) scale seeks to assess the presence or absence of sexual violence risk factors and the risk of future sexual violence. Sexual violence is defined broadly as "actual, attempted, or threatened sexual contact with a person who is nonconsenting or unable to give consent." The SVR-20 is an untimed, individual 20-item checklist for adults. The items were identified by a review of the literature on sex offenders (Douglas et al. 1997).

The SVR-20 sets out to make risk assessments with regard to sexual violence more systematic, to increase agreement among evaluators, to provide detailed guidelines that are grounded in the scientific literature, to assist in the planning and delivery of interventions (treatment and supervision), and to objectively evaluate the adequacy of risk assessments (i.e., evaluate the outcome of decisions based on this instrument). The SVR-20 manual provides specific information about how and when to conduct sexual violence risk assessments, the research on which the basic risk factors are based, and the key questions to address when judgments are to be made about risk. The SVR-20 specifies which risk factors should be assessed and also how the risk assessment should be conducted. The SVR-20 is structured so that the list of risk factors is 1) empirically related to future sexual violence, 2) useful in making decisions about the management of sex offenders, 3) nondiscriminatory, and 4) reasonably comprehensive without being redundant. The 20 factors in the comprehensive sexual violence risk assessment fall into three main categories: psychosocial adjustment, history of sexual offenses, and "future plans." The actual risk for sexual violence depends on the particular combination (not just the number) of risk factors present in a specific case. Coding of the SVR-20 involves determining the presence or absence of each factor and whether there has been any recent change in the status of the factor. This item-level information is integrated into a summary judgment of the level of risk (low, moderate, or high).

A most comprehensive actuarial study, the CPAI (McCarthy 1993), consists of several dozen items of what works for measuring recidivism among various rehabilitative strategies. The CPAI has been revised six times and has been used to assess the outcomes of more than 280 programs. It rates programs on program implementation, client preservice assessment, staff and program characteristics and practices, evaluation, and other categories. Recidivism reductions typically range from 25% to 60%, with the greater reductions found in community-based programs rather than their prison counterparts.

In summary, research and varied rehabilitative strategies have been developed in efforts to produce more reliable and valid measures to predict sexual and nonsexual offense recidivism. Difficulties range from adequately designing studies (given the inordinate number of variables for which one cannot possibly control) to undertaking the tremendous societal demands for improvement in predicting recidivism. Forensic clinicians need to continue to assess and record seemingly important data to increase gains in risk assessment. These findings may help direct more effective management, treatment, and rehabilitative strategies in reducing recidivism.

FUTURE DIRECTIONS FOR OUTCOME MEASUREMENTS IN FORENSIC PSYCHIATRY

Measures of evaluation and treatment outcome specific to forensic psychiatry and correctional psychiatry are in a relatively embryonic stage. Existing instruments need to be validated, nonforensic measures need to be adapted to forensic and correctional situations, and new measures need to be developed. Within the various subspecialty areas outlined in this chapter, the current state of outcome assessment development differs and the tasks ahead differ accordingly.

As noted in the section on forensic evaluations, the future directions in outcome assessments depend on the goals of the psychiatric service. Forensic psychiatrists may have some duties to the evaluation subjects, some duties to the courts, and some duties to society. It may be necessary to develop separate outcome assessment measures for these three categories of duties.

The duties to the subjects of the evaluation suggest the need for subject satisfaction surveys and assessments of the therapeutic effect of forensic evaluations. Both of these ideas may seem alien to most forensic psychiatrists, although many in the field note that evaluations do differ profoundly in their effect on the subject.

The duties to the court suggest the need for surveys of judges to assess their satisfaction with forensic psychiatric evaluations. Although such studies have been done in the past (Menzies et al. 1982; Owens et al. 1985), there are no universally established instruments to assess judiciary satisfaction with forensic evaluations. Other outcome assessment measurements of the duty of forensic psychiatrists to the court may be based on the duty of the psychiatrist to educate the court (Weinstock et al. 1994). Such measures might address the question of the degree to which a judge or a jury understands the relevant psychiatric issues after hearing expert testimony or after reading a report.

Perhaps the most ambitious duty of forensic psychiatrists is the duty to society. Not surprisingly, it is the hardest to assess because it requires an assessment of such terms as justice. One approach to this assessment may be the evaluation of postadjudicatory end points, such as whether subjects assessed to be dangerous do in fact engage in violent behaviors or whether individuals assessed to be mentally disabled later regain function.

The special problem of recidivism has already led to the development of valuable instruments, as noted previously. In this area, the primary task will be to assess the utility of these instruments.

The growing field of civil forensic evaluations will require special attention in the future. As with criminal forensic evaluations, there has been a proliferation of guidelines to aid in the assessment of the relevant legal standard (Shrier 1996; Simon 1995). The predictive value of such instruments may serve as the most meaningful assessment of the evaluation. However, the evaluation affects the outcome, and thus the predictive value of these evaluations cannot be meaningfully assessed unless the court, the subject, and other relevant parties are blind to the results. Again, as noted in the section on forensic evaluation, there can be a broad variety of end points for such studies. Do we want our assessments to accurately predict the decision of the court or do we want our assessments to predict some element of postadjudicatory course? Once the predictive value of such instruments has been established, it would then be possible to assess the quality of standard evaluations by comparison to the gold standard of these instruments.

For correctional psychiatry, the task continues to be adaptation of nonforensic measures. These modified instruments will need to be tested for reliability and validity. In addition, completely new instruments need to be developed to measure how treatment enables patients to adapt to the unique stressors of the correctional milieu. Such instruments would include measurements of victimization by other inmates, substance abuse, violence, disruptive behavior, transfer to hospitals, and suicide attempts. Although most of these end points have been studied in the past, an instrument that incorporates all of them into a single behavioral measure may serve a unique function.

Finally, it should be noted that existing forensic instruments can be administered serially over time to assess the stability of the measured traits or to measure the effect of specific interventions. Thus, existing instruments for recidivism, perceived coercion, psychopathy, competence, or disability may all serve as outcome assessment measures of forensic populations.

REFERENCES

Abel GG, Blanchard EB, Becker JV, et al: Differentiating sexual aggressives with penile measures. Criminal Justice and Behavior 5:315–332, 1978

Accreditation Council for Graduate Medical Education: Program Requirements for Residency Education in Forensic Psychiatry. Chicago, IL, Accreditation Council for Graduate Medical Education, 1996

American Academy of Psychiatry and the Law: Ethics Guidelines for the Practice of Forensic Psychiatry. Bloomfield, CT, American Academy of Psychiatry and the Law, 1991

American Psychiatric Association: Diagnostic and Statistical Manual of Mental Disorders, 4th Edition, Text Revision. Washington, DC, American Psychiatric Association, 2000

American Psychiatric Association: Practice Guidelines for the Treatment of Patients With Schizophrenia. Washington, DC, American Psychiatric Press, 1997

American Psychiatric Association: Psychiatric Services in Jails and Prisons. 2nd Edition. Washington, DC, American Psychiatric Press, 2000

Appelbaum PS: A theory of ethics for forensic psychiatry. J Am Acad Psychiatry Law 25:233–247, 1997

Barefoot v Estelle, 463 US 880, 1983

Blashfield R, Robbins L, Barnard G: An analogue study of the factors influencing competency decisions. Bulletin of the American Academy of Psychiatry and the Law 22(4):587–594, 1994

Carlson KA: Carlson Psychological Survey (CPS). Odessa, FL, Psychological Assessment Resources, 1999

Cooper D, Grisso T: Five year research update (1991–1995): evaluations for competence to stand trial. Behavioral Sciences and the Law 15:347–364, 1997

Douglas RB, Hart SD, Kropp PR, et al: Manual for the Sexual Violence Risk–20. Vancouver, BC, Institute Against Family Violence, 1997

Dusky v United States, 362 US 402, 1960

Edwards S, Lilford R, Thornton J, et al: Informed consent for clinical trials: in search of the "best method." Social Science and Medicine 47:1825–1840, 1998

Gendreau P, Andrews DA: Correctional Program Assessment Inventory (CPAI), 6th Edition. Fredericton, NB, Canada, University of New Brunswick, 1996

Grisso T: Competency to Stand Trial Evaluations. Sarasota, FL, Professional Resources Exchange, 1988, pp 81–88

Grisso T, Appelbaum P: Assessing Competence to Consent to Treatment. New York, Oxford University Press, 1998

Grisso T, Appelbaum P: The MacArthur Competence Assessment Tool for Treatment (MacCAT-T). Odessa, FL, Psychological Assessment Resources, 1999

Hanson RK, Bussiere MT: Predicting relapse: a meta-analysis of sexual offender recidivism studies. J Consult Clin Psychol 66:348–362, 1998

Hare R: Psychopathy Checklist. Law Hum Behav 15:625–637, 1991

Hare R: Without Conscience. New York, Simon & Shuster, 1993, pp 97–101

Hare R: Psychopathy as a risk factor for violence. Psychiatr Q 70:3, 1999

Hoge SK, Bonnie RJ, Poythress NG, et al: The MacArthur Competence Assessment Tool—Criminal Adjudication (MacCAT-CA). Odessa, FL, Psychological Assessment Resources, 1999

Janofsky J, Vandewalle M, Rappeport J: Defendants pleading insanity: an analysis of outcome. Bulletin of the American Academy of Psychiatry and the Law 17(2):203–211, 1989

Janofsky J, Dunn M, Roskes E, et al: Insanity defense pleas in Baltimore City: an analysis of outcome. Am J Psychiatry 153:1464–1468, 1996

Kaplan HI, Sadock BJ: Kaplan and Sadock's Synopsis of Psychiatry, 8th Edition. Baltimore, MD, Williams & Wilkins, 1998, pp 1314–1317

Katz M, Abbey S, Rydall A, et al: Psychiatric consultation for competency to refuse medical treatment. Psychosomatics 36(1):33–41, 1995

Lamb HR, Weinberger LE: Persons with severe mental illness in jails and prisons: a review. Psychiatr Serv 49:483–492, 1998

Leong GB: Dangerousness, in Principles and Practice of Forensic Psychiatry. Edited by Rosner R. New York, Chapman & Hall, 1994, pp 432–438

Leukefeld CG, Tims FM: Compulsory treatment of drug abuse. International Journal of the Addictions 25:621–640, 1990

Luettgen J: Preventing violent re-offending in not criminally responsible patients. An evaluation of a continuity of treatment program. Int J Law Psychiatry 21(1):89–98, 1998

McCarthy RE: Comprehensive Forensic Data Organization in Innovation in Clinical Practice: A Source Book. Sarasota, FL, Professional Resource Press, 1993, pp 387–402

Menzies R, Webster CD, Butler BT, et al: The outcome of forensic psychiatric assessment, a study of remands in six Canadian cities. Criminal Justice and Behavior 7(4):471–480, 1980

Menzies R, Jackson M, Glasberg R: The nature and consequences of forensic psychiatric decision making. Can J Psychiatry 27:463–470, 1982

Metzner JL: An introduction to correctional psychiatry: part III. J Am Acad Psychiatry Law 26:107–115, 1998

Miller R: Criminal competence, in Principles and Practice of Forensic Psychiatry. Edited by Rosner R. New York, Chapman & Hall, 1994, pp 174–197

Miller R, Ionescu-Pioggia R, Fiddleman P: The effect of witnesses, attorneys, and judges on civil commitment in North Carolina: a prospective study. J Forensic Sci 28:829–838, 1983

Nicholson RA, Robertson H, Johnson WG, et al: A comparison of instruments for assessing competency to stand trial. Law Hum Behav 12(3):313–321, 1988

Nicholson R, Norwood S, Enyart C: Characteristic and outcomes of insanity acquitees in Oklahoma. Behavioral Sciences and the Law 9:487–500, 1991

Nicholson RA, Briggs SR, Robertson HC: Instruments for assessing competency to stand trial: how do they work? Professional Psychology: Research and Practice 19(4):383–394, 1998

Olson DH, Mylan MM, Fletcher LA, et al: A clinical rating scale for response to civil commitment for substance abuse. Psychiatr Serv 48:1317–1322, 1997

Owens H, Rosner R, Harmon R: The judge's view of competency evaluations. Bulletin of the American Academy of Psychiatry and the Law 13(4):389–397, 1985

Packer I: Privatized managed care and forensic mental health services. J Am Acad Psychiatry Law 26(1):123–129, 1998

Robertson RG, Gupton T, McCabe S, et al: Clinical and demographic variables related to "fitness to stand trial" assessments in Manitoba. Can J Psychiatry 42:191–195, 1997

Rogers R: Rogers Criminal Responsibility Assessment Scales. Odessa, FL, Psychological Assessment Resources, 1984

Rogers R: Psychological measures in forensic practice, in Principles and Practice of Forensic Psychiatry. Edited by Rosner R. New York, Chapman & Hall, 1994, pp 473–479

Rogers R: Clinical Assessment of Malingering and Deception. New York, Guilford, 1997, pp 321–324

Rogers R, Gillis JR, Bagby RM, et al: Detection of malingering on the Structured Interview of Reported Symptoms (SIRS): a study of coached and uncoached simulators. Psychol Assess 3:673–677, 1991

Rogers R, Kropp PR, Bagby RM, et al: Faking specific disorders: a study of the Structured Interview of Reported Symptoms (SIRS). J Clin Psychol 48:643–648, 1992

Rosenfeld B, Ritchie K: Competence to stand trial: clinician reliability and the role of offense severity. J Forensic Sci 43(1):151–157, 1998

Sederer LI, Dickey B: Outcomes Assessment in Clinical Practice. Baltimore, MD, Williams & Wilkins, 1996

Shrier DK: Sexual Harassment in the Workplace and Academia. Washington, DC, American Psychiatric Press, 1996

Simon RI: Posttraumatic Stress Disorder in Litigation: Guidelines for Forensic Evaluation. Washington, DC, American Psychiatric Press, 1995

Steadman HJ: Insanity acquittals in New York State, 1965–1978. Am J Psychiatry 137:321–326, 1980

Steiner H: Personality traits in juvenile delinquents: relation to criminal behavior and recidivism. J Am Acad Child Adolesc Psychiatry 38:256–262, 1999

Stone A: Ethics of forensic psychiatry, in Law, Psychiatry and Morality. Washington, DC, American Psychiatric Press, 1984, pp 110–116

Strasburger LH, Gutheil TG, Brodsky A: On wearing two hats; role conflict in serving as both psychotherapist and expert witness. Am J Psychiatry 154:4, 1997

Travin S: Sex offenders: diagnostic assessment, treatment, and related issues, in Principles and Practice of Forensic Psychiatry. Edited by Rosner R. New York, Chapman & Hall, 1994, pp 528–536

Umapathy C, Ramchandani D, Lamdan R, et al: Competency evaluations on the consultation-liaison service. Psychosomatics 40(1):28–33, 1999

U.S. Bureau of Justice Statistics: Mental Health and Treatment of Inmates and Probationers. Washington, DC, U.S. Department of Justice, 1999

U.S. Food and Drug Administration: Compliance Policy Guidelines. 21 CFR 310. Washington, DC, U.S. Department of Health and Human Services, Associate Commission for Regulatory Affairs, 1980

Webster C, Douglas K, Eaves D, et al: HCR-2: Assessing Risk for Violence. Burnaby, BC, Canada, Mental Health, Law, and Policy Institute, 1997

Weinberger DA: The Weinberger Adjustment Inventory (WAI). Social-Emotional Adjustment in Older Children and Adults. I: Psychometric Properties of the Weinberger Adjustment Inventory. Unpublished manuscript, 1989

Weinstock R et al: Defining forensic psychiatry: roles and responsibilities, in Principles and Practice of Forensic Psychiatry. Edited by Rosner R. New York, Chapman & Hall, 1994, pp 7–12

Wheeldon TJ, Robertson C, Eagles JM, et al: Views and outcomes of consenting and non-consenting patients receiving ETC. Psychol Med 29(1):221–223, 1999

CHAPTER 8

Outcome Measurement in Patients Receiving Psychosocial Treatments

Paul Crits-Christoph, Ph.D.
Madeline Gladis, Ph.D.
Mary Beth Connolly, Ph.D.

Despite the increasing use of medication treatments in psychiatry, psychotherapy continues to be a widely practiced treatment for psychiatric disorders as well as for problems in living. Each year Americans make more than 80 million psychotherapy visits, at a cost of more than $4 billion (Olfson and Pincus 1994). Consumers, government agencies, and insurance companies that bear the cost of mental health treatments have increasingly called for accountability regarding psychotherapy, especially seeking of evaluation of treatment outcomes.

The evaluation of the outcomes of psychotherapy is often traced back to the well-known 1952 article by Hans Eysenck, which claimed that there is no evidence that psychotherapy is effective. Since that time, a rather extensive body of literature on the evaluation of psychotherapy outcomes has emerged, with over 1,000 studies conducted to date. Meta-analytical reviews of this psychotherapy outcome literature have provided evidence that psychotherapy generally is effective (Smith et al. 1980). Nevertheless, significant questions remain regarding the specific effectiveness of different psychotherapies for different patient problems and disorders.

How does one go about assessing the outcome of psychotherapy? There is no simple answer to this question. The methods used depend on the patient population, the specific treatments, and the goals of the assessment. In terms of patient populations, it is usually important to tailor the assessment battery to the particular types of presenting problems or psychiatric disorders characteristic of the population. For example, the assessment of outcomes for a population of substance abuse and dependence patients will generally require different measures than will a population of non–substance abusing outpatients. Similarly, with regard to treatment modalities, assessment of outcome in a marital/family/couples treatment program, for example, would also require specific instruments (i.e., evaluation of the functioning of the family unit) that would not be used in the evaluation of other treatments.

Summarizing the results of a conference on outcome assessment, Lambert et al. (1997) suggested eight criteria to apply when selecting measures:

- Measures should have clear, standardized procedures for scoring and administration.
- Norms for clinical and nonclinical samples should be available.
- Measures should have adequate reliability.
- Measures should have demonstrated validity.
- Measures should be brief and easy to use in clinical settings.
- Measures should be relevant to clinical needs.
- Measures should not be bound by theory.
- Measures should be applicable to multiple assessments (e.g., before, during, and after treatment).

Although such criteria are useful as a guide, no measure can meet all of these criteria.

In addition to the criteria listed above, the primary goal of the outcome assessment also influences the choice of outcome measures. A clear distinction can be made between an outcome assessment that is designed to answer a specific research question (e.g., does cognitive therapy have an impact on dysfunctional beliefs?) and an outcome assessment for clinical decision making. Whereas most research studies have rather extensive assessment batteries, for clinical purposes broad outcome measures that are brief and efficient are most highly valued. Thus, although it would be useful if a simple, cost-effective, core battery of measures could be recommended for the assessment of psychotherapy outcome, efforts by experts to arrive at such a core battery have not succeeded in producing a relatively small number of measures that could be applied across the variety of situations for which outcome assessment might be indicated.

Our own view is that it is not meaningful to ask the question, "How do you assess the outcome of psychotherapy?" However, within a domain of scientific inquiry (i.e., research on a specific disorder), or for a clearly articulated clinical decision-making process, it would be useful to achieve standardization of outcome assessment. Even here, however, new instruments are developed and old instruments are modified and improved over time, so outcome batteries will continue to change. Therefore, any specific recommendations will be useful only for a limited time. Another reason that it is difficult to standardize outcome assessment, even within a general domain, is that different investigators may hold different hypotheses about the process of psychotherapy or about theory-specific outcome measures. Therefore, although standardized recommendations about certain symptom and functioning measures can be proposed, process-specific and theory-specific measures will likely change depending on investigators' hypotheses.

However, what can be offered as recommendations is a range of measures that might be utilized for assessing psychotherapy outcome in different contexts. In this chapter, we first discuss the different potential domains of outcome assessment and provide a rationale for why each domain might be of importance to psychotherapy treatments. Second, we review a selected set of instruments within each domain. We conclude with a discussion of the methodological problems and issues inherent in the assessment of psychotherapy outcome. Because we attempt a broad survey of outcome measures, certain specialized areas—such as child, geriatric, and behavioral medicine—are not covered here.

Our selection of the domains of assessment was guided by the goals of psychotherapy as defined by the different stakeholders that have an interest in psychotherapy outcome. Managed care companies that ration access to psychotherapy are primarily interested in the medical necessity of treatments. Their focus is therefore on diagnosis, the severity of symptoms, and the extent to which the disorder is interfering with functioning (work and social relations). The National Institute of Mental Health, which funds most large-scale evaluations of psychotherapy outcome, has a public health mandate. Thus, its primary interests are also in clinical disorders, symptoms, and functioning. Patients are generally interested in their own subjective well-being. Psychotherapy researchers might have specific interests in the theoretical mechanism of action of a specific psychotherapy, and therefore they might be interested in going beyond measures of symptoms and functioning to examine theory-specific outcomes.

DOMAINS OF ASSESSMENT

Outcome

Diagnosis

From a public health point of view, identification of effective therapies for specific disorders is a priority in research and clinical psychiatry. This point of view assumes that an accurate and thorough assessment of these disorders is central to the evaluation process. Diagnosis is generally assessed during initial patient evaluation and sometimes at the termination of treatment.

Symptoms

With many disorders, the patient is not expected to be in remission at the termination of treatment. In fact, the time frames specified in the definitions of some disorders (e.g., 5 years for personality disorders) is longer than the durations of most treatments in either research or clinical settings. It is therefore more useful to use measures that consider symptoms as a continuum rather than the mere presence or absence of the disorder. Such continuous measures of the amount, timing, and nature of change are the primary outcomes of most intervention studies and are key elements in instruments developed for clinical applications. Assessment of symptoms includes ratings of a single construct representing a core feature of a disorder (e.g., a measure of worry for generalized anxiety disorder); scales that cover the range of symptoms present in a class of disorders (e.g., rating scales of depression for affective disorders or general anxiety for anxiety disorders); and measures that assess overall psychopathology or symptomatology that cuts across multiple disorders.

Functioning

Many mental illnesses are chronic and disabling. Some degree of symptoms related to the illness may be present over an extended period of time. It therefore becomes important to look beyond the symptoms of the disorder and to assess the patient's general life functioning. Moreover, in terms of costs to society, the patient's functioning in certain domains (e.g., work functioning) may be of relevance. A full evaluation of the effectiveness of a psychotherapeutic intervention should document effects on a number of specific domains, including social/interpersonal functioning, work functioning, quality of life, and utilization of health services.

Personality

Personality variables are utilized in evaluations of psychological treatment in multiple ways. For studies of psychotherapy for personality pathology, personality variables are used as primary outcomes. Studies of Axis I disorders often use personality variables as prognostic indicators or to describe the patient sample. Assessment of personality includes determination of the presence or absence of a DSM-IV-TR (American Psychiatric Association 2000) personality disorder as well as dimensional ratings of personality features.

Interpersonal Problems

Interpersonal problems are common complaints of patients initiating psychotherapy (Horowitz 1979). The assessment of social functioning (mentioned earlier) overlaps the assessment of interpersonal problems. However, measures of social functioning generally focus on the participation in social activities and the existence of relationships with friends and family members. In contrast, instruments to assess interpersonal problems focus on the specific types of interpersonal problems (e.g., problems with assertion or intimacy).

Measures of Self

Attitudes about one's self have been linked to the maintenance of behavioral change and therefore could be considered as outcome measures. Furthermore, for psychotherapy modalities that are explicitly oriented toward the improvement of self-esteem, self-concept, and self-confidence, it is relevant to assess the extent to which treatment successfully affects these constructs.

Process

Theory-Based Measures

Psychological treatments are based on a variety of theoretical models that hypothesize certain key psychological constructs as etiologic or relevant to change. Measures of such theory-based constructs can serve as outcome measures in their own right or as mediators of change in symptoms and functioning, thus as either outcome or process measures. For example, the cognitive model of depression (Beck et al. 1979) holds that distorted cognitions about the self and the world are partly responsible for generating and maintaining depression. In studies of cognitive therapy for depression, measures of distorted cognitions can serve as outcomes and mediators of change.

Therapeutic Alliance

One of the central ingredients in almost all schools of psychotherapy is the quality of the patient-therapist relationship (the therapeutic alliance). Alliance is typically conceived as a measure of the process of psychotherapy, as opposed to outcome. But because studies of the relation between the therapeutic alliance and treatment outcome have so consistently concluded that a positive alliance is associated with better outcomes (Horvath and Symonds 1991), it is reasonable to consider assessment of the alliance as a gauge of how well therapy is going, particularly in the early stages.

INSTRUMENTS

Specific instruments for the assessment of diagnosis, symptoms, and functioning are also reviewed in other chapters within this volume. These same instruments have utility in studies of psychosocial as well as pharmacologic treatments and are mentioned here only briefly. Further information on these instruments and others is available in a recent conference report on measuring the outcomes of mood, anxiety, and personality disorders. After offering suggestions for the assessment of diagnosis, symptoms, and functioning, we review in greater detail additional instruments (organized by outcome domain) that are often used for the evaluation of psychotherapy outcome.

Diagnosis, Symptoms, and Functioning

The most widely used instrument for assessing the major DSM-IV Axis I disorders and diagnoses in research settings is the Structured Clinical Interview for DSM-IV Axis II Personality Disorders (SCID-II) (First et al. 1994). Although this interview is widely used, concerns remain about the reliability and validity of some DSM diagnoses as assessed by this interview. Symptom measures usually include general measures as well as disorder-specific measures. For some disorders, single-item measures of target symptoms suffice. For example, to evaluate the outcome of treatment for panic disorder and bulimia, scales that rely on self-reporting of the number of episodes that occur in a well-defined interval such as the past week or the past month are used. For most disorders, however, core symptom measures of greater psychometric sophistication are needed to supplement simple single-item methods. An example is the Penn State Worry Questionnaire (Meyer et al. 1990), which assesses the posited central feature of generalized anxiety disorder.

Other examples from the anxiety disorder literature include the Yale-Brown Obsessive-Compulsive Scale (Goodman et al. 1989), the PTSD

Symptom Scale Self-Report (Foa et al. 1993), and the Fear Questionnaire (Marks and Mathews 1979). An example from depression research is the Inventory of Depressive Symptomatology (Rush 1986), which was developed as a continuous measure of the nine DSM symptoms for a major depressive episode. There are many other tools for assessing symptoms of depression, and some are widely used as outcome measures for both psychological and pharmacologic treatments. (For a review of these, see Basco et al. 1997).

In the assessment of substance use problems, the Addiction Severity Index (McLellan et al. 1980) is the most widely used instrument in both clinical and research settings. This measure has the advantage of providing comprehensive and detailed information on problem areas associated with abuse, and it yields scores that can be compared across individual patients or groups of patients.

A popular self-report measure of general psychopathology is the Symptom Checklist 90–Revised (SCL-90-R), or its 53-item abbreviated version, the Brief Symptom Inventory (BSI) (Derogatis and Derogatis 1996). This instrument yields nine symptom dimensions and three global indices of distress. However, evidence indicating that the nine subscales are highly intercorrelated has led some to conclude that the instrument is best used as a measure of overall distress (Morey and Kurtz 1995).

Another measure of general psychopathology is the Minnesota Multiphasic Personality Inventory (MMPI) (Hathaway and McKinley 1942), which remains one of the most popular of all psychological tests. However, the usefulness of the MMPI in clinical settings and efficacy studies is limited by its length, its use of obsolete diagnostic constructs, and its questionable psychometrics (Morey and Kurtz 1995).

Overall functioning can be assessed from the widely used Global Assessment of Functioning (GAF) scale (American Psychiatric Association 2000), which was derived from the Health-Sickness Rating Scale (Luborsky and Bachrach 1974) and was incorporated into the DSM system as a separate axis (Axis V). Limitations of the GAF include the confounding of symptom severity with functioning and the nonstandardized way in which scores are assigned.

A widely used scale for the assessment of social functioning is the Social Adjustment Scale (M.M. Weissman et al. 1974). This instrument was developed more than 20 years ago to document levels of functioning in six areas: work (as worker, homemaker, or student), social activities, relationship with extended family, relationship with spouse, parental responsibilities, and role as member of a family unit. The scale has been used with a wide range of adult outpatients, and there is considerable documentation of its psychometric properties.

Relatively little work has been done with regard to the assessment of work functioning. An exception is the Endicott Work Productivity Scale (Endicott and Nee 1997), a self-report instrument containing 25 items designed to be sensitive to subtle differences among patients in work attitudes and behavior. Initial testing of this instrument has provided evidence of its reliability, validity (concurrent and discriminant), and ability to detect change. However, wider use of this new scale is needed before conclusions can be made about its clinical utility.

Functioning can be also be examined in positive, rather than negative, aspects through the assessment of quality of life. The most promising quality-of-life measures are those based on a broad definition; they cover role functioning and social-material conditions as well as life satisfaction or well-being, and that can be applied across disorders and treatments. Examples of quality-of-life instruments, reviewed in detail elsewhere (Gladis et al. 1999), include the Quality of Life Enjoyment and Satisfaction Questionnaire (Endicott et al. 1993) and the Quality of Life Inventory (Frisch et al. 1992). One concern with these scales is that they are influenced by the patient's current mood. In part this problem is a definitional one regarding quality of life—should this construct rely completely on a respondent's subjective perception of the quality of his or her life, or should there be more objective characteristics of work and social life?

Personality Assessment

The SCID-II (First et al. 1994) is the most commonly used instrument for assessing the presence of Axis II diagnoses. An advantage of this instrument is its efficiency in eliciting the information required to assign Axis II diagnoses, particularly when used in conjunction with a preliminary self-report questionnaire.

A variety of dimensional methods of assessing personality have been developed. For example, the Five Factor Model (Costa and McCrae 1987) proposes that personality can be measured along five dimensions: neuroticism, extroversion, openness to experience, agreeableness, and conscientiousness. The instruments used to generate scores on these factors, including the self-report NEO Personality Inventory–Revised (Costa and McCrae 1992) and a semistructured interview (the Structured Interview of the Five-Factor Model of Personality) (Trull et al. 1998), have received substantial empirical support in both clinical and nonclinical samples. However, there are no studies to date on their sensitivity to treatment-induced change.

Self-reporting methods that yield dimensions targeted to the DSM Axis II categories also exist, such as the Wisconsin Personality Disorders

Inventory (WISPI) (Klein et al. 1993) and the Millon Clinical Multiaxial Inventory (Millon 1983). The WISPI may be particularly relevant to psychotherapy outcome assessment, because the items are generated from an interpersonal model of human behavior. The length of these instruments limits their use in settings that require a brief outcome battery. For more information, the reader is referred to Chapter 14 in this volume.

Interpersonal Problems

Two self-reporting instruments for assessing interpersonal problems can be recommended for psychotherapy evaluation: the Inventory of Interpersonal Problems (IIP) (Horowitz et al. 1988) and the Dyadic Adjustment Scale (DAS) (Spanier 1976). The IIP is a 127-item self-reporting scale with high test-retest and internal consistency reliability of each of the six subclasses: assertive, social, intimate, submissive, responsible, and controlling. Although the IIP in general has good psychometric properties, the total score correlates highly with general instruments of distress and symptoms, such as the SCL-90. The DAS is a 32-item scale designed specifically to assess the severity of relationship problems in married and unmarried cohabiting couples. The scale yields scores on dyadic consensus, dyadic cohesion, dyadic satisfaction, and affectional expression. An obvious limitation of this scale is that it can be completed only by patients who are currently in an ongoing relationship.

Measures of Self

One of the most widely used measures of self-esteem is the Rosenberg Self-Esteem Scale (Rosenberg 1965), an easily administered 10-item Likert-type scale, which yields a unidimensional indicator of global self-esteem. Additional scales to measure self-concept (the Beck Self-Concept Test; Beck et al. 1990) and self-discrepancy (the Selves Questionnaire; Higgins et al. 1986) have been developed. Although these scales are attractive as potential instruments to assess psychotherapy outcome, few studies employing them have been reported.

Theory-Specific

Instruments have been developed to assess the theoretically important constructs of specific psychotherapies. As mentioned earlier, these scales can be used as mediators of symptom change as well as outcome measures in their own right.

A variety of measures have been developed to assess change on theoretically important constructs of cognitive-behavioral therapy. The Dysfunctional Attitudes Scale (A.N. Weissman 1979) is a 40-item index of general attitudes and beliefs hypothesized to underlie a propensity for depressive thinking. The Automatic Thoughts Questionnaire (Hollon and Kendall 1980) covers 30 negative thoughts proposed to be part of a depressive syndrome. The Hopelessness Scale (Beck et al. 1974) is a 20-item self-reporting scale that assesses the hopelessness and pessimism that can sustain depression. Data on reliability, validity, and sensitivity to change from cognitive therapy have been reported. Whether these scales measure a dimension that can predict future changes in depressive symptoms, or simply a concomitant aspect of depression, has not yet been clarified.

Another measure that has been used to evaluate theory-specific mediation of change from cognitive therapy is the Attribution Style Questionnaire (ASQ) (Seligman et al. 1979). Changes in the ASQ from pretreatment to midtreatment have been found to predict subsequent change in depression from midtreatment to termination of treatment in depressed patients treated with cognitive therapy (DeRubeis et al. 1990).

With regard to psychodynamic psychotherapy, theory-specific mediators include measures of core conflicts (Luborsky and Crits-Christoph 1998) and self-understanding (Connolly et al. 1999). Measures of these constructs, however, are rather early in development and cannot yet be widely recommended for psychotherapy evaluation.

Studies of interpersonal psychotherapy have relied on the Social Adjustment Scale (M.M. Weissman et al. 1974). This scale, however, is not targeted to the specific interpersonal processes of Klerman's Interpersonal Psychotherapy (IPT). No scales have yet been developed to assess the specific interpersonal deficits, disputes, and role transitions that are the central elements of IPT.

Broad Scales for Clinical Applications

Several scales have been developed specifically for the assessment of outcome in clinical settings. Once again, these scales are relevant to pharmacotherapy as well as to psychotherapy. In fact, much of outpatient treatment in psychiatry consists of a combination of medication and psychotherapy. Two scales, the COMPASS Mental Health Index (MHI) (Sperry et al. 1996) and the Outcome Questionnaire (Lambert et al. 1996), have been developed by psychotherapy researchers and have been widely used for the measurement of outcome in clinical practice.

The MHI is brief self-report measure consisting of current life functioning, subjective well-being, and current symptom scales that are summed to create an overall index. The MHI has been reported to have an internal consistency reliability of 0.87 and a short-term test-retest reliability of 0.82. (Howard et al. 1996). Clinical uses of the scale include monitoring a patient's progress, comparing this progress with predicted progress generated from the average course of change for a large number of patients with similar initial clinical characteristics, and providing feedback on this comparison to the therapist, supervisor, or case manager. This feedback can be used as a basis for a case consultation or to change treatment modalities or providers.

Although this may be an appealing approach for managed care and other groups interested in evaluating clinical outcomes, no information has yet been published giving the rates of false positives and false negatives. Therefore, decisions to end or change treatment based on the MHI remain speculative. With practitioners' keeping the limitations of the system in mind, however, this instrument can be used to review progress in the context of other clinical considerations that may not be captured with either the prediction model or the outcome assessment.

The Outcome Questionnaire is a self-report instrument consisting of 45 items, each rated on a 1–5 scale. Most patients complete this scale is less than 10 minutes. Three subscales representing broad content areas are assessed: 1) symptom distress, 2) interpersonal relations, and 3) social role (dissatisfaction and distress in tasks related to work, family roles, and leisure life). However, questions remain regarding the extent to which these three subscales are independent. Using confirmatory factor analysis to examine the Outcome Questionnaire, Mueller et al. (1998) found that a one-factor model fit the data as well as multifactor models did. Umphress al. (1997) explored this issue further by examining whether each subscale of the Outcome Questionnaire was correlated with an alternative measure of each construct (e.g., social role subscale in relation to another measure of social functioning). Their results also did not support the uniqueness of the subscales.

Although the independence of the subscales of the Outcome Questionnaire is questionable, the psychometric characteristics of the total score appear promising. The internal consistency (Cronbach's α) of this total score has been reported to be 0.93, and test-retest reliability has been reported to be 0.84 (Burlingame et al. 1995). The total score also correlates highly with other measures of symptoms, interpersonal functioning, and social adjustment (Burlingame et al. 1995; Umphress al. 1997). Moreover, differences on the Outcome Questionnaire total score between clinical and community samples, and among clinical samples that vary in their degree of pathology, have been reported (Umphress al. 1997). Lambert et al. (1998) illustrate the use of the Outcome Questionnaire in clinical practice, comparing the progress and rate of recovery of patients treated by a private practice clinician.

Alliance

The California Psychotherapy Alliance Scale (CALPAS; Gaston 1991) is a 24-item self-report inventory designed to assess the client's and the therapist's separate contributions to the therapeutic alliance. The CALPAS has four subscales: patient commitment, patient working capacity, therapist understanding and involvement, and working strategy consensus. Each item is rated on a 7-point Likert scale. The CALPAS demonstrates good internal consistency ($\alpha=0.83$) for the total score (Gaston 1991) and has been associated with positive outcome in behavioral, cognitive, and brief dynamic therapies for depression (Gaston et al. 1991).

The Helping Alliance Questionnaire (HAQ-II) (Luborsky et al. 1996) is a self-report inventory designed to assess the helping alliance and collaborative aspects of the therapeutic relationship. The HAQ-II consists of 19 items, each rated on a 6-point Likert scale. This scale has demonstrated excellent internal consistency reliability (0.90–0.94) and good test-retest reliability over a period of 3 weeks (0.79 for the patient version) and has shown convergent validity with the CALPAS (Luborsky et al. 1996). Two complementary observer-rated measures have also been developed: the Helping Alliance Global Rating method and the Helping Alliance Counting Signs method (Luborsky et al. 1983).

The Working Alliance Inventory (WAI) (Horvath and Greenberg 1989) is a 36-item self-report inventory designed to capture Bordin's (1979) model of the working alliance. The scale assesses the bond between patient and therapist, mutual endorsement of treatment goals, and mutual responsibility for the tasks of therapy. The subscales, as well as the composite score, demonstrated good internal consistency, convergent validity, and discriminant validity (Horvath and Greenberg 1989). In addition, early-session WAI scores significantly predicted patient satisfaction and change across psychotherapy. Although there appears to be substantial overlap between the subscales, each subscale seems to predict a significant amount of unique outcome variance. The WAI has also been adapted to be rated by observers (Horvath and Greenberg 1986).

The CALPAS, WAI, and HAQ-II are all widely used measures of the therapeutic alliance. Each of these measures appears to be internally consistent and to be a valid representation of the alliance construct. These measures have been shown to be highly correlated (Hatcher and Barends 1996). Thus, there does not appear to be a basis for recommending one instrument over another. However, the consistent finding of a relationship between alliance and outcome suggests that it is essential to measure the alliance in almost any evaluation of psychotherapy outcome. Measures of alliance can serve as early indicators of good outcome and can be used to examine the mechanisms through which psychotherapy achieves its effects. Moreover, in studies that compare different psychotherapies, it is important to document that the different treatments were equivalent on the alliance to rule out this important factor as an explanation for differences in treatment outcome.

ISSUES IN MEASURING THE OUTCOME OF PSYCHOTHERAPY

As mentioned previously, there is no single method to assess the outcome of psychotherapy that is acceptable to all contexts. The specific domain or content area assessed will depend on the goals of the outcome assessment. There is also an obvious trade-off between efficiency and ease of use versus depth and breadth of assessment. A comprehensive assessment requires extensive time and patient cooperation that is typically not available in nonresearch clinical settings. In contrast, research studies require a detailed assessment with reliable and valid assessments, often of a range of dimensions.

There is some evidence that a thorough, systematic evaluation of symptoms can yield short-term psychological benefits for the patient (Scarvalone et al. 1996). Even in a research context, however, there is a limit to how much assessment can be accomplished without losing the patient's cooperation and consequently, perhaps, compromising validity. At a certain point, patients become tired or less attentive, and their responses tend to become less accurate. In addition, lengthy assessments can be performed only at initial assessment, treatment termination, and perhaps midtreatment. If outcome is to be assessed on a session-to-session basis (or every few sessions), a relatively short battery (5–15 minutes) is needed.

An important emerging distinction in research studies is between "efficacy" studies that focus on tight experimental control and internal validity, and "effectiveness" studies that maximize external validity (generalizability). Selection of outcome measures will depend in part on whether an investigator's primary intent leans more in the efficacy or effectiveness direction. Efficacy studies often focus primarily on symptom change under experimental conditions, whereas effectiveness studies are conducted in naturalistic settings and often assess broader outcomes that highlight the importance of functioning in the real world (e.g., social and work functioning).

In terms of pure clinical applications, several brief self-report scales (e.g., MHI, Outcome Questionnaire) appear to be promising. By combining a few key dimensions (e.g., symptoms and functioning) into an overall score, these instruments allow for easy tracking of patient progress. However, several limitations of this approach should be noted. First, this assessment approach will not be sensitive to measuring change in patients who have a focal problem (e.g., specific phobia) but who otherwise function well and have few symptoms. Most patients who seek psychotherapy, however, do have some degree of general symptoms, distress, and impairment in functioning, which makes these instruments relevant for most patients.

We expect to see continuing emphasis on the positive aspects of mental health, namely better quality of life. However, further development of self-reporting quality-of-life instruments is needed to help establish their utility and to help resolve a number of important measurement issues, including the value of more objective indices of quality of life and the relationship between symptoms and quality of life.

A final important issue is related to the interpretation of outcome assessments. Of course, an investigator or clinician has to be aware of the limitations of a particular assessment instrument (i.e., reliability, validity, sources of bias). In addition, the extent to which changes on a given measure reflect *clinically significant change* must be considered. Various suggestions for determining clinically significant change have been offered (Jacobson and Truax 1991) and provide statistical means for quantifying whether an individual patient, or group of patients, has achieved clinically meaningful change.

Because of the high level of current interest in outcome assessment, we expect notable developments in the coming years, including a better of understanding of the strengths and weaknesses of existing instruments as well as the advent of new measures. Although there will never be a simple solution to the complex task of assessing psychotherapy outcome, researchers and clinicians will likely have a range of useful alternatives for addressing the pressing questions that confront them.

REFERENCES

American Psychiatric Association: Diagnostic and Statistical Manual of Mental Disorders, 4th Edition, Text Revision. Washington, DC, American Psychiatric Association, 2000

Basco MR, Krebaum SR, Rush AJ: Outcome measures of depression, in Measuring Patient Changes in Mood, Anxiety, and Personality Disorders. Edited by Strupp HH, Horowitz LM, Lambert MJ. Washington, DC, American Psychological Association, 1997, pp 191–246

Beck AT, Weissman A, Lester D, et al: The measurement of pessimism: the Hopelessness Scale. J Consult Clin Psychol 42:861–865, 1974

Beck AT, Rush AJ, Shaw BF, et al: Cognitive Therapy of Depression. New York, Guilford, 1979

Beck AT, Steer RA, Epstein N, et al: Beck Self-Concept Test. Psychological Assessment 2:191–197, 1990

Bordin ES: The generalizability of the psychoanalytic concept of the working alliance. Psychotherapy: Theory, Research, and Practice 16:252–260, 1979

Burlingame GM, Lambert MJ, Reisinger CW, et al: Pragmatics of tracking mental health outcomes in a managed care setting. Journal of Mental Health Administration 22:226–236, 1995

Connolly MB, Crits-Christoph P, Shelton RC, et al: The reliability and validity of a measure of self-understanding of interpersonal patterns. Journal of Counseling Psychology 46:472–482, 1999

Costa PT, McCrae RR: Validation of the five-factor model of personality across instruments and observers. J Pers Soc Psychol 52:81–90, 1987

Costa PT, McCrae RR: The NEO Personality Inventory Manual. Odessa, FL, Psychological Assessment Resources, 1992

Derogatis LR, Derogatis MF: SCL-90-R and the BSI, in Quality of Life and Pharmacoeconomics in Clinical Trials, 2nd Edition. Edited by Spiker B. Philadelphia, PA, Lippincott-Raven, 1996, pp 323–335

DeRubeis RJ, Hollon SD, Evans MD, et al: How does cognitive therapy work? Cognitive change and symptom change in cognitive therapy and pharmacotherapy for depression. J Consult Clin Psychol 58:862–869, 1990

Endicott J, Nee J: Endicott Work Productivity Scale (EWPS): a new measure to assess treatment effects. Psychopharmacology Bulletin 33:13–16, 1997

Endicott J, Nee J, Harrison W, et al: Quality of Life Enjoyment and Satisfaction Questionnaire: a new measure. Psychopharmacology Bulletin 29:321–326, 1993

Eysenck HJ: The effects of psychotherapy: an evaluation. J Consult Clin Psychol 16:319–324, 1952

First MB, Spitzer RL, Gibbon M, et al: Structured Clinical Interview for DSM-IV Axis II Personality Disorders (SCID-II, version 2.0). Biometrics Research Department, New York State Psychiatric Institute, 1994

Foa EB, Riggs DS, Dancu CV, et al: Reliability and validity of a brief instrument for assessing post-traumatic stress disorder. J Trauma Stress 6:459–473, 1993

Frisch MB, Cornell J, Villanueva M, et al: Clinical validation of the Quality of Life Inventory: a measure of life satisfaction for use in treatment planning and outcome assessment. Psychol Assess 4:92–101, 1992

Gaston L: Reliability and criterion-related validity of the California Psychotherapy Alliance Scales: Patient Version. Psychol Assess 3:68–74, 1991

Gaston L, Marmar CR, Gallagher D, et al: Alliance prediction of outcome beyond in-treatment symptomatic change as psychotherapy process. Psychotherapy Research 1:104–112, 1991

Gladis MM, Gosch EA, Dishuk NM, et al: Quality of life: expanding the scope of clinical significance. J Consult Clin Psychol 67:320–331, 1999

Goodman WM, Price LH, Rasmussen SA, et al: The Yale-Brown Obsessive-Compulsive Scale. Arch Gen Psychiatry 46:1006–1011, 1989

Hatcher RL, Barends AW: Patients' view of the alliance in psychotherapy: exploratory factor analysis of three alliance measures. J Consult Clin Psychol 64:1326–1336, 1996

Hathaway SR, McKinley JC: A Multiphasic Personality Schedule (Minnesota); III: The measurement of symptomatic depression. J Psychol 14:73–84, 1942

Higgins ET, Bond RN, Klein R, et al: Self-discrepancies and emotional vulnerability: how magnitude, accessibility, and type of discrepancy influence affect. J Pers Soc Psychol 51:5–15, 1986

Hollon SD, Kendall PC: Cognitive self-statements in depression: development of an automatic thoughts questionnaire. Cognitive Therapy and Research 4:88–100, 1980

Horowitz LM: On the cognitive structure of interpersonal problems treated in psychotherapy. J Consult Clin Psychol 47:5–15, 1979

Horowitz LM, Rosenberg SE, Baer BA, et al: Inventory of Interpersonal Problems: psychometric properties and clinical applications. J Consult Clin Psychol 56:885–892, 1988

Horvath AO, Greenberg LS: The development of the Working Alliance Inventory, in The Psychotherapeutic Process: A Research Handbook. Edited by Greenberg LS, Pinsof WM. New York, Guilford, pp 529–566, 1986

Horvath AO, Greenberg LS: Development and validation of the Working Alliance Inventory. Journal of Counseling Psychology 36:223–233, 1989

Horvath AO, Symonds BD: Relation between working alliance and outcome in psychotherapy: a meta-analysis. Journal of Counseling Psychology 38:139–149, 1991

Howard KI, Moras K, Brill PL, et al: Evaluation of psychotherapy: efficacy, effectiveness, and patient progress. Am Psychol 51:1059–1064, 1996

Jacobson NS, Truax PA: Clinical significance: a statistical approach to defining meaningful change in psychotherapy research. J Consult Clin Psychol 59:12–19, 1991

Klein MH, Benjamin LS, Rosenfeld R, et al: The Wisconsin Personality Disorders Inventory: development, reliability, and validity. J Personal Disord 7:285–303, 1993

Lambert MJ, Burlingame GL, Umphress VJ, et al: The reliability and validity of the Outcome Questionnaire. Clinical Psychology and Psychotherapy 3:106–116, 1996

Lambert MJ, Horowitz LM, Strupp HH: Conclusions and recommendations, in Measuring Patient Changes in Mood, Anxiety, and Personality Disorders: Toward a Core Battery. Edited by Strupp HH, Horowitz LM, Lambert MJ. Washington, DC, American Psychiatric Press, 1997, pp 491–502

Lambert MJ, Okiishi JC, Johnson LD, et al: Outcome assessment: from conceptualization to implementation. Professional Psychology: Research and Practice 29:63–70, 1998

Luborsky L, Bachrach HM: Factors influencing clinicians' judgments of mental health: experiences with the health-sickness rating scale. Arch Gen Psychiatry 31:292–299, 1974

Luborsky L, Crits-Christoph P: Understanding Transference: The Core Conflictual Relationship Theme Method. Washington, DC, American Psychological Association, 1998

Luborsky L, Crits-Christoph P, Alexander L, et al: Two helping alliance methods for predicting outcomes of psychotherapy. J Nerv Ment Dis 171:480–491, 1983

Luborsky L, Barber JP, Siqueland L, et al: The revised Helping Alliance Questionnaire (HAQ-II): psychometric properties. J Psychother Pract Res 5:260–271, 1996

Marks IM, Mathews AM: Brief standard self-rating for phobic patients. Behav Res Ther 17:263–267, 1979

McLellan AT, Luborsky L, Woody GE, et al: An improved diagnostic evaluation instrument for substance abuse patients: the Addiction Severity Index. J Nerv Ment Dis 168:26–33, 1980

Meyer TJ, Miller ML, Metzger RL, et al: Development and validation of the Penn State Worry Questionnaire. Behav Res Ther 28:487–495, 1990

Millon T: Millon Clinical Multiaxial Inventory Manual, 3rd Edition. Minneapolis, MN, Interpretive Scoring Systems, 1983

Morey LC, Kurtz JE: Assessment of general personality and psychopathology among persons with eating and weight-related concerns, in Handbook of Assessment Methods for Eating Behaviors And Weight-Related Problems. Edited by Allison DB. Thousand Oaks, CA, Sage, 1995, pp 1–22

Mueller RM, Lambert MJ, Burlingame GM: Construct validity of the outcome questionnaire: a confirmatory factor analysis. J Pers Assess 70:248–262, 1998

Olfson M, Pincus HA: Outpatient psychotherapy in the United States: 1. Volume, costs, and user characteristics. Am J Psychiatry 151:1281–1288, 1994

Rosenberg M: Society and the Adolescent Self-Image. Princeton, NJ, Princeton University Press, 1965

Rush AJ, Giles DE, Schlesser MA, et al: The Inventory for Depressive Symptomatology (IDS): preliminary findings. Psychiatry Res 18:65–87, 1986

Scarvalone PA, Cloitre M, Spielman LA, et al: Distress reduction during the structured clinical interview for DSM-III-R. Psychiatry Res 59:245–249, 1996

Seligman MEP, Abramson LY, Semmel A, et al: Depressive attributional style. J Abnorm Psychol 88:242–247, 1979

Smith ML, Glass GV, Miller TI: The Benefits of Psychotherapy. Baltimore, MD, Johns Hopkins University Press, 1980

Spanier GB: Measuring dyadic adjustment: new scales for assessing the quality of marriage and similar dyads. J Marital Fam Ther 38:15–38, 1976

Sperry L, Brill P, Howard KI, et al: Treatment Outcomes in Psychotherapy and Psychiatric Interventions. New York, Brunner/Mazel, 1996

Trull TJ, Widiger TA, Useda JD, et al: A structured interview for the assessment of the five-factor model of personality. Psychol Assess 10:229–240, 1998

Umphress VJ, Lambert MJ, Smart DW, et al: Concurrent and construct validity of the outcome questionnaire. Journal of Psychoeducational Assessment 15:40–55, 1997

Weissman AN: The Dysfunctional Attitudes Scale: a validation study. Doctoral dissertation, Philadelphia, PA, University of Pennsylvania, 1979 [Dissertation Abstracts International 40:1389–1390, 1979]

Weissman MM, Klerman GL, Paykel ES, et al: Treatment effects in the social adjustment of depressed patients. Arch Gen Psychiatry 30:771–778, 1974

CHAPTER 9

Outcome Measurement in Serious Mental Illness

Lewis A. Opler, M.D., Ph.D.
Paul Michael Ramirez, Ph.D.
Vivian M. Mougios, M.A.

S erious mental illness (SMI), as operationalized by the Center for Mental Health Services (CMHS) of the U.S. Department of Health and Human Services, is a *disorder* with a *functional impairment* as defined below:

1. *Disorder:* Any DSM disorder diagnosed during a 12-month period, excluding V codes (conditions not attributable to a mental disorder that are a focus of attention or treatment, such as academic problems or malingering), substance use disorders, and developmental disorders.
2. *Impairment:* Substantial interference with one or more major life activities that include not only basic daily living skills such as eating and bathing, but also "instrumental living skills (e.g., maintaining a household, managing money, getting around the community, taking prescribed medication), and functioning in social, family, and vocational/educational contexts."

Criteria for functional impairment are also met if any of the following are true:

1. The disorder is schizophrenia, schizoaffective disorder, manic depressive disorder, autism, severe forms of major depression, panic disorder, or obsessive-compulsive disorder, given that all of these disorders almost always lead to serious impairment if not treated;
2. At some time during the past 12 months the disorder substantially interfered with vocational capacity, created serious interpersonal difficulties, or was associated with a suicide plan or attempt; or
3. At some time during the past 12 months functional impairment criteria would have been met without the benefit of treatment or other support services (Substance Abuse and Mental Health Services Administration 1993).

Using these CMHS definitions of disorder and impairment, Kessler and colleagues (1996) estimated that in the United States, the 12-month prevalence of SMI is 5.4%.

In this chapter, scales that can be used to measure functional impairment and assess treatment outcome in persons with SMI, regardless of diagnosis, are reviewed. In addition, because persons diagnosed with schizophrenia and schizoaffective disorder are, by definition, classified as having SMI, scales used for assessing changes in symptom severity as well as for measuring medication side effects in psychotic disorders are also discussed.

SCALES USED TO ASSESS FUNCTIONAL IMPAIRMENT

Global Assessment Scale and Global Assessment of Functioning Scale

The Global Assessment Scale (GAS) was developed by Endicott and colleagues (1976) by revising the Health-Sickness Rating Scale (Luborsky 1962). Further modification led to the Global Assessment of Functioning (GAF) Scale, used as Axis V to score an individual's overall level of functioning in DSM-III-R and DSM-IV-TR (American Psychiatric Association 2000).

The GAS and the GAF evaluate overall psychiatric functioning of a patient during a specified time period, usually up to 1 week before assessment, although ratings over longer periods of time may be useful in certain purposes. The scale ranges from 1 (most ill) to 100 (healthiest) and is

divided into 10 equal intervals. Each interval is defined by specific characteristics. For example, individuals rated between 91 and 100 are totally
asymptomatic and are considered to be very healthy while maintaining a
superior level of functioning throughout many areas of life. They are
socially competent and are sought out by others. Scores within the range
of 71–80 are generally assigned to individuals who show transient symptoms, which may reflect an expected reaction to psychosocial stressors and
lead to only slight impairment in functioning. Most individuals in need of
treatment are rated between 1 and 70. In general, outpatients are rated
between 31 and 70, whereas inpatients are most often rated somewhere
between 1 and 30. The scale is easy to use and is quite versatile, as it
includes the entire range of severity from very ill to very healthy. In addition, information needed to make a rating can be obtained from the patient,
a reliable informant, or case records.

A shortcoming of the scale is the fact that although several examples at
different levels of severity are provided, the GAF does not provide precise
anchoring within each of its 10-point increments. Thus, a patient who
exhibits behaviors that are listed within two 10-point increments may be
rated differently by different clinicians. Despite this shortcoming, the psychometric properties of the GAF have demonstrated sufficient reliability
and validity. Five studies were conducted to assess interrater reliability. In
each of the studies, raters were paired and were asked to simultaneously
rate the same patient, case record, and/or case vignette. The interrater correlation coefficient ranged between 0.61 and 0.91, indicating adequate
reliability. In addition, to assess the concurrent validity of the GAS, on
which the GAF was based, the scale was correlated with the Mental Status
Examination Record (MSER) and the Psychiatric Status Schedule (PSS).
These scales were used to assess the patient's overall degree of psychopathology at the time of admission and 6 months later. Correlations of the
GAS with the MSER and the PSS demonstrated good concurrent validity.
It should be noted that correlations for the GAS ratings were stronger at
6 months than at the time of admission. This was likely due to the greater
heterogeneity of the patient's severity of pathology (i.e., on admission,
patients are more similar in their pathology than they are 6 months after
treatment). It should be noted, however, that there is at least one study that
calls the validity of the GAF into question. Specifically, Roy-Byrne et al.
(1996) found that ratings of the GAF were more strongly correlated with
clinical symptoms rather than with the patient's overall level of functioning.

The GAF is suitable for all patient populations and requires about
5 minutes to score. Although it is used in clinical research studies, the GAF
is principally used to score Axis V in DSM-IV. The GAF scale can be found
in DSM-IV-TR (American Psychiatric Association 2000).

Nurses' Observation Scale for Inpatient Evaluation

The Nurses' Observation Scale for Inpatient Evaluation (NOSIE) was developed to provide a means whereby inpatient behavior could be evaluated on the basis of observation by nursing staff (Honigsfeld and Klett 1965; Honigsfeld et al. 1976). It comprises 30 items and can be completed in approximately 5–10 minutes.

The NOSIE is particularly useful in evaluating patients who cannot comply with the requirements of an interview. The NOSIE requires a minimum of training and is easy to score. Scoring is based on the frequency with which 30 behaviors have occurred during the 3 days immediately preceding a rating. Each of these behaviors is scored on a scale that ranges from 0 (never) to 4 (always). Interrater reliability of the NOSIE has been evaluated and has found to be high (Lentz et al. 1971). An advantage of the NOSIE is its objectivity, given that scores are based on simple observations that do not require inferences or interpretations on the part of the nursing staff. Although it has high interrater reliability, the NOSIE uses anchored ratings that are not defined, and therefore variability in scoring between adjacent rating points—for example, between 2 (often) and 3 (usually)—is to be expected. As is the case with many other rating scales, the NOSIE can be completed both before and after treatment regimens, or it can be completed on a weekly basis. Finally, the NOSIE is available within the public domain.

Behavior and Symptom Identification Scale

The Behavior and Symptom Identification Scale (BASIS-32) is a 32-item measure of symptoms and behavioral distress that is primarily used as an outcome assessment instrument for psychiatric inpatients. Originally, the scoring of the BASIS-32 was based on a 20- to 30-minute semistructured interview, with each of the 32 items being scored along a 5-point Likert-type scale ranging from 0 (no difficulty) to 4 (extreme difficulty). At present, however, the BASIS-32 is typically self-administered (Sederer and Dickey 1996). In addition, after a specified period of time (usually 6 months after the initial rating), patients can complete a self-administered follow-up questionnaire.

The items making up the BASIS-32 were empirically derived from open-ended inpatient reports of problems leading to hospitalization. Its validity was assessed in a study examining 387 patients in a psychiatric hospital (Eisen et al. 1994). In addition to changes in total score, the following five factors can be used for subscale ratings: relation to self and others, daily living and role functioning, depression and anxiety, impulsive and addictive behavior, and psychosis (Eisen et al. 1994).

Although the BASIS-32 was originally intended for psychiatric inpatients, it is now widely used in outpatient settings as well. Administration can take 20–30 minutes if a semistructured interview is used, or approximately 10 minutes if it is self-administered. A trained rater typically administers this measure. When self-administered, the BASIS-32 is subject to some of the same limitations inherent in any self-report measure. Specifically, truthfulness is an issue as well as individual variability in interpreting the differences between specific ratings of severity (e.g., "quite a bit of difficulty" and "extreme difficulty"). The issue of truthfulness can be addressed by having a significant other or an individual who spends a significant amount of time with the patient also complete the BASIS-32. Response variability, particularly among adjacent severity ratings, could be reduced if a brief description of each level of rating severity were to be added to the questionnaire. The BASIS-32 is available from the Evaluative Service Unit at McLean Hospital (115 Mill Street, Belmont, MA 02178).

Quality of Life Scale

The Quality of Life Scale (QLS) provides a means for assessing the life circumstances of individuals with SMI (Lehman 1983). Although the QLS has been modified to accommodate the needs of particular studies, the principal author has maintained a core version for evaluating quality-of-life issues relevant to all patients with a mental disorder. This core version provides an assessment of patients' recent and current life experiences in a variety of daily living experiences. In addition to a global measure of life satisfaction, it evaluates a patient's quality of life from both objective and subjective perspectives in the following eight areas of daily living: living situation, daily activities and functioning, family relations, social relations, finances, work and school (omitted in cases in which the patient is not involved in work or school), legal and safety issues, and health. Information is obtained on each of these domains to form an objective assessment, and then the patient's level of satisfaction in each area is assessed. Combining both objective and subjective quality-of-life indicators is a unique feature of the QLS.

The QLS consists of questions on the patient's objective life situation. Inquiries are then made regarding the patient's subjective experience of this life situation along the eight dimensions mentioned above, which are answered along a Likert-type scale ranging from 1 (terrible) to 7 (delighted). The internal consistency of these eight life-experience areas ranges from 0.77 for legal and safety issues to 0.87 for home living situation. One-week test-retest reliability ranges from 0.53 for leisure activities to 0.95 for work and school-related issues.

International Classification of Functioning and Disability

In a summary of the global burden of disease recently released by the World Health Organization (WHO) (Murray and Lopez 1996), an unexpected finding was that the burden of psychiatric conditions has been heavily underestimated. Of the 10 leading causes of disability worldwide in 1990, measured in years lived with a disability, 5 were psychiatric conditions: unipolar depression, alcohol use, bipolar affective disorder (manic-depressive), schizophrenia, and obsessive-compulsive disorder. Unipolar depression alone was responsible for more than 1 in every 10 years of life lived with a disability worldwide.

Although it is still being field tested and is subject to revision, the WHO is encouraging the use of the International Classification of Functioning and Disability (ICIDH-2). It was originally titled the International Classification of Impairments, Disabilities and Handicaps (ICIDH) in the evaluation of health status and of all medical disorders, including mental disorders (World Health Organization 1999). As psychiatry becomes better integrated into general health care, the ICIDH-2 is likely to become one of the main instruments used in evaluating functioning and disability in mental disorders in general and, in particular, in SMI.

The ICIDH-2 assesses three dimensions of functioning and disability: 1) body functions and structure, 2) activities at the individual level, and 3) participation in society. Ratings of specific areas of functioning (e.g., personal care) is rated from 0 (no disability) to 5 (gross disability).

The WHO is recommending that the ICIDH-2 be used in conjunction with the International Classification of Diseases, Tenth Revision (ICD-10) (World Health Organization 1992), because ICD-10 provides a diagnosis, and this information is enriched by the additional information obtained by ICIDH-2 on functioning at the bodily, individual, and societal levels. Information on both diagnosis and functioning provide a broader and more meaningful picture that describes the health status of individuals, which could be used for clinical decision making.

ASSESSMENT OF CHANGES IN SYMPTOM SEVERITY IN PSYCHOTIC DISORDERS

Schizophrenia and schizoaffective disorder are included in the CMHS operationalized definition of SMI, and persons with other psychotic disorders are frequently classified as having SMI as well. Therefore, scales developed for assessing changes in symptom severity in primarily psychotic disorders should be used as part of the assessment of persons with SMI.

Brief Psychiatric Rating Scale

The Brief Psychiatric Rating Scale (BPRS) (Overall and Gorham 1962) was developed as a quantitative measure for the assessment of an inpatient's mental state, and it has been widely used in evaluating the efficacy of antipsychotic medications. Ratings on the BPRS scale are made after a brief interview with the patient, usually lasting 15–20 minutes. Ratings on each item of the BPRS are based on information obtained solely during the interview. Assessment of treatment efficacy is based on changes in the total score across administrations. In addition, factor analytical studies have made obtaining additional factor scores possible in the areas of anergia, thought disturbance, activation, paranoia/belligerence, and anxiety/depression. More recently, with increased interest in assessing negative or deficit symptoms in contrast to positive or active symptoms, BPRS positive and negative factors have also been determined.

Four revisions of the BPRS have been made, with recent modifications providing operational definitions of items and anchoring scale points to improve interrater reliability (Woerner et al. 1988). Interrater reliability, assessed by comparing the ratings of five rater pairs, has yielded significant coefficients ranging from 0.50 to 0.58 (Hafkenscheid 1991).

Despite the widespread popularity of this measure (Hedlund and Vieweg 1980), it does not maintain clearly defined parameters for differences between various severity levels, and therefore overlapping may occur in scoring more broadly defined items. There have also been several attempts to develop semistructured as well as structured interviews for the BPRS (Rhoades and Overall 1988; Tarell and Schulz 1988).

Although it is primarily intended to assess patients with psychiatric disorders in general, the BPRS is most commonly used to evaluate patients with schizophrenia. Administration time is approximately 15–30 minutes. This scale is available within the public domain.

Scale for the Assessment of Negative Symptoms and Scale for the Assessment of Positive Symptoms

To provide a more focussed assessment of positive and negative symptoms, Andreasen (1983, 1984) developed the Scale for the Assessment of Negative Symptoms (SANS) and the Scale for the Assessment of Positive Symptoms (SAPS).

The SANS provides a methodology for rating 20 negative symptoms and 5 global symptoms: alogia, affective flattening, avolition/apathy, anhedonia/asociality, and attentional impairment. Each symptom is rated on a Likert scale ranging from 1 (no symptom) to 6 (severe manifestation).

These ratings are made by observations of the patient and interviews with reliable informants (e.g., nurses, ward personnel, and family members). Although no time frame is specified, investigators using the SANS are advised to use a time frame that covers the past month. Thus, they are able to monitor symptoms and to assess the degree of change. The most widely used scores are the 5 global ratings and the total SANS score.

The reliability of the SANS was assessed by comparing the ratings of pairs of investigators. Rating teams interviewed several patients and then rated each patient simultaneously. Correlations between raters ranged from 0.86 to 0.93, indicating high interrater reliability. Cronbach's α coefficient has been shown to range from 0.63 to 0.84, indicating strong internal consistency.

The SAPS is similar to the SANS in structure. This scale is composed of 38 items, of which 34 involve ratings of individual symptoms, with 4 items being global ratings for each of the 4 following symptom complexes: hallucinations, delusions, bizarre behavior, and formal thought disorder. Each symptom is rated on a Likert scale ranging from 1 (no symptom) to 6 (severe manifestation). These ratings are made by observations of the patient and interviews with reliable informants (e.g., nurses, ward personnel, and family members). Similarly to the SANS, the SAPS contains a global rating scale that summarizes all of the symptoms within a subscale category. The total score of the SAPS provides an overall index of positive symptoms. As is the case with the SANS, the investigator can calculate both the summary score (adding global rating scales) and the composite score (adding scores across specific symptoms).

Andreasen and colleagues (1994) have subjected the SAPS to factor analysis, which has yielded two factors: 1) thought disorder and bizarre behavior, and 2) delusions and hallucinations. The psychometric properties of the SANS and the SAPS have been repeatedly tested across several settings and have demonstrated adequate reliability and validity.

The SANS and the SAPS are intended for patients with schizophrenia and similar serious mental illnesses. Administration time is approximately 40 minutes for both scales. A clinician or trained rater can administer these scales.

Positive and Negative Syndrome Scale

The Positive and Negative Syndrome Scale (PANSS), originally designed as a modification and expansion of the BPRS, evolved into a new scale as additional psychometric features were added (Kay et al. 1992). The PANSS was developed by clinicians, is easy to learn, and can be readily adapted to a wide range of clinical settings (Opler and Ramirez 1998). The PANSS was developed by supplementing the 18-item BPRS with 12 items selected from the Psychopathology Rating Schedule (PRS). The 12 PRS items were added to the BPRS to provide an adequate assessment of negative symptoms and other phenomenological features believed to be inadequately represented in the BPRS.

The PANSS is a 30-item scale in which each item is rated on a Likert-type severity scale ranging from 1 (absent) to 7 (extreme). Each item in the PANSS is accompanied by an item definition as well as detailed anchoring criteria, which are used to score item severity. It yields three scores: a positive scale score, a negative scale score, and a general psychopathology scale score. The positive and negative scales include 7 items each, and the remaining 16 items constitute the general psychopathology scale. A factor analytical study of 1,233 schizophrenic patients from five different sites carried out by the PANSS Study Group (White et al. 1997) yielded the derivation of a five-factor or pentagonal model of schizophrenic symptoms. Items targeted the following five factors: "negative," "positive," "activation," "dysphoria," and "autistic preoccupation factors."

The Structured Clinical Interview for the PANSS (SCI-PANSS) (Opler et al. 1992) was developed to standardize the assessment procedure while ensuring the collection of all information needed to score the presence and severity of all PANSS items. The SCI-PANSS, which can be completed in 30–40 minutes, provides a decision-tree sequence in such a way that a patient's previous answer leads into the next question. Fourteen of the PANSS items require input from an outside informant familiar with the patient's behavior during the specified period of time (usually the preceding week). To ensure that PANSS raters obtain all of the necessary information from nursing staff, family members, or significant others, the Informant Questionnaire for the PANSS (IQ-PANSS) was introduced (Opler and Ramirez 2000).

The PANSS has been demonstrated to be both reliable and valid and to have high internal consistency. Interrater reliability coefficients between 0.83 and 0.87 have been obtained, and α coefficients of 0.73 for the positive subscale, 0.83 for the negative subscale, and 0.79 for the general psychopathology subscale have been obtained.

Symptom Checklist-90–Revised

The Symptom Checklist-90–Revised (SCL-90-R) is a 90-item self-administered symptom inventory used to assess patterns of psychological symptoms among patients (Derogatis 1994). The SCL-90-R uses a Likert scale to assess degree of distress ranging from "not at all" (0) to "extremely" (4). The inventory contains nine subscales or symptom dimensions and three global indices of psychological distress. The nine subscales are somatization, obsessive-compulsive, interpersonal sensitivity, depression, anxiety, hostility, phobic anxiety, paranoid ideation, and psychoticism. The three global indices, which provide for an overall assessment of the patient's psychopathological status (Derogatis 1994), are global severity index, positive symptoms distress index, and positive symptom total.

Adequate psychometric properties for the SCL-90-R have been established. Internal consistency of the nine symptom dimensions was assessed in two studies using coefficient α. Coefficients from both studies were satisfactory, ranging from 0.70 to 0.90. Test-retest reliability was evaluated in a study using 94 heterogeneous psychiatric outpatients. These patients were assessed during an initial evaluation and then a week later. Test-retest reliability coefficients ranged from 0.80 to 0.90. Additional studies have shown test-retest reliability ranging from 0.68 to 0.83. Several studies have also demonstrated adequate construct validity and convergent-discriminant validity.

The SCL-90-R is suitable for all patient populations in either clinical or research settings. Administration time is usually between 15 and 20 minutes; however, this time may vary depending on the reading and educational background of the patient. To ensure validity of the responses, a minimum sixth-grade reading level is required. The referent time set for the SCL-90-R is also important. Patients are asked to rate the severity of their symptoms based on the past 7 days including the present day.

Schedule of Affective Disorders and Schizophrenia

The Schedule for Affective Disorders and Schizophrenia (SADS) provides a detailed description of current episodes of illness, a description of the level of severity of phenomenological manifestations of major dimensions of psychopathology, and a progression of questions and criteria providing information relevant to making diagnoses. The SADS also provides for detailed descriptions of past psychopathology as well as functioning, which are relevant to evaluations of diagnosis, prognosis, and overall severity of disturbance (Endicott and Spitzer 1978). It was specifically developed to reduce the information variance among investigators using the Research Diagnostic Criteria by providing clinicians with an interviewing guide and data recording form. As an interview, the full SADS is conducted in two parts, one focusing on the present and/or last year and the other focusing on the past. The initial application of the SADS was in clinical studies in which accurate diagnosis was essential to treatment evaluation studies. The 120 items on the SADS are primarily rated on a Likert scale. Eight summary scales are derived from the SADS: depressive mood and ideation, endogenous features, depressive-associated features, suicidal ideation and behavior, anxiety, manic syndrome, delusions-hallucinations, and formal thought disorder.

The psychometric properties of the SADS appear to be sufficient. Intraclass correlation coefficients of reliability for the 120 scaled items were 0.60 or better (Endicott and Spitzer 1978). Similar reliability has been established for the summary scales.

The SADS is primarily intended for schizophrenic patients. This interview should be conducted by well-trained clinicians. Total administration time is 1.5–2 hours, depending on the severity of the symptoms.

Social Adjustment Scale–II

The Social Adjustment Scale–II (SAS-II) (Weissman et al. 1981) is an adaptation of the Social Adjustment Scale interview developed by Weissman and Bothwell (1976) and is intended to assess the social adjustment of schizophrenic patients. The SAS-II contains 52 questions, which are administered in a semistructured interview format. Assessment includes work role, relationships with a "principal household member," sexual adjustment, romantic involvement, parental role, extended family relationships, social leisure activities, and personal well-being. The SAS-II is sensitive to the unique living arrangements typical for the chronically mentally ill.

A study of 56 ambulatory schizophrenic patients and their partners was conducted to assess the reliability of the SAS-II. Overall agreement among informants yielded a Spearman's rank correlation coefficient of 0.98 (Weissman et al. 1981). The SAS-II is limited to assessing schizophrenic patients, and it can facilitate assessment of social functioning in a wider variety of social situations. Typically, this scale is administered by a trained clinician. The interview takes approximately 1 hour to complete.

ASSESSMENT OF MEDICATION SIDE EFFECTS

Simpson-Angus Scale

The Simpson-Angus Scale was developed to provide an objective method for rating extrapyramidal motor side effects of neuroleptic agents (Simpson and Angus 1970). The Simpson-Angus Scale contains 10 items: gait, arm dropping, shoulder shaking, elbow rigidity, wrist rigidity, leg pendulousness, head dropping, glabella tap, tremor, and salivation. Each item is rated on a 5-point Likert-type scale ranging from 0 (no symptoms) to 4 (symptom in extreme form). Adding the numbers endorsed on each item and dividing by 10 tabulates the final score, hence the mean.

Psychometric properties include sufficient reliability and validity. Clinical validity was assessed by examining the manifestations of symptoms in patients receiving varying doses of neuroleptic medications. In addition, factor analysis revealed four principal components. The first factor included the following symptoms: rigidity, shoulder shaking, elbow rigidity, wrist rigidity, and leg pendulousness. The second factor included gait, salivation, and head dropping. The third factor included the glabella tap, and the fourth factor included tremors. Interrater reliability was assessed in patients receiving varying doses of neuroleptics, who were rated by two physicians in a double-blind study. The correlation coefficients of the two investigators ranged from 0.71 to 0.96.

This scale is intended to assess extrapyramidal symptoms of patients with drug-induced parkinsonism. One of the disadvantages of this scale is its failure to include ratings for akinesia and bradykinesia. The Simpson-Angus Scale is typically administered by physicians and takes 10 minutes to administer. It is available within the public domain.

Abnormal Involuntary Movement Scale

The Abnormal Involuntary Movement Scale (AIMS) is a 10-item rating instrument that assesses abnormal movements, which are either related to the disease itself or to treatment with antipsychotic medication. It also includes 2 additional items provided to correct for buccolingual movements that may be due to the patient's dental status (Alcohol, Drug Abuse, and Mental Health Administration 1985).

The AIMS evaluates symptoms related to tardive dyskinesia, tardive dystonia, and tardive akathisia. The AIMS examination consists of rating the presence and severity of movement disorders involving the face, mouth, extremities, and trunk on a 5-point scale ranging from 0 (none) to 4 (severe). There are also three items that provide for a global judgment of the severity of abnormal movements, incapacitation due to these abnormal movements, and the patient's awareness of these abnormal movements. The AIMS can be completed quickly and is relatively easy to learn.

Adequate interrater reliability for the AIMS has been established (Lane et al 1985; Munetz and Benjamin 1988). The AIMS can be administered by clinicians, with administration time being approximately 5–10 minutes. This measure is available within the public domain.

Extrapyramidal Symptom Rating Scale

The Extrapyramidal Symptom Rating Scale (ESRS) was developed to assess extrapyramidal motor symptoms. The ESRS consists of a questionnaire on parkinsonian symptoms, a physician's examination for parkinsonian and dyskinetic movements, and a clinical global impression of tardive dyskinesia. The parkinsonian questionnaire is composed of nine items to assess the type of symptoms the patient reports experiencing (e.g., restlessness, balance difficulties, tremors). The physician's examination for parkinsonian movements consists of eight items to assess the patient's parkinsonism during the examination. Tardive dyskinesia is evaluated by utilizing a standard procedure aimed at activating dyskinetic symptoms that may be less overtly apparent and rating them accordingly. Finally, the physician also assesses the frequency and amplitude of dyskinetic movements involving the tongue, jaw, lips, trunk, and extremities.

Psychometric properties of the ESRS were assessed, and it demonstrated sufficient reliability and validity. The ESRS was validated in eight double-blind studies. In all eight studies, the ESRS was able to detect changes in both parkinsonian and dyskinetic symptoms. The ESRS has also demonstrated concurrent validity with other standard scales, such as the AIMS. In addition, the ESRS has been found to correlate significantly with biological measures of drug action (e.g., prolactin levels). Interrater reliability coefficients were calculated for each item of the scale by comparing independent ratings conducted by physicians on 89 schizophrenic patients. These coefficients ranged from 0.80 to 0.97.

In general, the ESRS is a sensitive and reliable instrument that is useful in clinical practice and research settings where the evaluation of parkinsonian and dyskinetic phenomenological presentation is an important issue.

Barnes Akathisia Scale

Akathisia is a syndrome of motor and subjective restlessness often caused by neuroleptic medications. The Barnes Akathisia Scale (Barnes et al. 1989) was designed to provide criteria that would allow for a more reliable differential diagnosis of akathisia from other drug-induced movement disorders (e.g., dystonia, parkinsonism, and tardive dyskinesia) as well as from mannerisms and stereotypical movements. This scale is composed of items that evaluate restless movements, subjective awareness of restlessness, and any distress associated with the akathisia.

Reliability coefficients have been shown to be sufficient, ranging from 0.74 to 0.96. Validity of the scale is based on signs and symptoms identified in previous studies involving schizophrenic outpatients receiving antipsychotic medication.

This scale is primarily used for patients with drug-induced akathisia and is typically administered by a physician. Total administration time is approximately 15 minutes. The Barnes Akathisia Scale is available within the public domain.

CONCLUSION

Psychiatric disorders in general and SMI in particular are receiving more attention as public health problems in light of emerging evidence that psychiatric illness accounts for a large percentage of disability. Scales assessing functional impairment, symptom severity, and medication side effects will become increasingly important as clinicians, researchers, and health planners allocate resources to improve services and treatments available for persons with SMI.

REFERENCES

Alcohol, Drug Abuse, and Mental Health Administration: NIMH Treatment Strategies in Schizophrenia Study (Publ No ADM-117). Washington, DC, U.S. Department of Health and Human Services, Public Health Service, 1985

American Psychiatric Association: Diagnostic and Statistical Manual of Mental Disorders, 4th Edition, Text Revision. Washington, DC, American Psychiatric Association, 2000

Andreasen NC: Scale for the Assessment of Negative Symptoms (SANS). Iowa City, IA, University of Iowa, 1983

Andreasen NC: Scale for the Assessment of Positive Symptoms (SAPS). Iowa City, IA, University of Iowa, 1984

Andreasen NC, Nopoulos P, Schultz S: Positive and negative symptoms of schizophrenia: past, present, and future. Acta Psychiatr Scand 90:51–59, 1994

Barnes TRE: A rating scale for drug-induced akathisia. Br J Psychiatry 154:672–676, 1989

Derogatis L: SCL-90-R Symptom Checklist-90–R: Administration, Scoring, and Procedures Manual. Minneapolis, MN, National Computer Systems, 1994

Eisen SV, Dill DL, Grob MC: Reliability and validity of a brief patient report instrument for psychiatric outcome evaluation. Hospital and Community Psychiatry 45:242–247, 1994

Endicott J, Spitzer RL: A diagnostic interview: the schedule for Affective Disorders and Schizophrenia. Arch Gen Psychiatry 35:837–844, 1978

Endicott J, Spitzer RL, Fleiss JL, et al: The Global Assessment Scale: a procedure for measuring overall severity of psychiatric disturbance. Arch Gen Psychiatry 33:776–771, 1976

Hafkenscheid A: A psychometric evaluation of a standardized and expanded brief psychiatric rating scale. Acta Psychiatr Scand 84:294–300, 1991

Hedlund JL, Vieweg BW: The Brief Psychiatric Rating Scale (BPRS): a comprehensive review. Journal of Operational Psychiatry 11:48–65, 1980

Honigsfeld G, Klett CJ: The Nurses' Observation Scale for Inpatient Evaluation: the new scale for measuring improvement in chronic schizophrenia. J Clin Psychol 21:65–71, 1965

Honigsfeld G, Gillis RD, Klett CJ: The Nurses' Observation Scale for Inpatient Evaluation, in ECDEU Assessment Manual for Psychopharmacology (DHEW Publ No ADM 76-338). Edited by Guy W. Rockville, MD, U.S. Department of Health, Education, and Welfare, 1976, pp 265–273

Kay SR, Opler LA, Fiszbein A: The Positive and Negative Syndrome Scale (PANSS) Manual. Toronto, ON, Canada, Multi-Health Systems, 1992

Kessler RC, Berglund PA, Zhao S, et al: The 12-month prevalence and correlates of serious mental illness (SMI), in Mental Health, United States, 1996. Edited by Manderscheid RW, Sonnenschein MA. Washington, DC, U.S. Government Printing Office, 1996, pp 59–70

Lane RD, Glazer WM, Hansen TE, et al: Assessment of tardive dyskinesia using the abnormal involuntary movement scale. J Nerv Ment Dis 173:353–357, 1985

Lehman AF: The well being of chronic mental patients: assessing their quality of life. Arch Gen Psychiatry 40:369–373, 1983

Lentz RJ, Paul GL, Calhoun JF: Reliability and validity of three measures of functioning with "hard-core" chronic mental patients. J Abnorm Psychol 78:69–76, 1971

Luborsky L: Clinicians' judgments of mental health. Arch Gen Psychiatry 7:407–417, 1962

Munetz MR, Benjamin S: How to examine patients using the Abnormal Involuntary Movement Scale. Hospital and Community Psychiatry 39:1172–1177, 1988

Murray CJL, Lopez AD (eds): The Global Burden of Disease: Summary. Geneva, World Health Organization, 1996

Opler LA, Ramirez PM: Use of the Positive and Negative Syndrome Scale (PANSS) in clinical practice. Journal of Practical Psychiatry and Behavioral Health 4:157–162, 1998

Opler LA, Ramirez PM: The Informant Questionnaire for the PANSS (IQ-PANSS). Toronto, ON, Canada, Multi-Health Systems, 2000

Opler LA, Kay SR, Fiszbein A, et al: The Structured Clinical Interview for the Positive and Negative Syndrome Scale (SCI-PANSS). Toronto, ON, Canada, Multi-Health Systems, 1992

Overall JE, Gorham DR: Brief Psychiatric Rating Scale. Psychol Rep 10:799–812, 1962

Rhoades HM, Overall JE: The semi-structured interview and rating guide. Psychopharmacology Bulletin 24(1):101–104, 1988

Roy-Byrne P, Dagadakis C, Unutzer J: Evidence for limited validity of the revised Global Assessment of Functioning Scale. Psychiatr Serv 47(8):864–866, 1996

Sederer LI, Dickey B: Outcome Assessment in Clinical Practice. Baltimore, MD, Williams & Wilkins, 1996

Simpson GM, Angus JWS: A rating scale for extrapyramidal side effects. Acta Psychiatr Scand 212 (suppl):11–19, 1970

Substance Abuse and Mental Health Services Administration: Final notice establishing definitions for (1) children with a serious emotional disturbance and (2) adults with a serious mental illness. Federal Register 58(96):29422–29425, 1993

Tarell JD, Schulz SC: Nursing assessment using the BPRS: a structured interview. Psychopharmacology Bulletin 24(1):105–111, 1988

Weissman MM, Bothwell S: Assessment of social adjustment by patient self-report. Arch Gen Psychiatry 33(9):1111–1115, 1976

Weissman M, Sholomskas D, John K: The assessment of social adjustment: an update. Arch Gen Psychiatry 38:1250–1258, 1981

White L, Harvey PD, Opler LA, et al: Empirical assessment of the factorial structure of clinical symptoms in schizophrenia. A multisite, multimodel evaluation of the factorial structure of the Positive and Negative Syndrome Scale. The PANSS Study Group. Psychopathology 30:263–274, 1997

Woerner MG, Mannuzza S, Kane JM: Anchoring the BPRS: an aid to improved reliability. Psychopharmacology Bulletin 24(1):112–117, 1988

World Health Organization: International Statistical Classification of Diseases and Related Health Problems, 10th Revision. Geneva, Switzerland, World Health Organization, 1992

World Health Organization: International Statistical Classification of Functions and Disability (ICIDH-2). Geneva, Switzerland, World Health Organization, 1999

10

Outcome Measurement in Mood Disorders

Tal Burt, M.D.
Waguih William IsHak, M.D.

Mood disorders include bipolar I, bipolar II, major depression, dysthymia, cyclothymia, mood disorders due to a general medical condition, substance-induced mood disorders, and adjustment disorders. These disorders are characterized by an episodic course and often rapid fluctuations in symptoms. Effective management, to a large extent, is contingent on the accurate detection of shifts in clusters of symptoms. Although in the past two decades a large number of studies have been aimed at standardization of assessment tools, the continuous evolution in the definitions of mood disorders has led to difficulty in using earlier outcome measures created before the current definitions and diagnostic criteria were established. In fact, the validity of these measures has been questioned.

Outcome instruments used in the assessment of patients with mood disorders are used primarily to evaluate the severity of a particular episode. Longitudinal aspects of the disorder—such as frequency of episodes, their duration, and rapidity of onset—are not assessed by these instruments, which can miss critical information regarding the course of these disorders.

This chapter covers a few of the many outcome measurement tools that have been developed for the assessment of patients with mood disorders. Unfortunately, no other psychiatric diagnostic category has the plethora of available instruments or the potential for challenges to standardization. The scales were chosen based on their prevalence in the peer-reviewed literature as found in PsychINFO and MEDLINE searches. The Hamilton Rating Scale for Depression; the Beck Depression Inventory, second version; and the Young Mania Rating Scale receive more comprehensive discussion than the other tools because of their widespread use.

PARAMETERS TO MEASURE

Most mood assessment tools cover many of the DSM-IV-TR criteria for mood disorders (American Psychiatric Association 2000a). Some tools measure additional symptoms not covered in DSM-IV. Other tools, on the other hand, fall short of covering all DSM-IV criteria for the specific disorder to be assessed. These discrepancies are a potential source of inconsistencies in outcome assessment. For example, it is possible that some patients will experience some of these non-DSM-IV symptoms while no longer meeting the diagnostic criteria for the disorder or episode.

Non-DSM-IV symptoms of depression include crying spells, social withdrawal, helplessness, anxiety (psychic and somatic), somatic or hypochondriachal symptoms, gastrointestinal symptoms, sympathetic arousal, paranoid ideation, obsessional and compulsive symptoms, depersonalization, derealization, irritability, interest in sex, menstrual disturbances, diurnal variation, and insight.

Non-DSM-IV symptoms of mania include aggressiveness, altered appearance and grooming, and insight.

In addition, nonmood features pertinent to the assessment of mood disorders (covered elsewhere in this book) include functioning, cognition, quality of life, physical health, and side effects.

Measurement of Suicidality

Several scales have been developed to assess suicidality. Most have been used only in research settings and have been found to have limited clinical applicability. Only one scale, the Beck Hopelessness Scale (BHS), has been found to have moderate predictive validity regarding only future attempt of suicide 5–10 years after administration. This prediction is of limited clinical value because most interventions could be realistically implemented in a span of only days to weeks after the assessment. In addition, there is a poor correlation between attempt and completion of suicide. In view of these criticisms, this chapter does not cover scales assessing suicide. The interested reader in referred elsewhere (American Psychiatric Association 2000b).

COMMONLY USED OUTCOME MEASUREMENT TOOLS

Measures of Depression

Clinician-administered scales for depression include the following:

- Hamilton Rating Scale for Depression (HRSD or Ham-D) (Hamilton 1960)
- Montgomery-Asberg Depression Rating Scale (MADRS) (Montgomery and Asberg 1979)
- Raskin Scale (or the Three Area Severity of Depression Scale) (Raskin 1988)
- Geriatric Depression Scale (GDS) (please see Chapter 6, in this volume)

Patient-administered (self-report) scales for depression include the following:

- Beck Depression Inventory, second version (BDI-II) (Beck et al. 1996a)
- Zung Self-Rating Depression Scale (SRDS) (Zung 1965)
- Center for Epidemiologic Studies Depression Scale (CES-D) (Radloff 1977)
- Profile of Mood States (POMS) (McNair et al. 1971)

Scales for depression that are *administered by both patient and clinician* include the following:

- Inventory for Depressive Symptomatology (IDS) (Rush et al. 1996)
- Depression Outcome Module (DOM) (Smith et al. 1995)

Measures of Mania and Hypomania

Clinician-administered scales for mania and hypomania include the following:

- Young Mania Rating Scale (YMRS) (Young et al. 1978)
- Clinician-Administered Rating Scale for Mania (CARS-M) (Altman et al. 1994)

Patient-administered (self-report) scales for mania and hypomania include the following:

- Altman Self-Rating Mania Scale (ASRM) (Altman et al. 1997)

Measures of Both Depression and Mania/Hypomania

Clinician-administered scales for both depression and mania/hypomania include the following:

- Schedule for Affective Disorders and Schizophrenia–Change Version (SADS-C) (Endicott and Spitzer 1978)

Patient-administered (self-report) scales for both depression and mania/hypomania include the following:

- Internal State Scale (ISS) (Bauer et al. 1991)

Graphic Measures of Mood Disorders

Graphic measures of mood disorders include the following:

- Visual analog scale (VAS)
- National Institute of Mental Health Prospective Life-Chart Methodology (NIMH LCM-p) (Denicoff et al. 1997)

CRITICAL REVIEWS OF SPECIFIC OUTCOME MEASURES

Clinician-Administered Measures of Depression

Hamilton Rating Scale for Depression

Table 10–1 provides an overview of the Hamilton Rating Scale for Depression (HRSD).
Psychometric properties of the HRSD are summarized below:

- *Reliability:* The HRSD was found to be reliable in adult and adolescent populations (Clark and Donovan 1994). Hooijer et al. (1991) studied the effect of training on HRSD scores and found that raters' scores increased significantly during HRSD training. Interrater reliability ranges from 0.65 to 0.9 (Rehm et al. 1985).
- *Validity:* Correlations between the HRSD and clinician-rated instruments range between 0.8 and 0.9 (American Psychiatric Association

Table 10–1. Hamilton Rating Scale for Depression

Author and reference	Max Hamilton, M.D. (Hamilton 1960)
Mode of administration	Clinician administered
Total number of items	24
Scoring	12 items are rated 0–4 and 12 are rated 0–2; total score range, 0–72
Cutoff score	16 (for moderate to severe depression)
Target group	Originally designed for patients with primary depression
Time to administer	15–20 minutes
Period covered	Past week
Training requirements	Preferable (Hooijer et al. 1991)
Cost	No fee
Languages	English, Spanish, Chinese, French, German, Italian, Russian, Greek (and other languages)
Other versions	The 24-item version is the most frequently used; 6-, 10-, 17-, and 28- item versions exist (the 10- and 6-item versions are not widely used). In addition, there are numerous versions with modifications of the original 17-item scale.

2000b). Principal-components analysis of the HRSD yielded a four-factor solution: core depression, anxiety, insomnia-hypochondriasis, and cognitive-ideational symptoms (Samuels et al. 1996). In a factor analysis, only one dimension of depressive symptoms appeared to be well defined and associated with global depression severity. These symptoms were depressed mood, guilt, suicide, work and interests, agitation, psychic anxiety, somatic anxiety, and loss of libido. This suggests that the HRSD total score is a weak index of depressive syndrome severity (Gibbons et al. 1993). Comorbidity does not appear to affect the core factor of depression in the 17-item HRSD (Fleck et al. 1995), but overall the validity of the HRSD is affected by medical comorbidity, especially in the elderly population (Linden et al. 1995). The HRSD was found to be valid in the adolescent population (Clark and Donovan 1994). Validity is low in older patients and in patients with medical illness (Linden et al. 1995).

The HRSD is the most widely used depression scale in both clinical and research settings. It covers both primary and secondary depression. It is a reliable scale and has a high validity (Bech 1993). The presence of several versions has led to some confusion in reports of outcome studies (Grundy 1994; Snaith 1996). Lambert et al. (1986) performed meta-analyses comparing the HRSD, the Zung Self-Rating Depression Scale, and the BDI regarding their use as outcome measurement tools. They reported that the HRSD showed more change in depression than did the BDI and the Zung. Hamilton suggested that two raters be involved in each assessment, thereby reducing cost-effectiveness. The HRSD is designed to collect data representative of the past 7 days. However, in some items the clinician is asked to rate the observed state exclusively at the time of the interview (e.g., item 8 on psychomotor agitation). In addition, some items leave the option of rating symptoms before the past 7 days (e.g., rating the loss of job due to the current depressive episode). It is not clear when during the course of the episode to stop rating the loss of job. Also, some items (e.g., item 1, depressed mood) allow the rating to be based either on patient reporting over the past week (e.g., "these feelings spontaneously reported verbally") or on the clinician's observation at the time of the interview (e.g., "communicates feeling states nonverbally [i.e., through facial expression, posture, voice, and tendency to weep]"). These options are not necessarily mutually exclusive, but the rater has to choose between them. In addition, the clinician's observation, in this case, gets a score of 3 and the patient's report a score of 2. It is not clear what the basis is for this preference. This example also emphasizes another important limitation of the HRSD: it does not specify whether severity of symptoms should be based on their intensity at any one point during the past week (e.g., as observed during the interview) or on their duration and frequency over the past week, opening the possibility for different interpretations by different raters (Ciarlo et al. 1986).

The HRSD defines depressed mood differently than does the DSM-IV-TR. It describes it as sadness, hopelessness, helplessness, and worthlessness, whereas the DSM-IV defines depression as a subjective feeling of sadness or emptiness or tearfulness observed by others (American Psychiatric Association 2000a).

- Essential DSM-IV-TR features covered in the 24-item HRSD are depressed mood and diminished interest.
- Associated features covered in DSM-IV-TR and included in the 24-item HRSD are weight changes, sleep changes, psychomotor agitation or retardation, fatigue or loss of energy, worthlessness, guilt, suicidal ideation, and psychotic and melancholic features.
- Features in the 24-item HRSD not covered in DSM-IV-TR include anxiety, sexual interest, hypochondriasis, insight, depersonalization, obsessive and compulsive symptoms, helplessness, and hopelessness.
- DSM-IV-TR features not covered in the 24-item HRSD include concentration difficulties.
- Non-DSM-IV-TR features not covered in the 24-item HRSD include social withdrawal and atypical core features (included in the 28-item version of the HRSD).

Figure 10–1 illustrates the relative representation of items in the HRSD compared with DSM-IV-TR.

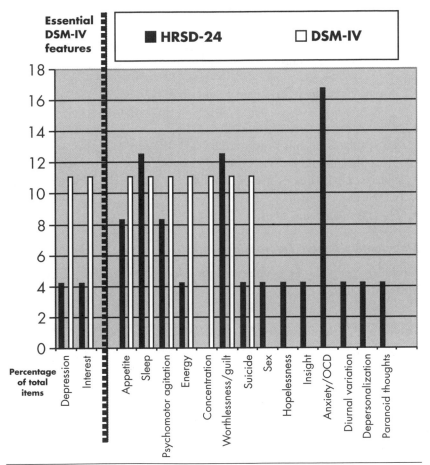

Figure 10–1. Relative representation of items in the 24-item Hamilton Rating Scale for Depression (HRSD-24) compared with DSM-IV. OCD=obsessive-compulsive disorder.

Weaknesses of the Ham-D are summarized below:

- There are discrepancies between the DSM-IV-TR definition of depression and the symptoms covered in the HRSD (as detailed above).
- The HRSD, unlike the BDI (see below), does not examine one feature per each rated item. For example, item 2 in the HRSD (feelings of guilt) includes assessment of both guilt and psychotic symptoms (e.g., "experiences threatening visual hallucinations").

- In items 1 (depressed mood), 22 (helplessness), 23 (hopelessness), and 24 (worthlessness), a great emphasis is given to the spontaneous expression of symptoms (based on the assumption that spontaneity implies greater severity). That assumption has little support in the literature or in clinical experience.
- Some items on the HRSD reflect symptoms that might not be related to depression (e.g., fatigue, hypochondriasis, insight).

Strengths of the Ham-D are summarized below:

- It has high interrater reliability.
- It is standardized and widely used.
- It is applicable and has been studied in a wide variety of subjects (control subjects, inpatients, outpatients, medically ill, elderly, adolescent, various cultural groups).
- There is no cost for its use.

Montgomery-Asberg Depression Scale

Table 10–2 provides an overview of the Montgomery-Asberg Depression Scale (MADRS).

Table 10–2.	Montgomery-Asberg Depression Scale
Author and reference	Stuart Montgomery, M.D., and Marie Asberg, M.D., Ph.D. (Montgomery and Asberg 1979)
Mode of administration	Clinician administered
Total number of items	10
Scoring	Scale from 0 to 6 anchored at 2-point intervals (0, 2, 4, 6); total score range, 0–60
Cutoff score	18 (for moderate to severe depression) (Mittmann et al. 1997)
Time to administer	15 minutes
Period covered	Not specified
Training requirements	Minimal and can be used by non–mental health professionals (Montgomery and Asberg 1979)
Copyright	Stuart Montgomery, *British Journal of Psychiatry*
Languages	English, Spanish, French

The MADRS was originally designed to be particularly sensitive to treatment effects. Unlike the HRSD, the MADRS does not rely heavily on the presence of physical symptoms. Thus the MADRS is considered specific for the assessment of depression. Of 17 most commonly occurring symptoms in primary depressive illness, the 10 that demonstrated the largest changes from antidepressant treatment were selected to create this scale (Montgomery and Asberg 1979).

Psychometric properties of the MADRS are summarized below:

- *Reliability:* Interrater reliability is 0.97 between psychiatrists and general practitioners (Montgomery and Asberg 1979).
- *Validity:* Scores on the scale correlated significantly with scores on the HRSD, indicating its validity in assessing general severity (Montgomery and Asberg 1979).
- *Sensitivity to change:* The capacity of the MADRS to differentiate between those who did and did not respond to antidepressant treatment was better than that of the HRSD, indicating greater sensitivity to change (Davidson et al. 1986).

Weaknesses of the MADRS are summarized below:

- The MADRS does not adequately match current definitions of depression. For example, the item on inner tension measures a symptom of anxiety rather than depression.
- The time frame for assessment was not defined by the authors, which leaves open the possibility for inconsistencies in documentation.

Strengths of the MADRS are summarized below:

- It can be used by a variety of clinicians, including nurses and general practitioners, with high interrater reliability.
- It is standardized and widely used.
- It is applicable and has been studied in a wide variety of subjects (control subjects, inpatients, outpatients, the medically ill, the elderly, adolescents, and various cultural groups)

Raskin Scale (the Three Area Severity of Depression Scale)

Table 10–3 provides an overview of the Raskin Scale (the Three Area Severity of Depression Scale).

Very little data are available on the psychometric properties of the Raskin Scale. Known psychometric properties are summarized below:

- *Reliability:* The author reported intraclass reliability of 0.88 (Raskin 1988).
- *Validity:* The scale demonstrates high face validity, but psychometric data are limited (Ciarlo et al. 1986).

Table 10–3.   Raskin Scale

Author and reference	Allen Raskin, Ph.D. (Raskin 1988)
Mode of administration	Clinician administered
Total number of items	3
Scoring	5-point Likert scale (1–5) ranging from "not at all" to "very much"; total score range, 3–15
Cutoff score	9, in the original publication; 7, in subsequent studies
Target group	Originally designed as a screening tool for depressed outpatients participating in medication studies
Time to administer	5 minutes
Period covered	Not specified
Training requirements	Not specified
Cost	None (in public domain)
Other versions	Raskin-Covi version for assessment of both depression and anxiety

Weaknesses of the Raskin Scale are summarized below:

- More psychometric data are needed to support the general use of the Raskin Scale.
- The scale does not fully cover DSM-IV-TR criteria for depression.
- Changes in specific depression symptoms cannot be detected.

Strengths of the Raskin Scale are summarized below:

- It is quick to administer.
- There is no cost for its use (public domain).

Patient-Administered Measures of Depression

Beck Depression Inventory II

Table 10–4 provides an overview of the Beck Depression Inventory II (BDI-II)

Psychometric properties of the BDI-II are summarized below:

- *Reliability:* Internal consistency was 0.93 in college students and 0.92 in outpatients (Beck et al. 1996a). Ahava et al. (1998) studied test-retest reliability of the original BDI in a nonclinical sample of college students. Results show a 40% decline in weekly BDI scores over a period of 8 weeks, in the absence of any intervention. Similar findings have also been reported by Sharpe and Gilbert (1998). Richter et al. (1997) showed that the BDI is very sensitive to change in inpatients and should be administered at time intervals of several weeks.

Table 10–4. Beck Depression Inventory II

Author and reference	Aaron Beck, M.D. (Beck et al. 1996b)
Mode of administration	Self-report
Total number of items	21 items with 4 answer options
Scoring	Equally scored 0–3; total score range, 0–63
Cutoff score	For the BDI-II: Not-depressed, 0–12; dysphoric, 13–19; dysphoric-depressed, 20+ (Dozois et al. 1998)
	For the original BDI the following cutoff scores for depression were recommended: primary care, 16 (Zich et al. 1990); college students, 20 (Pace and Trapp 1995); geriatric population, 22 (Kogan et al. 1994)
Target group	Depressed adults, adolescents, elderly persons, inpatients, outpatients, primary care patients, patients with medical conditions
Time to administer	15–20 minutes
Period covered	BDI: "right now"; BDI-IA: past 1 week+today; BDI-II: past 2 weeks+today
Cost	$1.20 per copy (copyright, Psychological Corporation 2000)
Languages	English, Spanish, Chinese, Arabic, French, German, 11 other languages
Versions	BDI (Beck et al. 1961); BDI 13-item short form (Beck et al. 1974); BDI-IA (Beck and Steer 1993); BDI-II (Beck et al. 1996a); BDI-PC (primary care) (Beck et al. 1997); automated (scannable) version also available

- *Validity:* The construct validity of the BDI-II showed correlation of 0.76 with the depression subscale of the Symptom Checklist 90–Revised and 0.60 with the depression subscale of the Minnesota Multiphasic Personality Inventory. Like many self-rated scales, the BDI is vulnerable to feigning symptoms. Lees-Haley (1989) found that 96% of untrained subjects were able to fake depression, and 58% were able to fake extremely severe depression. Similar findings were reported by Scafidi et al. (1999). Rudd and Rajab (1995) suggested that the specificity of the BDI might be affected by comorbid conditions, resulting in higher or lower scores.
- *Sensitivity* of the original BDI was 100%, and specificity was 89% at a cutoff score of 16 (Zich et al. 1990).

The BDI-II is an easily administered instrument that has been standardized and studied in a wide variety of subjects (control subjects, inpatients, outpatients, the medically ill, and those in different age, gender, and cultural groups). It is the most commonly used self-reporting scale for depression. An issue that faces patients taking the BDI-II is their difficulty in assessing their mood over a period of time in which symptoms may have been quite variable in severity. In addition, some patients need assistance in taking self-administered tests. Griffin and Kogut (1988) found that reading the test (versus giving the patient the form to complete) to low-functioning patients may yield scores that are better correlated with DSM criteria for depression. The scale cannot be used with uncooperative patients or those who cannot understand the questions. It is also subject to patients' denial, minimization, and exaggeration or faking of symptoms. Dahlstrom et al. (1990) studied the effect of randomizing the response items, because it was noted that subjects who are aware that a score of 3 on each item corresponds to "most severe" tend to minimize their symptoms. The random-order administration of the original version of the BDI resulted in a significantly higher depression score. A number of these criticisms were addressed in the BDI-II version. For example, the original BDI covered only insomnia and decreased appetite. Sleep and appetite-disturbance spectrum are now covered in the BDI-II (insomnia–hypersomnia and decreased–increased appetite). Dozois et al. (1998) concluded that the BDI-II is a stronger instrument than the BDI in terms of its factor structure.

The relative weight of items in the BDI-II that assess worthlessness, hopelessness, and guilt (7 of 21 items) surpasses that of items assessing the essential DSM-IV-TR features of depressed mood and anhedonia (3 of 21 items) (American Psychiatric Association 2000a).

- Essential DSM-IV-TR features covered in the BDI-II are sadness and loss of interest or pleasure.
- Associated features covered in DSM-IV-TR and included in the BDI-II are worthlessness and guilt, appetite (weight is not covered), sleep, psychomotor agitation (but not retardation), fatigue or loss of energy, concentration and indecisiveness, and suicide.
- BDI-II features not covered in the DSM-IV-TR include crying, hopelessness, and sexual symptoms.
- DSM-IV-TR features not covered in the BDI-II include psychotic, melancholic, and atypical features (mood reactivity is a supplemental question in the BDI-II that is not included in the total score).

Figure 10–2 illustrates the relative representation of items in the BDI-II compared with DSM-IV-TR.

Relationship of rated features to the disorder. Many questions in the BDI-II require the subject to report symptoms that might not necessarily be related to depression. Item 3 ("as I look back I see a lot of failures") may be

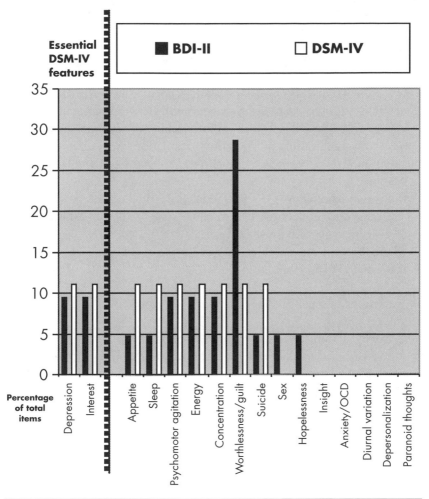

Figure 10–2. Relative representation of items in the Beck Depression Inventory II (BDI-II) compared with DSM-IV. OCD=obsessive-compulsive disorder.

related to realistic life circumstances. Item 20 ("I am too tired or fatigued to do most of the things I used to do") could be related to medical illness or its treatment (e.g., cancer or chemotherapy) (Schneider 1998).

In 16 of the 21 items, the BDI-II compares current symptoms to baseline by using statements such as "more or less than usual," "than ever," or "used to be." Comparison to baseline is problematic in chronic illness or in disorders dating since early childhood, such as chronic depression and dysthymia.

Language and phrasing. The following provide examples of item vagueness. Item 10 (crying): "I feel like crying but I can't" is to be scored as the most severe degree of crying. There is no evidence to support such an evaluation. Item 9 (suicide) does not ask specifically about suicidal plan or attempt.

Weaknesses of the BDI-II are summarized below:

- It has the general weaknesses of a self-reporting measure, such as vulnerability to minimization or exaggeration of symptoms, subjectivity, interference of the illness with subjects' ability to accurately rate themselves (disorganization, psychomotor retardation, memory impairment, attention and concentration difficulties, lack of insight, and lack of motivation)
- It diverges from DSM-IV-TR criteria, as detailed earlier.
- The scale does not consistently measure severity of symptoms in terms of their intensity or frequency.
- There is significant variability in test-retest studies.
- It is expensive ($1.20 per copy).

Strengths of the BDI-II are summarized below:

- It is easily administered and requires minimal instructions.
- It is widely used and has been standardized in diverse clinical and demographic populations.
- It has the advantage of limiting the questions to asking about one feature per each item, for example, item 1 covers the severity of sadness only. Many other scales do not follow this basic rule (see HRSD review).

Zung Self-Rating Depression Scale

Table 10–5 provides an overview of the Zung Self-Rating Depression Scale (SRDS).

The SRDS measures three factors: cognitive, affective, and somatic symptoms (Sakamoto et al. 1998).

Psychometric properties of the SRDS are summarized below:

- *Reliability and validity* have been established across cultures and age groups (Jegede 1976). Biggs et al. (1978) demonstrated adequate validity of the SRDS in depressed patients. Schotte et al. (1996) raised a question regarding the construct validity of the SRDS due to the presence of negatively keyed items (e.g., with items such as "I feel hopeful about the future," the more positive the response, the lower the score).
- *Sensitivity* was found to be 97% and specificity 63% at the cutoff score of 50 (Zung et al. 1990).

Table 10–5. Zung Self-Rating Depression Scale

Author and reference	William W.K. Zung, M.D. (Zung 1965).
Mode of administration	Self-report
Total number of items	20 items with 4 answer options
Scoring	Equally scored 1–4; the score represents the frequency of symptoms ranging from little to most of the time; total score range, 20–80
Cutoff score	50 (Zung et al. 1990)
Target group	Depressed adults, adolescents, elderly persons, inpatients, outpatients, primary care patients, patients with medical conditions
Time to administer	15–20 minutes
Period covered	"Past several days"
Cost	Free (public domain)
Languages	English, Spanish, French, German, Italian, Finnish, Dutch, Chinese, Polish

Weaknesses of the SRDS are summarized below:

- DSM-IV-TR features not covered in the SRDS include suicidal ideation and psychotic and atypical features.
- The SRDS covers features not included in the DSM-IV-TR, such as palpitation, constipation, crying, hopelessness, and sexual desire.
- The scale compares many current symptoms to baseline by using statements such as more or less "than usual," "I used to…," or "used to be." Comparison to baseline is problematic in chronic illness.

Strengths of the SRDS are summarized below:

- It is an easily administered instrument.
- It has short and clear statements.
- There is no cost to administer it (in the public domain).

Center for Epidemiologic Studies Depression Scale

Table 10–6 provides an overview of the Center for Epidemiologic Studies Depression Scale (CES-D).

A unique feature of the CES-D is that it uniformly rates all items using the frequency of symptom occurrence as a measure of severity as follows: 0=rarely or none of the time (less than 1 day); 1=some or little of the time (1–2 days); 2=occasionally or moderate amount of the time (3–4 days); 3=most or all of the time (5–7 days). There are four reverse items (4, 8, 12, and 16), which measure positive mood and are used to control for response bias.

Table 10–6. Center for Epidemiologic Studies Depression Scale

Author and reference	Lenore Radloff (Radloff 1977)
Mode of administration	Self-report
Total number of items	20
Scoring	All items are scored on a 0–3 scale; total score range, 0–60
Cutoff score	16 (Boyd et al. 1982)
Target group	Originally designed for assessment of depression in the general population
Time to administer	5–10 minutes
Period covered	Past week
Cost	No fees (public domain)
Languages	English, Spanish, Chinese, French, German, Italian, Dutch, Swedish, Japanese, and Cambodian
Other versions	10-item version (CESD-10) (Andresen et al. 1994)

Psychometric properties of the CES-D are summarized below (American Psychiatric Association 2000b):

- *Reliability:* Internal consistency ranged from 0.85 in the general population to 0.9 in a psychiatric population.
- *Validity:* Correlation with the HRSD ranged from 0.49 to 0.85. Correlation with the Zung SRDS was 0.69. Correlation with the Symptom Checklist–90 ranged from 0.73 to 0.89.
- *Sensitivity and specificity* measures varied widely across studies at a cutoff score of 16. Sensitivity ranged from 64% to 99%, and specificity from 59% to 94%.

Weaknesses of the CES-D are summarized below:

- The CES-D rates severity of depression by using only the frequency/duration of symptoms. The patient is not given choices that vary in intensity. Furthermore, quantifying the frequency by number of days does not account for the frequency or duration within a given day or days. As an extreme example, depression might occur for 1 hour a day for 5 days and receive the same score as overwhelming depression all day every day of the week.
- The scale does not cover some key DSM-IV-TR features of depression such as anhedonia, suicidal ideation, guilt, and psychomotor agitation or retardation. The CES-D does not cover most atypical symptoms of depression (e.g., increased appetite and sleep, rejection sensitivity).

Strengths of the CES-D are summarized below:

- It takes minimal time to complete.
- It is standardized and is widely used for screening
- It is applicable to and has been studied in a wide variety of subjects (e.g., control subjects, inpatients, outpatients, the medically ill, the elderly, adolescents, various cultural groups)
- There is no cost for its use.

Profile of Mood States

Table 10–7 provides an overview of the Profile of Mood States (POMS).

Table 10–7. Profile of Mood States

Author and reference	Douglas McNair, Maurice Lorr, and Leo Droppleman (McNair et al. 1971)
Mode of administration	Self-report
Total number of items	65
Scoring	All items scored on a 5-point scale ranging from "not at all" to "extremely"
Cutoff score	Not specified
Target group	Recommended for adult outpatient population with at least high school education; applicable in adolescent and geriatric populations; used in sports medicine
Time to administer	15 minutes
Period covered	Past week, but the scale also specifically measures mood on the day of administration and within the last 3 minutes
Cost	No fees for purchase or scoring
Languages	English, Spanish, French, German, Dutch, Swedish, Italian, Japanese, Polish
Other versions	Shortened version (37 items) by S. Shacham 1983

There are six mood factors built into the POMS: "tension-anxiety" (T), "depression-dejection" (D), "anger-hostility" (A), "vigor-activity" (V), "fatigue-inertia" (F), and "confusion-bewilderment" (C). A total mood disturbance score is calculated (Ciarlo et al. 1986). Raw scores are plotted as a profile. The POMS has been used to assess mood states in sports and exercise psychology.

Psychometric properties of the POMS are summarized below:

- *Reliability:* Internal consistency ranged from 0.84 to 0.95 in psychiatric outpatients (McNair et al. 1971).

- *Validity:* There are no data comparing the POMS to the BDI or the HRSD. However, correlations with the Hopkins Symptom Distress Scale ranged widely from 0.21 to 0.86 in psychiatric outpatients. The authors report that the six mood factors could be identified, measured reliably, and replicated in male Veterans Administration patients, college men, and outpatients. They also report significant reduction in POMS scores after psychotherapy and medication treatment (McNair et al. 1971).

Weaknesses of the POMS are summarized below:

- The POMS has not been studied adequately in psychiatric inpatients (although it has been studied in inpatients with alcohol dependence).
- Its internal consistency ranged widely (see previous).
- There are no validity or reliability data on the total mood disturbance score (even though they exist for the six mood factors).
- The "anger-hostility" and "tension-anxiety" symptoms are frequently associated with depressed mood; however, it is not clear whether their measurement increases the validity of a depression scale. In fact, these factors may reduce the validity of depression assessment because patients may receive significant rating in the absence of depressive symptoms.
- Rasmussen and Jeffrey (1995) warned that single assessment of mood states using the POMS may lead to inaccuracies and recommended multiple assessments over several days.

Strengths of the POMS are summarized below:

- There is no cost for its use.

Patient- and Clinician-Administered Measures of Depression

Inventory for Depressive Symptomatology

The Inventory for Depressive Symptomatology (IDS) includes a clinician-administered (IDS-C) and a patient self-reporting version (IDS-SR). Both versions have the same items (i.e., ask the same questions).

Table 10–8 provides an overview of the IDS.

Corruble et al. (1999) compared the IDS-C and the IDS-SR with the MADRS, Symptom Checklist–90-R regarding sensitivity to change. They concluded that the high sensitivity to change of the IDS-C might be an advantage for this scale compared with the MADRS.

Psychometric properties of the IDS are summarized below (Corruble et al. 1999; Rush et al. 1996):

Table 10–8. Inventory for Depressive Symptomatology

Author and reference	John Rush, M.D. (Rush et al. 1996)
Mode of administration	Clinician administered and self-report
Total number of items	30 for both clinician and patient versions
Scoring	All items scored on a 0–3 scale; only one of items 11–12 (increase or decrease in appetite) and 13–14 (increase or decrease in weight) is scored; total score range, 0–84
Cutoff score	Clinician version: 14–22, mild depression; 23–30, moderate; 31–38, moderate to severe; 39+, severe Patient version: 16–24, mild depression; 25–32, moderate; 33–40, moderate to severe; 41+, severe (Rush et al. 1996)
Target group	Inpatient and outpatient depressed
Time to administer	Clinician version: 30 minutes Patient version: 15–20 minutes
Period covered	Past week
Cost	No fees (copyright, John Rush)
Languages	English, Spanish, French, Japanese, Italian, Dutch, Rumanian, German
Other versions	Original version, 28 items (Rush et al. 1986); Quick IDS (Q-IDS) with 16 items (Rush et al. 2000)

- *Reliability:* Internal consistency of the clinician version is 0.77 and for the patient version is 0.81 for patients with major depression. With inpatients, most of the IDS-C and IDS-SR items were significantly correlated with the final score, and the Cronbach's α coefficients were high (0.75 for the IDS-C and 0.79 for the IDS-SR).
- *Validity:* Correlation with the HRSD was 0.95. Correlation with the BDI was 0.93. Correlation between the clinician and patient versions of the IDS was 0.91. In inpatients, concurrent validity of the IDS-C with the MADRS was high ($r=0.81$), as well as concurrent validity of the IDS-SR with the Symptom Checklist–90-R depression factor ($r=0.84$).
- *Sensitivity* was 0.997 for both the clinician and the patient versions.
- *Specificity* was 0.958 for the clinician version and 0.941 for the patient version.

Weaknesses of the IDS are summarized below:

- Four items are not included in DSM-IV-TR criteria and are nonspecific to depression (change in bowel habits, aches and pains, other bodily symptoms, panic and phobic symptoms).
- It has not been widely used and tested in clinical practice and research studies.

Strengths of the IDS are summarized below:

- It covers all DSM-IV-TR criteria for depression, including melancholic and atypical subtypes.
- It has excellent psychometric properties.
- It has been studied in large groups of symptomatic patients as well patients in remission.
- Clinician and patient versions are available with identical questions and scoring.
- A reliable, shortened, 9-item version (Q-IDS) is available.
- There is no cost for its use.

Depression Outcome Module

Table 10–9 provides an overview of the Depression Outcome Module (DOM).

The DOM was originally based on DSM-III-R criteria and later modified to match DSM-IV-TR criteria for depression. The DOM assesses both process and outcome of care.

Psychometric properties of the DOM are summarized below:

- *Reliability:* Test-retest reliability measured 1 week apart was 0.87.
- *Validity:* Internal consistency was 0.87. The DOM correlated with the HRSD (r=0.41), the depression symptoms on the SCID (r=0.60), and the depression symptoms on the Diagnostic Interview Schedule (DIS) (r=0.56). Changes in depressive symptoms correlated with change in bed days (r=0.56), change in social functioning (r=–0.52), and change in emotional functioning (r=–0.47). Intraclass correlation is 0.82–0.85 for depressive symptom severity (Rost et al. 1992).
- *Sensitivity* was found to be 100%, and specificity was 77.8% in a specialty care population.

Weaknesses of the DOM are summarized below:

- The DOM is lengthy to administer and complicated to score.
- Data are not available on the reliability and validity of the DOM in special clinical and demographic populations.

Strengths of the DOM are summarized below:

- It is based on DSM-IV-TR criteria.
- It assesses both process and outcome of care.
- Prognostic case-mix adjustments (taking into account demographic variabilities) are included.

Table 10–9.   Depression Outcome Module

Author and reference	Richard G. Smith, M.D. (Rost et al. 1992; Smith et al. 1995)
Mode of administration	Clinician administered and self-report
Total number of items and scoring	The scale is composed of 4 different forms:
	Patient baseline assessment: 80 items; combination of yes/no questions (1=yes, 2=no); duration questions ranging from "not at all" (1) to "nearly every day" (4); and demographic questions incorporated into scoring algorithms
	Clinician baseline assessment: 20 items, 1=yes, 2=no, 3=unsure
	Patient follow-up assessment: 83 items, scored as the baseline assessment
	Medical record review (by a trained clerical worker): 11 items for general information purposes, not scored
Target group	Adult outpatients and inpatients with depression
Time to administer	Patient baseline assessment: 25 minutes
	Clinician baseline assessment: 5 minutes
	Patient follow-up assessment: 25 minutes
	Medical record review: 10 minutes
Period covered	Patient baseline assessment: past 2 weeks
	Clinician baseline assessment: past 2 weeks
	Patient follow-up assessment: past 4 weeks to 4 months
	Medical record review: past 4 months
Cost	Unlimited free use for clinical purposes (copyright, Richard Smith)
Languages	English only
Other versions	A 3-item patient screener

- A scoring manual is available.
- There is no cost for clinical use.
- A computerized version is available.

Clinician-Administered Measures of Mania/Hypomania

Young Mania Rating Scale

Table 10–10 provides an overview of the Young Mania Rating Scale (YMRS).

Psychometric properties of the YMRS are summarized below (Young et al. 1978):

- *Reliability:* Interrater reliability was 0.93 (range, 0.66 for item 9 [disruptive aggressive behavior] to 0.95 for item 4 [sleep]). Correlations between individual items and total score ranged from 0.41 for item 10

Table 10–10.   Young Mania Rating Scale

Author and reference	Robert Young, M.D. (Young et al. 1978)
Mode of administration	Clinician administered
Total number of items	11
Scoring	7 items are scored 0–4; 4 items are scored 0–8; score range, 0–60; half points can be given by experienced raters
Cutoff	11 was the lowest score in patients who met Feighner's criteria for a manic episode; 20.5 was the highest score in patients who did not meet criteria for a manic episode
Target group	Adult, adolescent, and child populations (Fristad et al. 1995)
Time to administer	15–20 minutes
Period covered	Past 48 hours
Training requirements	Minimal training required
Cost	None (copyright, *British Journal of Psychiatry*)
Languages	English, Spanish

(appearance) to 0.85 for item 7 (language-thought disorder).

- *Validity:* The correlation of the YMRS with the Beigel-Murphy Scale (Sajatovic and Ramirez 2001) was 0.71, and 0.89 with the Petterson Rating Scale (Sajatovic and Ramirez 2001).
- *Sensitivity* was 96%, and specificity 100% at a cutoff point of 28 in a Spanish-speaking population (Apiquian et al. 1997).

The YMRS is the most commonly used rating scale for mania in research studies. It is easy to use and quick to administer and covers most manic symptoms. However, it has some limitations. The assessment period of the past 48 hours is problematic. Relevant symptoms may be eliminated from consideration by this time limit. The instruction to use all available respondents in rating might lead to variability among raters, and conflicting reports among patients, family members, and medical records might make rating more difficult. Scores may vary widely depending on the amount of information available about the patient's behavior outside the interview. The rating could be affected by the setting, especially in inpatient units where, for example, appearance (item 10) is regulated.

- Essential DSM-IV-TR features covered in the YMRS are elevated, expansive, and irritable mood (abnormally and persistently) (American Psychiatric Association 2000a).
- Associated features covered in DSM-IV-TR and included in the YMRS are inflated self-esteem or grandiosity, decreased need for sleep, talk-

ativeness, racing thoughts or flight of ideas, distractibility, increased goal-directed activity or psychomotor agitation, excessive involvement in pleasurable activities (limited to sexual acts in the YMRS), and psychotic features.

- YMRS features not covered in DSM-IV-TR include increased humor, inappropriate laughter, rhyming, echolalia, incoherence, disruptive and aggressive behavior, appearance and grooming, insight, and paranoid ideation.
- DSM-IV-TR features not covered in the YMRS include excessive involvement in pleasurable activities that have a high potential for painful consequences (unrestrained buying sprees, foolish business investments) and catatonic features.
- Non-DSM-IV-TR features not covered in the YMRS include depressed mood, suicidal ideation, anxiety, guilt, mood lability, intrusiveness, and congruency of psychotic features (Cassidy et al. 1998; Loudon et al. 1977; Tohen et al. 1992).

Figure 10–3 illustrates the relative representation of items in the YMRS compared with DSM-IV-TR.

Regarding relationship of the rated features to the disorder, appearance (item 10) and insight (item 11) are not specific to mania because they may be caused by a variety of other disorders. Similarly, in item 4 (sleep), the first two options are not specific to mania (reduction of sleep might be caused by depression, anxiety, etc.). Also, in item 9 (disruptive-aggressive behavior), sarcasm is given 2 points and being demanding is given 4 points; however, there is no evidence of the relationship of these behaviors to mania or their relative severity.

The YMRS does not limit the questions to asking about one feature for each rated item. Item 8 includes grandiosity (score of 6) and hallucinations (score of 8). The requirement to give the highest score may leave grandiosity unaccounted for in the presence of hallucinations.

The sleep item (item 4) requires rating sleep pattern according to the patient's assessment of "less than normal." Manic patients often have erratic sleep patterns as their baseline, and they may find it difficult to identify a "normal" duration of sleep.

Some items are repetitive and overlap, forcing the rater to add more points for the same behavior, for example, if the patient is "hostile, uncooperative" (item 5) and "threatens interviewer, shouting" (item 9), the patient will not only get 8 points but another 6.

Item 11 (insight) assesses two parameters simultaneously. One is admission of illness and the other is recognition of behavioral change. Denial of behavior change might not be necessarily be the most severe form of lack

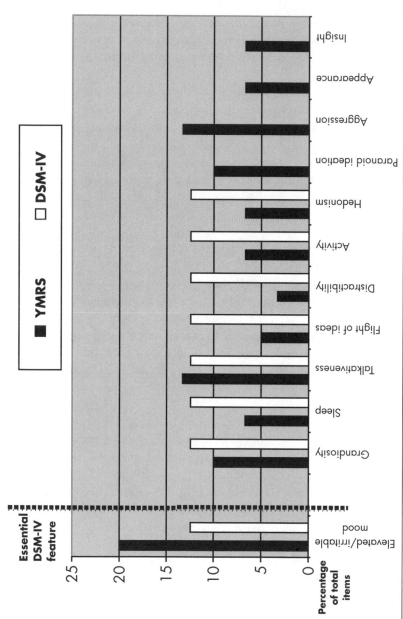

Figure 10–3.   Relative representation of items in the Young Mania Rating Scale (YMRS) compared with DSM-IV.

of insight. Some patients continue to deny behavior change but still recognize their illness and pursue treatment.

Weaknesses of the YMRS are summarized below:

- No items account for depressive symptoms. Considering the prevalence of mixed states and dysphoric mania, the absence of items for the rating of depression may lead to overlooking important aspects of the clinical presentation.
- There are discrepancies with DSM-IV-TR criteria for mania as detailed above.
- Intensity is the only basis for rating severity, discounting frequency of symptoms.

Strengths of the YMRS are summarized below:

- Reliability and validity have been demonstrated, although larger samples of raters and patients are needed.
- It is widely used in research studies.
- There is no cost for its use.

Clinician-Administered Rating Scale for Mania

The Clinician-Administered Rating Scale for Mania (CARS-M) is composed of two subscales: the mania subscale (items 1–10), and the psychosis subscale (items 11–15).

Table 10–11 provides an overview of the CARS-M.

Table 10–11. Clinician-Administered Rating Scale for Mania

Author and reference	Edward Altman, Psy.D., et al. (Altman et al. 1994)
Mode of administration	Clinician administered
Total number of items	15
Scoring	6-point Likert scale, rated from 0–5 (0=absent; 1=slight; 2=mild; 3=moderate; 4=severe; 5=extreme); total score range, 0–74
Cutoff score (applies to the Mania subscale only)	0–7 is questionable to mild mania; 8–15 is mild; 16–25 is moderate; 26 or greater is severe
Time to administer	15–30 minutes
Period covered	Past week
Training requirements	Required. Interrater reliability should be established in a sample of at least 7–10 patients; videotapes available
Copyright	Edward Altman (Altman et al. 1994)
Languages	English, Spanish

Psychometric properties of the CARS-M are summarized below (Altman et al. 1994):

- *Reliability:* Internal consistency was 0.88 for the mania subscale and 0.63 for the psychosis subscale. Interrater reliability was established across multiple raters viewing 14 videotaped interviews and comparing agreement among individual items and total scores. Principal-components analysis of items revealed two factors: mania and psychosis. Test-retest reliability was 0.77 for the mania subscale and 0.95 for the psychosis subscale.
- *Validity:* Correlation between the CARS-M and the YMRS is 0.94. Internal validity, comparing each item with its respective total factor score, revealed significant correlations for all items.

Weaknesses of the CARS-M are summarized below:

- The CARS-M focuses almost exclusively on measuring the intensity of symptoms and does not take into account their frequency.
- The scale covers items that are not included in the DSM-IV criteria (such as insight and orientation).
- Considering the prevalence of mixed states and dysphoric mania, the absence of items for the rating of depression may lead to overlooking important aspects of the clinical presentation.
- This is a new scale that yet has to demonstrate clinical utility. In particular, the relative weighting to be attached to the individual items needs further study (Poolsup et al. 1999).

Strengths of the CARS-M are summarized below:

- It covers all DSM-IV criteria.
- There are clear instructions on how to administer the scale, with recommended questions, standardized manual, and videotapes.

Patient-Administered Measures of Mania/Hypomania

Altman Self-Rating Mania Scale

Table 10–12 provides an overview of the Altman Self-Rating Mania Scale (ASRM).

Psychometric properties of the ASRM are summarized below (Altman et al. 1997):

Table 10–12. Altman Self-Rating Mania Scale

Author and reference	Edward Altman, Psy.D., et al. (Altman et al. 1997)
Mode of administration	Self-report
Total number of items	5 items with 5 answer options
Scoring	Items are rated 0–4 (0=not present; 4=present all the time or constantly); total score range, 0–20
Cutoff score	6 or above indicates the presence of manic symptoms
Target group	Originally tested in inpatients with mania
Time to administer	5 minutes
Period covered	Past week
Copyright	Biological Psychiatry

- *Reliability:* Test-retest reliability is 0.86.
- *Validity:* ASRM correlation with the YMRS total score was 0.72, and 0.77 with the CARS-M mania subscale.
- *Sensitivity and specificity:* At a cutoff score of 6 or more, sensitivity was 85.5% and specificity was 87.3%.

Weaknesses of the ASRM are summarized below:

- The ASRM is a newly introduced scale that requires further validation in indifferent settings and populations.
- Insight is not assessed (unlike the YMRS).
- It cannot be used for the assessment of mixed states.
- Distractibility and lack of insight in manic patients may interfere with accurate self-assessment. With extreme mania the scale cannot be used.
- It focuses exclusively on the frequency of symptoms, rather than intensity.

Strengths of the ASRM are summarized below:

- The ASRM contains most DSM-IV-TR criteria for mania (except distractibility, racing thoughts, and psychotic symptoms).
- The scale is brief and easy to complete, an important aspect for a scale that is to be completed by manic patients.

Clinician-Administered Measures of Both Depression and Mania/Hypomania

Schedule for Affective Disorders and Schizophrenia–Change Version

Table 10–13 provides an overview of the Schedule for Affective Disorders and Schizophrenia–Change Version (SADS-C).

Table 10–13. Schedule for Affective Disorders and Schizophrenia–
Change Version

Author and reference	Jean Endicott, Ph.D., and Robert L. Spitzer, M.D. (Endicott and Spitzer 1978)
Mode of administration	Clinician administered
Scoring	Scale from 0 to 6 (0=no information; 1=none at all; 6=most extreme)
Cutoff score	3 or greater on the individual items is considered clinically significant
Time to administer	20 minutes
Period covered	Past week
Training requirements	Requires extensive training; manual and videotapes available (from Dr. Endicott)
Cost	No cost
Languages	10 languages
Other versions	K-SADS for assessment of children

Psychometric properties of the SADS-C are summarized below:

- *Reliability:* The SADS-C was found to be a reliable instrument. Johnson et al. (1986) found it capable of differentiating between psychopathological groups such as nonparanoid and paranoid schizophrenic, bipolar manic, and unipolar depressed patients and subjects without such disorders.
- *Validity:* An extracted HRSD score based on depression items from the SADS-C was shown to have high correlation with the original HRSD (Endicott et al. 1981).

Weaknesses of the SADS-C are summarized below:

- The SADS-C is based on Research Diagnostic Criteria rather than DSM-IV-TR criteria.
- The training process is labor intensive.

Strengths of the SADS-C are summarized below:

- It is standardized and widely used.
- It applicable and has been studied in a wide variety of subjects (control subjects, inpatients, outpatients, the medically ill, the elderly, adolescents, and various cultural groups).
- There is no cost for its use.

Patient-Administered Measures of Both Depression and Mania/Hypomania

Internal State Scale

Table 10–14 provides an overview of the Internal State Scale (ISS).

Table 10–14. Internal State Scale

Author and reference	Mark Bauer, M.D. et al. (Bauer et al. 1991)
Mode of administration	Self-report
Total number of items	17
Scoring	Each visual analog is rated from 0 to 100 (0=not at all or rarely, 100=very much so or much of the time). Score is calculated using four subscales: activation (0–500), perceived conflict (0–500), well-being (0–300), and depression (0–200)
Cutoff	Cutoff for depression: score less than 125 on the well-being subscale
	Cutoff for hypomania/mania: score of 125 or higher on the well-being subscale and a score of 200 or more on the activation subscale
	Cutoff for remission: score of 125 or higher on the well-being subscale and a score of less than 200 on the activation subscale
Time to administer	10–15 minutes
Period covered	Past 24 hours
Cost	No fee (copyright, Mark Bauer)
Versions	ChronoBook, a booklet for recording a month's worth of sleep-wake, medication, and event logs and daily ratings of the ISS

The ISS is composed of visual analogs in which each statement (e.g., "Today I feel restless") is accompanied by a horizontal line and the patient is asked to rate the severity of symptom by making a mark on the line.

Psychometric properties of the ISS are summarized below (Bauer et al. 1991):

- *Reliability:* Internal consistency was 0.84 for the activation subscale, 0.81 for the perceived conflict subscale, 0.87 for the well-being subscale, and 0.92 for the depression subscale.
- *Validity:* The activation subscale was the only subscale that correlated with the YMRS (0.6). The correlation of the depression subscale with the HRSD was 0.84. Discriminant-function analysis showed that the subscales assigned 88% of subjects to the correct diagnostic groups.

Weaknesses of the ISS are summarized below:

- The ISS does not cover all DSM-IV-TR criteria for mania (omitting pressured speech, sleep changes, and distractibility) and does not cover most of the criteria for depression (covers only depressed mood and lack of energy).
- Validity and reliability data for depression ratings are better than those for mania ratings.

Strengths of the ISS are summarized below:

- It is easy to administer.
- It is sensitive to daily changes in mood state.
- Availability of the ChronoBook allows for documentation of mood changes over periods greater than 24 hours.
- There is no fee for its use.

Graphic Measures of Mood Disorders

Visual Analog Scales

There are various forms of visual analog scales. In its simplest form, a visual analog scale (VAS) consists of a horizontal line 100 mm long anchored at each end with a quantitative statement (Figure 10–4).

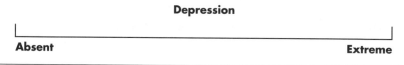

Figure 10–4.   Example of a visual analog scale for depression.

Psychometric properties of visual analog scales are summarized below:
Ahearn (1997) reviewed studies of various visual analog scales and reported the following findings:

- *Reliability:* Test-retest reliability ranged from 0.3 to 0.89.
- *Validity:* The Visual Analogue Mood Scale (VAMS) correlated highly with the Zung SRDS (Folstein and Luria 1973). In studies of different mood analog scales, correlation with the HRSD ranged between 0.14 and 0.84 (for the ISS). Correlation with the BDI ranged from 0.3 to 0.76. Correlation with the Zung SRDS ranged from 0.37 to 0.63.

Weaknesses of VASs are summarized below:

- VASs are not standardized. Many versions, often locally developed, are available.
- VASs are subject to symptom exaggeration and minimization.
- The extremes of mood states are subjective and may change during the course of an individual mood episode and may vary across patients.

Strengths of VASs are summarized below:

- Subjective mood experience is not always easy to articulate into words, which makes VASs a powerful alternative to verbal questionnaires (Zealley and Aitken 1969).
- They are simple to complete.
- They have a high rate of compliance.
- There is no fee for their use.

National Institute of Mental Health
Prospective Life-Chart Methodology

The National Institute of Mental Health Prospective Life-Chart Methodology (NIMH LCM-p) is a scale that uses graphic representation of daily ratings of mood symptoms and functioning (Denicoff et al. 1997). It is a modification of Kraepelin's (1921) Life Course Rating of depressive and manic episodes. Patients are given a computer-scannable form each month to take home to perform daily self-ratings. Both mania and depression are rated by the length of a vertical bar above and below the time line. In cycling bipolar patients, a monthly HRSD missed six of eight moderately severe depressions over a 1-year period compared with the NIMH LCM-p.

Psychometric properties of the NIMH LCM-p are summarized below (Denicoff et al. 1997):

- *Reliability:* The interrater reliability was between 0.61 and 0.8.
- *Validity:* On average severity for depression, the correlation of the LCM-p with the HRSD was 0.86, and with the BDI was 0.73. On average severity for mania, the correlation between the LCM-p and the YMRS was 0.61. The correlation of average severity between the LCM-p and the Global Assessment Scale (GAS) was −0.81.

Weaknesses of the NIMH LCM-p are summarized below:

- Manic patients are less reliable in completing the LCM-p than are depressed patients.

- Ratings of dysfunction due to depression show higher construct validity than those of mania (Meaden et al. 2000).
- The ratings provide only a general measure of severity.

Strengths of the NIMH LCM-p are summarized below:

- It provides continuous documentation of mood episodes between office visits, an advantage in rapid-cycling bipolar patients.
- It is easy to administer.
- It is sensitive to daily and seasonal changes in mood state.
- It has psychoeducational value for patients and their families.
- There is no fee for its use.

CONCLUSION

This review highlights the extraordinary developments that have taken place in assessment measures for mood disorders in the past few decades. Many tools have good psychometric properties, are in widespread use, and reflect changes in the definitions of mood disorders. However, the plethora of mood scales and the lack of standardization in the field are obstacles to the routine use of these scales in clinical and research settings. Professional organizations may be the most appropriately positioned to undertake the task of standardizing the use of scales for mood disorders. An ideal scale would assess both manic and depression symptoms, would include assessment of both intensity and frequency of symptoms, would integrate both clinician and patient self-report ratings, and would be in accordance with current definitions of mood disorders.

REFERENCES

Ahava GW, Iannone C, Grebstein L, et al: Is the Beck Depression Inventory reliable over time? An evaluation of multiple test-retest reliability in a nonclinical college student sample. J Pers Assess 70:222–231, 1998

Ahearn EP: The use of visual analog scales in mood disorders: a critical review. J Psychiatr Res 31:569–579, 1997

Altman EG, Hedeker DR, Janicak PG, et al: The Clinician-Administered Rating Scale for Mania (CARS-M): development, reliability, and validity. Biol Psychiatry 36:124–134, 1994

Altman EG, Hedeker D, Peterson JL, et al: The Altman Self-Rating Mania Scale. Biol Psychiatry 42:948–955, 1997

American Psychiatric Association: Diagnostic and Statistical Manual of Mental Disorders, 4th Edition, Text Revision. Washington, DC, American Psychiatric Association, 2000a

American Psychiatric Association: Handbook of Psychiatric Measures. Washington, DC, American Psychiatric Press, 2000b

Andresen EM, Malmgren JA, Carter WB, et al: Screening for depression in well older adults: evaluation of a short form of the CES-D (Center for Epidemiologic Studies Depression Scale). Am J Prev Med 10:77–84, 1994

Apiquian R, Paez F, Tapia R, et al: Validez y confiabilidad de la Escala para la Evaluacion de la Mania. Salud Mental 20:23–29, 1997

Bauer MS, Crits-Christoph P, Ball WA, et al: Independent assessment of manic and depressive symptoms by self-rating. Scale characteristics and implications for the study of mania [see comments]. Arch Gen Psychiatry 48:807–812, 1991

Bech P: The Hamilton disorders. Psychother Psychosom 60:113–115, 1993

Beck AT, Steer RA: Manual for the Beck Depression Inventory. San Antonio, TX, Psychological Corporation, 1993

Beck AT, Ward CH, Mendelson M, et al: An inventory for measuring depression. Arch Gen Psychiatry 4:561–571, 1961

Beck AT, Rial WY, Rickels K: Short form of Depression Inventory: cross-validation. Psychol Rep 34:1184–1186, 1974

Beck AT, Steer RA, Ball R, et al: Comparison of Beck Depression Inventories-IA and -II in psychiatric outpatients. J Pers Assess 67:588–597, 1996a

Beck AT, Steer RA, Brown GK: BDI-II, Beck Depression Inventory Manual, 2nd Edition. San Antonio, TX, Psychological Corporation, 1996b

Beck AT, Steer RA, Ball R, et al: Use of the Beck Anxiety and Depression Inventories for primary care with medical outpatients. Assessment 4:211–219, 1997

Biggs JT, Wylie LT, Ziegler VE: Validity of the Zung Self-Rating Depression Scale. Br J Psychiatry 132:381–135, 1978

Boyd JH, Weissman MM, Thompson WD, et al: Screening for depression in a community sample. Understanding the discrepancies between depression symptom and diagnostic sales. Arch Gen Psychiatry 39:1195–1200, 1982

Cassidy F, Forest K, Murry E, et al: A factor analysis of the signs and symptoms of mania. Arch Gen Psychiatry 55:27–32, 1998

Ciarlo JA, Brown TR, Edwards DW, et al: Assessing Mental Health Treatment Outcome Measurement Techniques. Washington, DC, U.S. Government Printing Office, 1986

Clark DB, Donovan JE: Reliability and validity of the Hamilton Anxiety Rating Scale in an adolescent sample. J Am Acad Child Adolesc Psychiatry 33:354–360, 1994

Corruble E, Legrand JM, Duret C, et al: IDS-C and IDS-SR: psychometric properties in depressed in-patients. J Affect Disord 56:95–101, 1999

Dahlstrom WG, Brooks JD, Peterson CD: The Beck Depression Inventory: item order and the impact of response sets. J Pers Assess 55:224–233, 1990

Davidson J, Turnbull CD, Strickland R, et al: The Montgomery-Asberg Depression Scale: reliability and validity. Acta Psychiatr Scand 73:544–548, 1986

Denicoff KD, Smith-Jackson EE, Disney ER, et al: Preliminary evidence of the reliability and validity of the prospective life-chart methodology (LCM-p). J Psychiatr Res 31:593–603, 1997

Dozois DJA, Dobson KS, Ahnberg JL: A psychometric evaluation of the Beck Depression Inventory-II. Psychol Assess 10:83–89, 1998

Endicott J, Spitzer RL: A diagnostic interview: the schedule for affective disorders and schizophrenia. Arch Gen Psychiatry 35:837–844, 1978

Endicott J, Cohen J, Nee J, et al: Hamilton Depression Rating Scale: extracted from regular and change versions of the schedule for affective disorders and schizophrenia. Arch Gen Psychiatry 38:98–103, 1981

Fleck MP, Poirier-Littre MF, Guelfi JD, et al: Factorial structure of the 17-item Hamilton Depression Rating Scale. Acta Psychiatr Scand 92:168–172, 1995

Folstein MF, Luria R: Reliability, validity, and clinical application of the Visual Analogue Mood Scale. Psychol Med 3:479–486, 1973

Fristad MA, Weller RA, Weller EB: The Mania Rating Scale (MRS): further reliability and validity studies with children. Ann Clin Psychiatry 7:127–132, 1995

Gibbons RD, Clark DC, Kupfer DJ: Exactly what does the Hamilton Depression Rating Scale measure? J Psychiatr Res 27:259–273, 1993

Griffin PT, Kogut D: Validity of orally administered Beck and Zung depression scales in a state hospital setting. J Clin Psychol 44:756–759, 1988

Grundy CT: Assessing clinical significance: Application to the Hamilton Rating Scale for Depression. Doctoral dissertation, Provo, UT, Brigham Young University, 1994 [Dissertation Abstracts International 55:592B, 1994]

Hamilton M: A rating scale for depression. J Neurol Neurosurg Psychiatry 23:56–62, 1960

Hooijer C, Zitman FG, Griez E, et al: The Hamilton Depression Rating Scale (HDRS): changes in scores as a function of training and version used. J Affect Disord 22:21–29, 1991

Jegede RO: Psychometric properties of the Self-Rating Depression Scale (SDS). J Psychol 93:27–30, 1976

Johnson MH, Magaro PA, Stern SL: Use of the SADS-C as a diagnostic and symptom severity measure. J Consult Clin Psychol 54:546–551, 1986

Kogan ES, Kabacoff RI, Hersen M, et al: Clinical cutoffs for the Beck Depression Inventory and the Geriatric Depression Scale with older adult psychiatric outpatients. Journal of Psychopathology and Behavioral Assessment 16:233–242, 1994

Kraepelin E: Manic-Depressive Insanity and Paranoia. Edinburgh, E & S Livingstone, 1921

Lambert MJ, Hatch DR, Kingston MD, et al: Zung, Beck, and Hamilton Rating Scales as measures of treatment outcome: a meta-analytic comparison. J Consult Clin Psychol 54:54–59, 1986

Lees-Haley PR: Malingering traumatic mental disorder on the Beck Depression Inventory: cancerphobia and toxic exposure. Psychol Rep 65:623–626, 1989

Linden M, Borchelt M, Barnow S, et al: The impact of somatic morbidity on the Hamilton Depression Rating Scale in the very old. Acta Psychiatr Scand 92:150–154, 1995

Loudon JB, Blackburn IM, Ashworth CM: A study of the symptomatology and course of manic illness using a new scale. Psychol Med 7:723–729, 1977

McNair DM, Lorr M, Droppleman LF: Profile of Mood States Manual. San Diego, CA, Educational and Industrial Testing Service, 1971

Meaden PM, Daniels RE, Zajecka J: Construct validity of life chart functioning scales for use in naturalistic studies of bipolar disorder. J Psychiatr Res 34:187–192, 2000

Mittmann N, Mitter S, Borden EK, et al: Montgomery-Asberg severity gradations [letter]. Am J Psychiatry 154:1320–1321, 1997

Montgomery SA, Asberg M: A new depression scale designed to be sensitive to change. Br J Psychiatry 134:382–389, 1979

Pace TM, Trapp M: A psychometric comparison of the Beck Depression Inventory and the Inventory for Diagnosing Depression in a college population. Assessment 2:167–172, 1995

Poolsup N, Li Wan Po A, Oyebode F: Measuring mania and critical appraisal of rating scales. J Clin Pharm Ther 24:433–443, 1999

Radloff LS: The CES-D Scale: a self report depression scale for research in the general population. Applied Psychological Measurement 1:385–401, 1977

Raskin A: Three-Area Severity of Depression Scale, in Dictionary of Behavioral Assessment Techniques. Edited by Hersen M, Bellack AS. New York, Pergamon, 1988, pp 336–345

Rasmussen PR, Jeffrey AC: Assessment of mood states: biases in single-administration assessments. Journal of Psychopathology and Behavioral Assessment 17:177–184, 1995

Rehm LP, O'Hara MW: Item characteristics of the Hamilton Rating Scale for Depression. J Psychiatr Res 19(1):31–41, 1985

Richter P, Werner J, Bastine R, et al: Measuring treatment outcome by the Beck Depression Inventory. Psychopathology 30:234–240, 1997

Rost K, Smith GR, Burnam MA, et al: Measuring the outcomes of care for mental health problems. The case of depressive disorders. Med Care 30 (5 suppl):MS266–MS273, 1992

Rudd MD, Rajab MH: Specificity of the Beck Depression Inventory and the confounding role of comorbid disorders in a clinical sample. Cognitive Therapy and Research 19:51–68, 1995

Rush AJ, Giles DE, Schlesser MA, et al: The Inventory for Depressive Symptomatology (IDS): preliminary findings. Psychiatry Res 18:65–87, 1986

Rush AJ, Gullion CM, Basco MR, et al: The Inventory of Depressive Symptomatology (IDS): psychometric properties. Psychol Med 26:477–486, 1996

Rush AJ, Carmody T, Reimitz P-E: The Inventory of Depressive Symptomatology (IDS): clinician (IDS-C) and self-report (IDS-SR) ratings of depressive symptoms. International Journal of Methods in Psychiatric Research 9:45–59, 2000

Sajatovic M, Ramirez LF: Rating Scales in Mental Health. Hudson, OH, Lexi-Comp, 2001, pp 109–110

Sakamoto S, Kijima N, Tomoda A, et al: Factor structures of the Zung Self-Rating Depression Scale (SDS) for undergraduates. J Clin Psychol 54:477–487, 1998

Samuels SC, Katz IR, Parmelee PA, et al: Use of the Hamilton and Montgomery-Asberg Depression Scales in institutionalized elderly patients. Am J Geriatr Psychiatry 4:237–246, 1996

Scafidi FA, Field T, Prodromidis M, et al: Association of fake-good MMPI-2 profiles with low Beck Depression Inventory scores. Adolescence 34:61–68, 1999

Schneider RA: Concurrent validity of the Beck Depression Inventory and the Multidimensional Fatigue Inventory-20 in assessing fatigue among cancer patients. Psychol Rep 82:883–886, 1998

Schotte CK, Maes M, Cluydts R, et al: Effects of affective-semantic mode of item presentation in balanced self-report scales: biased construct validity of the Zung Self-Rating Depression Scale. Psychol Med 26:1161–1168, 1996

Shacham S: A shortened version of the Profile of Mood States. J Pers Assess 47:305–306, 1983

Sharpe JP, Gilbert DG: Effects of repeated administration of the Beck Depression Inventory and other measures of negative mood states. Personality and Individual Differences 24:457–463, 1998

Smith GR, Burnam MA, Burns BJ: The Depression Outcomes Module. Little Rock, AR, University of Arkansas for Medical Sciences, 1995

Snaith RP: Present use of the Hamilton Depression Rating Scale: observations on method of assessment in research of depressive disorders. Br J Psychiatry 168(5):594–597, 1996

Tohen M, Tsuang MT, Goodwin DC: Prediction of outcome in mania by mood-congruent or mood-incongruent psychotic features. Am J Psychiatry 149:1580–1584, 1992

Young RC, Biggs JT, Ziegler VE, et al: A rating scale for mania: reliability, validity and sensitivity. Br J Psychiatry 133:429–435, 1978

Zealley AK, Aitken RC: Measurement of mood. Proceedings of the Royal Society of Medicine 62:993–996, 1969

Zich JM, Attkisson CC, Greenfield TK: Screening for depression in primary care clinics: the CES-D and the BDI. Int J Psychiatry Med 20:259–277, 1990

Zung WW: A self-rating depression scale. Arch Gen Psychiatry 12:63–70, 1965

Zung WW, Magruder-Habib K, Velez R, et al: The comorbidity of anxiety and depression in general medical patients: a longitudinal study. J Clin Psychiatry 51 (suppl):77–80; discussion 81, 1990

CHAPTER 11

Outcome Measurement in Anxiety Disorders

Eric D. Peselow, M.D.

During the past 20 years much has been learned about anxiety disorders. The concept of diagnosis has shifted from a psychodynamic formulation to a group of disorders with reliable and recognizable criteria. The DSM-IV-TR criteria (American Psychiatric Association 2000a) identify 12 disorders: panic disorder without agoraphobia, panic disorder with agoraphobia, agoraphobia, social and specific phobia, obsessive-compulsive disorder (OCD), posttraumatic stress disorder (PTSD), generalized anxiety disorder (GAD), anxiety disorder due to a general medical condition, substance-induced anxiety disorder, acute stress disorder, and anxiety disorder not otherwise specified (NOS). The appendix of DSM-IV-TR also contains criteria for a research set designated as mixed anxiety-depressive disorder.

Many of the older anxiety scales were developed before the publication of DSM-IV. In addition, there is a high degree of comorbidity among the various anxiety disorders (Kessler et al. 1994) along with a high degree of comorbidity between various anxiety states and depression. Indeed, three of the nine DSM-IV criteria for depression (fatigue, poor concentration, and sleep difficulty) are also among the six criteria for GAD. Because there are 12 different anxiety disorders, and because panic, phobias, fears and obsessions, and compulsive behavior are sufficiently different from GAD, independent rating scales for each disorder are warranted. This chapter presents a review of the utility of the various scales for outcome measurement in many anxiety disorders.

GENERALIZED ANXIETY DISORDER

The scales described below are the ones most commonly used to assess generalized anxiety. van Riezen and Segal (1988) described more than 30 scales that have been used in the assessment of anxiety disorders. The problem with these other scales is that there is much overlap among patients with different anxiety disorders (e.g., GAD, social phobia, OCD), and none of these scales is specific to generalized anxiety disorder.

Hamilton Anxiety Scale

The Hamilton Anxiety Scale (HAS) (Hamilton 1959) is the oldest and most frequently used anxiety scale. It is a 14-item scale broken down into seven psychic components (anxious mood, tension, fear, insomnia, concentration, fears, and nervous behavior) and seven somatic components (muscular, sensory, cardiovascular, respiratory, gastrointestinal, genitourinary, and autonomic). The items are rated on a scale of 1–4. Usually scores of 18–20, with scores of at least 2 for both anxious mood and tension, are considered severe enough for inclusion into drug studies. The main flaw of this scale (as with most scales for anxiety disorders) is that it is almost entirely dependent on the subjective responses of the patient as opposed to observed behavior or signs. The HAS is intended primarily for patients with GAD; however, its utility in other disorders remains to be established. In fact, because of the overlap with depression, patients with primary depressive illness may have very high scores on this scale. Weekly ratings are useful, and decreases in scores correlate with improvement in the symptoms of GAD. The scale has high 1-week test-retest reliability ($r=0.96$). There are high correlations with the Covi (r range, 0.63–0.75) and the Beck ($P=0.56$) anxiety inventories.

Beck Anxiety Inventory

Similar to the Beck self-reporting scale for depression, the Beck Anxiety Inventory (BAI) (Beck et al. 1988) is a 21-item self-report measure, with items rated on a scale of 0–3, that assesses the severity of generalized anxiety symptoms. Symptoms are rated on their presence or absence and intensity over the past week. The test has been shown to have reasonably good test-retest reliability and is a good measure of change. The internal consistency of the BAI ranged from 0.90 to 0.94. Test-retest reliability after 1 week ranged from 0.67 to 0.93, and there is a high correlation of this scale with the anxiety subscale of the Symptom Checklist-90 ($r=0.81$).

Covi Anxiety Scale

The Covi Anxiety Scale (CAS) (Covi et al. 1981) is a three-item scale, with each item scored on a scale of 1–5 (not at all, somewhat, moderately, considerably, and very much), hence the scale has a 5- to 15-point range. The three items are the patient's verbal report (feeling shaky, jittery, jumpy), observed behavior consistent with anxiety during the interview (e.g., appearing frightened, shaky, restless), and somatic complaints (e.g., sweating, trembling, heart pounding). The CAS is often used in conjunction with the three-item Raskin depression scale (Raskin et al. 1969) (for more details see Chapter 10, in this volume). It is scored along similar lines, and it is used in pharmacologic trials not only as a change measure but also to assess whether anxiety predominates over depression (and vice versa) in individuals who have comorbid symptoms (Dunbar et al. 1991).

Other Anxiety Scales

Zung Anxiety Status Inventory

The Zung Anxiety Status Inventory (ASI) (Zung 1974) is a clinician-rated scale of 20 items that are rated on a 0–3 scale (none, mild, moderate, severe). The items rated are anxiousness, fear, panic, mental disintegration, apprehension, tremors, pains, fatigue and weakness, restlessness, palpitations, dizziness, faintness, dyspnea, paresthesias, nausea/vomiting, urinary frequency, sweating, face flushing, initial insomnia, and nightmares. In this measure, observed as well as elicited behaviors are scored. Intensity, frequency, and duration of the symptom over the specified period for the symptom are included in the scoring. If the symptom is present but causes no distress, it is rated as zero.

Zung Self-Rating Anxiety Scale

The Zung Self-Rating Anxiety Scale (SAS) (Zung 1969) is a patient-rated scale of 20 statements that are rated on a 0–3 scale (none or a little of the time, some of the time, a good part of the time, all of the time). It is parallel in design to the ASI, and its ratings are usually lower at the beginning and end of a specific treatment period.

SOCIAL PHOBIA

Liebowitz Social Anxiety Scale

The Liebowitz Social Anxiety Scale (LSAS) (Liebowitz 1987) was the first clinician-administered scale to evaluate the many social situations that patients with social phobia have difficulty encountering; it is probably the most widely used scale for social phobia. It consists of 24 items: 13 for performance situations (e.g., telephoning in public, participating in small groups, eating in public) and 11 for social interaction (e.g., meeting strangers, being the center of attention). Each item is rated twice: on a scale of 0–3 for fear (none, mild, moderate, severe), and on a scale of 0–3 for avoidant behavior (0=never, 0% of the time; 1=occasionally, 10% of the time; 2=often, 33%–67% of the time; 3=usually, 67%–100% of the time). The total score ranges from 0 to 144 points, with scores for four separate subscales: performance fear, performance avoidance, social fear, and social avoidance. Although it is clinician rated (and not intended for self-reporting), the LSAS is worded in a manner similar to that of a self-rated instrument, which has led to its use in pharmacologic research (Greist et al. 1995). The LSAS has been successfully used to monitor improvement in many studies of pharmacologic and cognitive-behavioral treatment. A total score of 70 or greater indicates significant pathology. Reliability, based on a sample of 312 patients enrolled in clinical trials, ranged from 0.82 to 0.92. The scale has high correlations with the Brief Social Phobia Scale ($r=0.87$) and the Social Phobia Scale ($r=0.76$).

Brief Social Phobia Scale

The Brief Social Phobia Scale (BSPS) (Davidson et al. 1991) is an 11-item observer-rated assessment of symptom severity. Its principal function is to measure changes due to treatment over time. The scale consists of 7 items measuring specific phobic situations (speaking in public or in front of others, talking to people in authority, talking to strangers, being embarrassed or humiliated, being criticized, attending social gatherings, and doing something while being watched). These items are scored twice on a scale of 0–4: once with respect to fear (none, mild, moderate, severe, extreme) and once with respect to avoidance (never, rarely, sometimes, frequently, always). In addition, the BSPS has 4 additional physiologic items usually experienced while in contact with or thinking about the phobic situation—including blushing, palpitations, trembling, and sweating—which are rated on a 0–4 scale (none, mild, moderate, severe, extreme). Thus both a total score and three subscale scores (fear, avoidance, and physiologic) are generated and can be assessed at various times.

Fear Questionnaire

The Fear Questionnaire (Marks and Mathews 1979) is a 23-item scale of various fears and a 24th item that relates to the overall global distress from these symptoms. The fears are rated on a 0–8 scale, with 0 noting no fear, 2 noting fear that is slightly troublesome, 4 noting definitely troublesome fear, 6 noting markedly troublesome fear, and 8 noting significantly troublesome fear. Within this 23-item framework is a 5-item social phobia subscale that is rated on the same parameters and that takes into account degrees of avoidance. Social phobic items included in this scale are eating and drinking with other people, being watched or stared at, talking to people in authority, being criticized, and speaking or acting to an audience. The discriminant validity of the Fear Questionnaire was highest for patients experiencing phobic anxiety. The subscales measuring agoraphobic and social phobias are reliable and valid measures and are believed to be better indicators of change than the total phobia score (Moylan and Oei 1992).

Social Phobia and Anxiety Inventory

The Social Phobia and Anxiety Inventory (SPAI) (Turner et al. 1989) includes 45 items with two subscales: 13 items are for social phobia, and 32 items are for agoraphobia. The total range of scores is 0–192, with a score above 60 being consistent with a diagnosis of social phobia. Test-retest reliability was high at 0.86. The SPAI was able to distinguish between individuals with social phobia, those with other anxiety disorders, and nonanxious control subjects. Despite the fact that it is a reasonably good measure of change, it is a very long instrument and is time consuming to administer. Its scoring is also very complex.

Social Phobia Scale and Social Interaction Anxiety Scale

The Social Phobia Scale (SPS) and the Social Interaction Anxiety Scale (SIAS) (Heimberg et al. 1992) are companion self-reporting scales of 20 items each rated on a scale of 0–4. The SPS items concern situations in which the patient is scrutinized by others (e.g., eating in a restaurant). The SIAS basically describes the individual's emotional and behavioral responses to the phobic situation. Validity and reliability data were stronger for the SIAS compare with the SPS.

Social Anxiety (Avoidance) and Distress Scale

The Social Anxiety (Avoidance) and Distress (SAD) Scale (D. Watson and Friend 1969) is a 28-item true-false scale that contains bidirectional statements (e.g., "I feel relaxed in unfamiliar social situations"; "I often find social occasions upsetting"). The SAD Scale can distinguish between social phobia and simple phobia or panic disorder but cannot distinguish between social phobia and panic disorder with agoraphobia or GAD (Oei et al. 1991).

Fear of Negative Evaluations Scale

The Fear of Negative Evaluations (FNE) Scale (D. Watson and Friend 1969) is a bidirectional, 30-item true-false scale that assesses a subject's expectation of being evaluated negatively by others (e.g., if someone is evaluating me, I tend to expect the worst). A shorter 12-item scale is also available (Leary 1983). The FNE Scale can discriminate patients with social phobia from those with simple phobia but not from those with panic disorder, panic disorder with agoraphobia, or GAD (Oei et al. 1991).

Social Phobic Disorders Severity and Change Form

The Social Phobic Disorders Severity and Change Form (SPDSC) (Liebowitz et al. 1986) evaluates five domains associated with having a social phobic disorder. These include anxiety episodes (rated on intensity and frequency), overall functional impairment, phobic avoidance, anticipatory anxiety, and overall severity of illness. Items are rated on a scale of 1–7 (normal, slight impairment, mild impairment, moderate impairment, marked impairment, severe impairment, extreme impairment). The SPDSC also allows for change scores on a scale of 1–7 (1–3 = marked, moderate, and mild improvement; 4 = no change; 5–7 = mild, moderate, and marked worsening). The SPDSC is a global scale that evaluates the consequences of having the disorder and is useful in clinical trials to measure change.

Liebowitz Disability Self Rating Scale

The Liebowitz Disability Self Rating Scale (Liebowitz et al. 1992) is an 11-item scale that assesses various quality-of-life issues with respect to having a social phobia. The baseline screen provides a 2-week and lifetime rating of 0–3 points (none, mild, moderate, severe). Items include use of alcohol and drugs and effect of symptoms on education, employment, family relations, romantic relations, social network, leisure interests, activities of daily living, and desire to live.

OBSESSIVE-COMPULSIVE DISORDER

Yale-Brown Obsessive Compulsive Scale and Symptom Checklist

Although it was originally developed as a research tool (Goodman et al. 1989), the Yale-Brown Obsessive Compulsive Scale (Y-BOCS) has excellent clinical utility. The clinician begins the interview by defining the terms *obsession* and *compulsions* for the interviewee. He or she then inquires about past or present history of 39 obsessive and 25 ritualistic traits. Examples of obsessive fears include aggression, contamination, sex, saving/hoarding, and symmetry. Examples of rituals include cleaning/washing, repeating, and checking behaviors.

The Y-BOCS contains 10 items rated on a scale of 0–4. Five involve obsessions, with 3 of these items assessing time spent on obsessions, interference from obsessions, and distress with obsessions. These items are rated 0–4 (none, mild, moderate, severe, extreme). Resistance to the obsessions is rated from 0 (patient strongly resists) to 4 (patient completely yields). Control over obsessions is rated 0–4 (complete control, much control, moderate control, little control, no control). A 5-item subset on compulsions is rated in much the same way as the obsessions subset. A score of 17–18 on these items indicates significant pathology. Additional items rate insight into the obsessive-compulsive symptoms, scored from 0 (complete) to 4 (absent); global severity (none, mild, moderate, severe, extreme); and global improvement. Despite the time required to administer (at least 30 minutes) the Y-BOCS, many consider it extremely useful not only for the researcher but also for the clinician in quantifying patients' response to treatment.

Maudsley Obsessional-Compulsive Inventory

The Maudsley Obsessional-Compulsive Inventory (MOC) (Hodgson and Rachman 1977) is a 30-item true-false inventory that is bidirectional and concerned with specific symptoms. It is scored with a total obsessional score (all 30 items) along with five subscales: checking (9 items), washing (11 items), slowness repetition (7 items), doubling-conscientious (7 items), and ruminations (which is not scored because it contains only 2 items). Although it is useful for assessing change, the MOC does not take into account many other symptoms associated with OCD (e.g., mental rituals). Thus a total obsessional score may be low despite severe incapacitating symptoms.

Compulsive Activity Checklist

Originally designed as a 62-item list (Philpott 1975), the Compulsive Activity Checklist (CAC) has been revised to a briefer 28 items. (Steketee and Freund 1993). The CAC assesses compulsive impairment in 28 daily activities by the following 0- to 3-point scoring module: 0=I have no problem with this activity; 1=This activity takes me twice as long as most people or I have to do it twice or I tend to avoid it; 2=This activity takes me three times as long as most people or I have to do it three times or I usually avoid it; and 3=I am unable to complete or attempt this activity. Although it is not as comprehensive as the Y-BOCS, the CAC allows for the detection of specific clinical problems that may not emerge in a clinical interview.

Padua Inventory

The Padua Inventory, a self-report measure, was developed in a 60-item original version (Sanavio 1988) and more recently a 39-item revised version (Burns et al. 1996). Severity of symptoms is rated on a 5-point Likert-type scale: 0=not at all, 1=a little, 2=quite a lot, 3=a lot, and 4=very much. Total score is calculated, as well as five subscale scores for contamination obsessions and washing compulsions, dressing and grooming compulsions, checking compulsions, obsessional thoughts of harm to self and others; and obsessional impulses of harm to self and others. The internal consistency of the Padua Inventory ranged from 0.80 to 0.94, and its test-retest reliability ranged from 0.71 to 0.83. Correlations of the total score of the Padua Inventory with self-reporting measures of OCD such as the MOC ranged from 0.70 to 0.75. According to the American Psychiatric Association *Handbook of Psychiatric Measures* (American Psychiatric Association 2000b), the Padua Inventory is considered to be the best available self-report measure of severity of OCD as determined by DSM-IV criteria.

Leyton Obsessional Inventory

The Leyton Obsessional Inventory (LOI) (Cooper 1970) was one of the most widely used OCD instruments until it was more or less supplanted by the Y-BOCS. The LOI is a 69-item inventory measuring the subjective assessment of obsessional traits and compulsions. Patients first respond "yes" or "no" to the statements. They then consider the "yes" answers and place each into one of five categories: "sensible to do"; "habit"; "not necessary"; "I try to stop it"; and "I try very hard to stop it." The next inquiry is the degree of interference with daily routines. There are five subscale scores to the LOI (clean and tidy, indecisive, checking, orderliness, and sensitization), with much interdependence between these scales. The LOI takes about an hour to administer; some consider the instrument inadequate for assessing intrusive thoughts and washing rituals.

PANIC DISORDER (WITH OR WITHOUT AGORAPHOBIA)

Panic Disorder Severity Scale

The Panic Disorder Severity Scale (PDSS) (Shear et al. 1997) was modeled after the Y-BOCS. It is a seven-item scale that assesses the seven key dimensions of panic disorder: panic frequency; distress during the panic attack; anticipatory anxiety; situational fear and avoidance; fear and avoidance of sensations; interference or impairment in work; and interference or impairment in social functioning. Administration of the PDSS takes 5–10 minutes. The items are rated on a 4-point range from none to extreme. The composite score represents an average score of the seven items. The internal consistency of the PDSS was 0.65, and interrater reliability ranged from 0.74 to 0.88. Correlation of the PDSS with the Anxiety Disorders Interview Schedule was 0.55 (Shear et al. 1997). Despite the fact that it was developed to be a clinician-rated instrument, the PDSS can be applied as a patient-rated instrument (Penava et al. 1998).

Acute Panic Inventory

The Acute Panic Inventory (API) (Gorman et al. 1983) is an instrument for assessing various domains of panic disorder. It can be used to assess both full-blown and limited symptoms and both unexpected and situational panic attacks over a specified time period. In the API the intensity of the attack is rated on a scale of 0–10 and the duration of attacks (in minutes) is estimated. The percentage of the time the patient has anticipatory anxiety is recorded, as is the intensity of the anticipatory anxiety on a scale of 0–10. The number of feared situations entered is also assessed, as well as the percentage of time the feared situation is entered. Also assessed globally, on a scale of 1–7, are the severity and improvement of the panic attacks, phobic avoidance, and anticipatory anxiety as well as overall functional impairment and overall severity of illness. The patient is also allowed to rate these global measures (Otto et al. 1998). The API has been used widely in experimental research studies on lactate and carbon dioxide–induced panic attacks.

Mobility Inventory for Agoraphobia

The Mobility Inventory for Agoraphobia (MI) (Chambless et al. 1985) is a seven-item self-reporting scale (with one item assessing panic frequency) that measures avoidance of a wide range of situations. Each item is rated on a 5-point Likert scale (from 1, never avoid, to 5, always avoid). Administration of the MI takes about 20 minutes. The patient rates avoidance of situations while accompanied by a trusted companion (to calculate the MI-AAC subscale, ranging from 1 to 5) and while alone (to calculate the MI-AAL subscale, also ranging from 1 to 5). The latter is considered an indicator of a more severe degree of avoidance. MI-AAC and MI-AAL scores had a correlation of 0.67 with each other. Both subscales had an internal consistency that ranged from 0.91 to 0.97, with test-retest reliability ranging from 0.56 to 0.90. The correlation of the MI with the agoraphobia subscale of the Fear Questionnaire ranged from 0.44 to 0.63 for the MI-AAC and from 0.68 to 0.84 for the MI-AAL. This scale has shown good discrimination between agoraphobia and social phobia and is sensitive to change in pathology. According the American Psychiatric Association *Handbook of Psychiatric Measures,* the MI is considered to be the best available measure of agoraphobic avoidance (American Psychiatric Association 2000b).

Fear Questionnaire

As discussed previously, in addition to the five-item social phobia subscale, the Fear Questionnaire contains a five-item scale for agoraphobia, and it is believed that these two subscales discriminate social phobia from agoraphobia.

As noted, the subscales measuring agoraphobia and social phobias are reliable and valid measures and are believed to be better indicators of change than the total phobia score. (Moylan and Oei 1992).

Anxiety Sensitivity Index and Brief Panic Disorder Screen

The Anxiety Sensitivity Index (ASI) (Reiss et al. 1986) is a 16-item self-report to evaluate fear of anxiety symptoms. Two additional versions were developed: one is an 18-item scale for children, and the other is a 4-item panic screening scale (Brief Panic Disorder Screen [Apeldorf et al. 1994]). The items are rated on a 5-point Likert scale (from 0, not at all, to 4, severe). The internal consistency of the ASI ranged from 0.84 to 0.90, with test-retest reliability of 0.75. The ASI correlation with the Fear Survey Schedule ranged from 0.59 to 0.71. The ASI discriminated control subjects from individuals with agoraphobia and other anxiety disorders and has been shown to predict the development of panic disorder in college students. Of note, the 4-item Brief Panic Disorder Screen had a sensitivity of 78% and a specificity of 73% at a cutoff score of 11 for panic disorder. Considering the facts that they are brief and possess the psychometric properties outlined above, both scales are useful for assessment at baseline and during treatment.

QUALITY-OF-LIFE SCALES IN ANXIETY DISORDERS

Sheehan Disability Scale

The Sheehan Disability Scale (SDS) (Leon et al. 1992) is a four-item scale that measures on a scale of 0–10 whether symptoms cause problems at work, with social life leisure, with family life, and with home responsibilities. There is also a 0- to 5-point global scale assessing work and social activities. The instrument can be used with any anxiety disorder but has been shown to have validity in panic disorder with respect to changes from treatment. The SDS also can discriminate symptomatic from asymptomatic anxiety disorders.

Quality of Life Enjoyment and Satisfaction Questionnaire

The Quality of Life Enjoyment and Satisfaction Questionnaire (Q-LES-Q) (Endicott et al. 1993) is a 105-item questionnaire that is rated on a scale of 1–5 (none, rarely, sometimes, often or most of the time, frequently or all of the time). The instrument assesses eight areas of functioning rather than the specific symptoms of the disorder. The areas investigated are physical health, subjective feelings of well-being, work, household duties, school, leisure-time activities, social relationships, and overall general condition. In addition, there are questions asked about satisfaction with medication and overall satisfaction with life. Although this questionnaire can be used for most psychiatric disorders, it is particularly useful for panic disorder, because it has been shown that improvement in clinical symptoms correlates with improvement in quality of life.

Other Useful Scales for Panic Disorder

Body Sensations Questionnaire

The Body Sensations Questionnaire (BSQ) (Chambless et al. 1984) is an instrument that is used to rate fears of body sensation on a 5-point scale from "not frightened or worried by this sensation" to "extremely worried or frightened by this sensation." Higher scores indicate a higher degree of fear. This scale has been found to distinguish between control subjects without panic disorder and individuals with agoraphobia and was shown to be sensitive to change.

Agoraphobic Cognitions Questionnaire

The Agoraphobic Cognitions Questionnaire (ACQ) (Chambless et al. 1984) is a 14-item scale assessing the frequency of thoughts about the negative consequences of anxiety. It is rated on a scale of 1–5, with the total score being the average of the 14 items. This scale has shown good discrimination between patients with panic disorder and control subjects without panic disorder and has shown good sensitivity to change.

POSTTRAUMATIC STRESS DISORDER

The number of self-reporting forms and clinician-rated measures for the various types of traumas (childhood sexual, combat-related exposures) that give rise to PTSD is beyond the scope of this chapter. The reader is referred to Wilson and Keane (1997) for a more complete description of more than 60 self-reporting and clinician-administered scales. The more frequently used scales are reviewed below.

Clinician-Administered PTSD Scale

The Clinician-Administered PTSD Scale (CAPS-I) (Blake et al. 1995) is a new and frequently used scale that can be used by clinicians and nonclinicians. It is essentially a structured interview that examines both lifetime and current symptoms. The first 17 items are taken straight from the DSM-IV criteria and are rated on a scale of 0–4 with respect to frequency (never, rarely, occasionally, frequently, constantly) and intensity (none, mild, moderate, severe, extreme). Three items assess impact on social functioning, occupational functioning, and global severity, which are rated on a scale of 0–4 (none, slight, moderate, severe, extreme). Another question assesses global improvement since the first visit on a scale of 0–4 (asymptomatic, very much improvement, moderate improvement, slight improvement, no improvement or insufficient information). There is also an item for rating validity (excellent, good, fair, poor, invalid or faking). Finally, there are eight symptoms associated with PTSD rated on a scale of 0–4 (never, rarely, occasionally, frequently, constantly). The symptoms include guilt over acts of commission or omission, survivor guilt, homicidality, disillusionment with previously esteemed authority or authority figures, feelings of hopelessness, memory impairment or forgetfulness, sadness and depression, and feelings of being overwhelmed.

The administration of the CAPS-I is labor intensive. Despite good test-retest reliability ($\kappa = 0.84$), it has mainly been used in Vietnam War veterans and not others with trauma experiences. It is based on the presumption that a traumatic event has occurred rather than being designed to elicit it. An important advantage of the scale is that it allows for a categorical assessment of diagnosis plus a dimensional evaluation of the degree of PTSD. There are good validity correlations with the Mississippi Scale (0.73) and the Impact of Events Scale (0.62).

Mississippi Scale for Combat-Related PTSD and Revised Civilian Mississippi Scale for PTSD

The original Mississippi Scale for Combat-Related PTSD (Keane et al. 1988) contained 39 items (35 plus 4 subsequently added) rated on a scale of 0–4 (not true at all, rarely true, sometimes true, frequently true, very frequently true). The original 35 items tap four areas associated with PTSD: 11 items for reexperiencing the event, 11 for withdrawal and numbing, 8 for arousal, and 5 for self-persecution (guilt and suicidality). A form of the scale for assessing PTSD in civilians was developed by Keane et al. (1988). The scale has been able to detect differences between trauma victims and those with no trauma history.

The Revised Civilian Mississippi Scale for PTSD (Norris and Perilla 1996) has 30 items, of which 24 are similar to those in the original scale. The first 18 items assess the symptoms based on the specific trauma, whereas the remaining 12 items are general and are not related to the event. Items are rated from 1 (not at all true) to 5 (extremely true). The Revised Civilian Mississippi Scale is shorter and easier to administer than the combat-related scale and is as reliable. It has good correlation with a diagnosis of PTSD, with scores and diagnoses of PTSD higher for life-threatening injuries than for personal loss injuries.

Combat Exposure Scale and Military Stress Scale

The Combat Exposure Scale (CES) and the Military Stress Scale are useful in evaluating combat-related PTSD by examining stressors in war zone settings. The CES (Lund et al. 1984) has eight items. The first question is whether the patient has ever gone out on combat patrols or other dangerous duties (1=none, 5=more than 50 times). The second question is whether the patient was ever under enemy fire (1=never, 5=more than 6 months). Questions 3,4, and 8 (rated on a scale of 1–4) are whether the patient was ever surrounded by the enemy, whether he was involved in handling dead bodies, and what percentage of members of his unit were killed. In questions 5 and 7 (rated on a scale of 1–5) the patient is asked to note how many times he fired rounds of ammunition at the enemy, how often rounds were fired at him, and how often the patient felt he was in danger of being killed or maimed.

The Military Stress Scale (C.G. Watson et al. 1988), often administered with the CES, contains six situations that are rated either "no experience," "heard about it," "witnessed it," or "participated in it." These situations include torturing of prisoners of war, torturing of civilians, killing of prisoners of war, killing of civilians, mutilation of corpses, and killing of children.

CONCLUSION

Although many scales for anxiety disorders have been used primarily for research and many of the scales address symptoms as opposed to quality of life, clinicians find that a schedule of items that covers a variety of observable events and patients' attitudes, feelings, and behaviors helps to ensure a more complete psychiatric evaluation. The existence of specific, quantifiable scales for each anxiety disorder makes it less likely that significant phenomena may be omitted or overlooked and allows for better communication among clinicians. The anxiety rating scales described in this chapter allow for a systematic and common format that can be used by mental health professionals. Moreover, a reliable and valid scale allows not only the assessment of symptoms (disease) but also a systematic way of assessing behavioral or other trends indicative of change during the course of treatment or ongoing reassessment after successful treatment (remission). In short, the scales for anxiety disorders now not only assess efficacy of various treatments (as in research trials) but also permit a better assessment of clinical treatment in everyday practice.

REFERENCES

American Psychiatric Association: Diagnostic and Statistical Manual of Mental Disorders, 4th Edition, Text Revision. Washington, DC, American Psychiatric Association, 2000a

American Psychiatric Association: Handbook of Psychiatric Measures. Washington, DC, American Psychiatric Press, 2000b

Apeldorf WJ, Shear MK, Leon AC, et al: A brief screen for panic disorder. J Anxiety Disord 8:71–78, 1994

Beck AT, Epstein N, Brown G, et al: An inventory for measuring clinical anxiety-psychometric properties. J Consult Clin Psychol 56:893–897, 1988

Blake DD, Weathers FW, Nagy LM, et al: The development of the clinician administered PTSD scale. J Trauma Stress 8:75–90, 1995

Burns GL, Keortge SG, Formea GM, et al: Revision of the Padua Inventory of obsessive compulsive disorder symptoms: distinctions between worry, obsessions, and compulsions. Behav Res Ther 34:163–173, 1996

Chambless DL, Caputo GC, Bright PN, et al: Assessment of fear of fear in agoraphobics. The Body Sensations Questionnaire and the Agoraphobic Cognitions Questionnaire. J Consult Clin Psychol 52:1090–1097, 1984

Chambless DL, Caputo GC, Jasin SE, et al: The Mobility Inventory for Agoraphobia. Behav Res Ther 23:35–44, 1985

Cooper JE: The Leyton Obsessional Inventory. Psychol Med 1:48–64, 1970

Covi L, Rickels K, Lipman OS: Effects of psychotropic agents on primary depression. Psychopharmacology Bulletin 100–101, 1981

Davidson JRT, Potts NLS, Richichi EA, et al: The Brief Social Phobia Scale. J Clin Psychiatry 52:48–51, 1991

Dunbar GC, Cohn JB, Fabre LF, et al: A comparison of paroxetine, imipramine and placebo in depressed outpatients. Br J Psychiatry 159:394–398, 1991

Endicott J, Nee J, Harrison W, et al: Quality of Life Enjoyment and Satisfaction Questionnaire: a new measure. Psychopharmacology Bulletin 29:321–326, 1993

Goodman WK, Price LH, Rasmussen SA, et al: The Yale-Brown Obsessive Compulsive Scale; II: Validity. Arch Gen Psychiatry 46:1012–1016, 1989

Gorman J, Levy GF, Liebowitz MR, et al: Effect of acute beta-adrenergic blockade on lactate induced panic. Arch Gen Psychiatry 40:1079–1082, 1983

Greist JH, Kobak KA, Jefferson JW, et al: The clinical interview, in Social Phobia—Diagnosis, Assessment and Treatment. Edited by Heimberg RG, Liebowitz MR, Hope DA, et al. New York, Guilford, 1995, pp 183–201

Hamilton M: The assessment of anxiety states by rating. Br J Med Psychol 32:50–55, 1959

Heimberg RG, Mueller G, Holt CS, et al: Assessment of anxiety in social interaction and being observed by others. The Social Interaction Anxiety Scale and the Social Phobia Scale. Behavior Therapy 23:53–73, 1992

Hodgson RJ, Rachman M: Obsessional-compulsive complaints. Behav Res Ther 15:389–395, 1977

Keane TM, Cadell JM, Taylor KL: Mississippi Scale for Combat Related PTSD. Three studies in reliability and validity. J Consult Clin Psychol 52:888–891, 1988

Kessler RA, McGonagle KA, Zhao S, et al: Lifetime and 12 month prevalence of DSM-III-R psychiatric disorders in the United States. Arch Gen Psychiatry 51:8–19, 1994

Leary MR: The brief version of the Fear of Negative Evaluations Scale. Personality and Social Psychology Bulletin 9:371–375, 1983

Leon A, Shear MK, Portera L, et al: Assessing impairment in patients with panic disorder. The Sheehan Disability Scale. Soc Psychiatry Psychiatr Epidemiol 27:78–82, 1992

Liebowitz MR: Social phobia. Mod Probl Pharmacopsychiatry 22:141–173, 1987

Liebowitz MR, Fyer AJ, Gorman JM, et al: Phenelzine in social phobia. J Clin Psychopharmacol 6:93–98, 1986

Liebowitz MR, Schnieier FR, Campeas R, et al: Phenelzine vs atenolol in social phobia. A placebo controlled comparison. Arch Gen Psychiatry 44:669–677, 1992

Lund M, Foy D, Sipprelle C, et al: The Combat Exposure Scale: a systematic assessment of trauma in the Vietnam War. J Clin Psychol 6:1323–1328, 1984

Marks IM, Mathews AM: Brief standard rating for phobic patients. Behav Res Ther 17:267–273, 1979

Moylan A, Oei TP: Is the Fear Questionnaire (FQ) a useful instrument for patients with anxiety disorders? Behaviour Change 9:138–149, 1992

Norris F, Perilla J: Reliability, validity, and cross-language stability of the Revised Civilian Mississippi Scale for PTSD. J Trauma Stress 9:285–298, 1996

Oei TP, Kenna D, Evans L: The reliability, validity and utility of the SAD and FNE scales for anxiety disorder patients. Personality and Individual Differences 12(2):111–116, 1991

Otto MW, Penava SJ, Pollack MH: Diagnostic and symptom assessment of panic disorder, in Panic Disorder and Its Treatment. Edited by Rosenbaum JF, Pollack MH. New York, Marcel Dekker, 1998, pp 323–340

Penava SJ, Otto MW, Maki KM, et al: Rate of improvement during cognitive-behavioral group treatment for panic disorder. Behav Res Ther 36:665–673, 1998

Philpott R: Recent advances in the behavioral measurement of obsessional illness: difficulties common to these and other instruments. Scott Med J 20 (suppl 1):33–40, 1975

Raskin A, Schulterbrandy J, Rettig N: Replication of factors of psychopathology in interview, ward behavior, and self report ratings of hospitalized depressed patients. J Nerv Ment Dis 148:87–98, 1969

Reiss S, Peterson RA, Gursky DM, et al: Anxiety sensitivity, anxiety frequency, and the prediction of fearfulness. Behav Res Ther 24:1–8, 1986

Sanavio E: Obsessions and compulsions: the Padua Inventory. Behav Res Ther 26:169–177, 1988

Shear MK, Brown TA, Barlow DH, et al: Multicenter Collaborative Panic Disorder Severity Scale. Am J Psychiatry 154:1571–1575, 1997

Steketee CS, Freund B: Psychometric properties of the Compulsive Activity Checklist. Behavioural Psychotherapy 21:13–25, 1993

Turner SM, Biedel DC, Dancu CV, et al: An empirically derived inventory to measure social fears and anxiety. The Social Phobia and Anxiety Inventory. Psychol Assess 1:35–40, 1989

van Riezen H, Segal M (eds): Comparative Evaluation of Operating Scales for Clinical Psychopharmacology. New York, Elsevier, 1988

Watson CG, Kucala T, Manifold V, et al: Differences between post-traumatic stress disorder patients with delayed and undelayed onsets. J Nerv Ment Dis 176:568–572, 1988

Watson D, Friend R: Measurement of social evaluatory anxiety. J Consult Clin Psychol 33:448–457, 1969

Wilson JP, Keane TM: Assessing Psychological Trauma and PTSD. New York, Guilford, 1997

Zung WW: A rating instrument for anxiety disorders. Psychosomatics 12:371–379, 1969

Zung WW: The measurement of affects: depression and anxiety. Mod Probl Pharmacopsychiatry. 7:170–188, 1974

CHAPTER 12

Outcome Measurement in Substance Use Disorders

Monika E. Kolodziej, Ph.D.
Shelly F. Greenfield, M.D., M.P.H.
Roger D. Weiss, M.D.

Abuse of substances such as alcohol, illicit drugs, and prescription medications is associated with substantial individual and societal costs. The types and effectiveness of treatments provided for persons with substance use disorders (SUDs) vary greatly, and accurate measures of treatment outcome are needed for both clinical and research purposes. In this chapter indicators and consequences of substance use are presented, measures commonly used to assess SUD treatment outcomes are described, and challenges and recent developments in this area are pointed out.

This chapter was supported by Grants DA00407, DA00326, and DA09400 from the National Institute on Drug Abuse; Grant AA11756 from the National Institute on Alcohol Abuse and Alcoholism; and a grant from the Dr. Ralph and Marian C. Falk Medical Research Trust.

When considering treatment outcome measures for SUDs, it is important to keep in mind the considerable heterogeneity among individuals who abuse substances. The sources of this heterogeneity include gender and other sociodemographic characteristics, the number and type of substances used, the severity of the disorder, the degree of functional impairment, the presence or absence of comorbid medical and psychiatric conditions, personal strengths and vulnerabilities, and the social and environmental context (American Psychiatric Association 1995). The heterogeneity of this population is considered in the following discussion of the indicators and consequences of substance use and in the subsequent description of relevant outcome measures.

INDICATORS AND CONSEQUENCES OF SUBSTANCE USE

Assessment of substance use may be categorized into two broad perspectives: the unidimensional perspective centered on quantity and frequency of use, and the multidimensional perspective focused on life-functioning domains in addition to substance use (Tonigan 1995). The choice of assessment perspective depends on the context of the assessment. Although the unidimensional perspective may suffice in forensic and worksite settings, the multidimensional perspective is needed to more thoroughly measure SUD treatment outcomes. This point is clear when one considers the goals of treatment as specified by the practice guidelines of the American Psychiatric Association in 1995: "goals of treatment include reduction in the use and effects of substances or achievement of abstinence, reduction in the frequency and severity of relapse, and improvement in psychological and social functioning" (p. 1). Using these guidelines, we identified the following indicators and consequences of substance use: 1) quantity and frequency of use, 2) physical health and psychosocial functioning, and 3) frequency and severity of relapse. These characteristics are described as follows.

Quantity and Frequency of Use

Although some patients with SUDs are able to reduce their use to a non-problematic level, the optimal outcome for the vast majority of patients with SUDs is total cessation of substance use. However, many patients are unable or unmotivated to reach this goal, particularly in the early phase of treatment. This may be especially true for individuals with other co-occurring psychiatric disorders (Drake et al. 1998). In these cases, reduction in the amount or frequency of substance use may be considered an important *intermediate* goal of treatment. It is possible that the initial reduction in use may eventually lead to acceptance of the goal of total abstinence.

Severity and Frequency of Relapse

For patients who achieve abstinence, reduction in the frequency and severity of relapse is the second goal of treatment. A major goal of relapse prevention is to help patients identify situations that place them at high risk for relapse and to develop alternative responses to such situations other than substance use. As these abilities improve, the patient is more likely to refrain from substance use for longer periods of time. Thus, one measure of relapse-related outcome consists of measurement of time elapsed between episodes of substance use (e.g., length of time between cessation and resumption of use); this measure may be integrated with assessments of frequency of use.

Physical Health and Psychosocial Functioning

SUDs may be associated with problems in psychological development, social adjustment, school or work performance, financial and legal status, and general health. Hence, important outcomes of SUD treatments include improvements in physical health and psychosocial functioning. Attainment and maintenance of these improvements may depend on the quality and amount of therapeutic and environmental supports. Thus, in addition to assessing patients' functioning, it is important to assess treatment and social support variables as they relate to outcome.

Definitions of successful treatment outcomes may vary according to the emphasis that is being placed on each of the characteristics described earlier. If the emphasis is on abstinence, then measuring quantity and frequency of use is an important outcome indicator. However, many SUDs have a chronic, relapsing nature, and improvements in psychosocial functioning are important characteristics of treatment success in addition to decrease in frequency and severity of relapse. Specific instruments used to assess frequency and quantity of use and psychosocial functioning are described as follows.

ASSESSMENT INSTRUMENTS

A variety of assessment tools have been developed to measure the parameters of substance use. The tools can be categorized as either interview and self-administered measures or biological markers. Interview and self-administered measures provide information about quantity and frequency of use as well as about psychosocial functioning. Biological markers may detect the presence (and at times quantity) of various substances, or they may indicate physiologic changes (e.g., liver dysfunction) often associated with recent substance use. Biological markers are used primarily to improve the validity of interview and self-administered measures.

Interview and Self-Administered Measures

Interviews and self-administered measures are the most commonly used techniques by which substance use outcomes are assessed. Data gathered from these forms of assessment are often subject to doubt and scrutiny because respondents are asked to provide information about behaviors that are undesirable, stigmatized by society, or illegal. When inquiring about substance use, it is important to keep in mind the following factors that enhance valid reporting: 1) the respondent is not experiencing intoxication or withdrawal symptoms, 2) information is gathered in a setting designed to promote honest reporting, 3) questions are worded clearly and comprehensibly, and—perhaps the most important—4) there are no negative consequences attached to reporting substance use. Described below are instruments that are generally considered to provide satisfactory outcome information in clinical and research settings.

Addiction Severity Index

The Addiction Severity Index (ASI), developed by McLellan and colleagues in 1980, and most recently revised in 1992 (McLellan et al. 1992b), is a structured interview that assesses problem severity in seven areas frequently affected by SUDs. The ASI thus provides information about recent and lifetime alcohol and drug use, legal history, employment history, family and social functioning, and medical and psychiatric status. A summary score for each of these domains indicates areas in which treatment is needed.

The ASI has several advantages. First, it has been shown to have excellent psychometric properties. Second, normative values are available for a variety of treatment groups, including patients with psychiatric disorders, homeless persons, probationers, and clients of employee assistance programs (McLellan et al. 1992b). Third, several versions of the ASI have been adapted for use with adolescents. One of the adapted versions is the Teen-ASI (TASI) by Kaminer and colleagues (1991). Like the ASI, the TASI is a structured interview that inquires about drug and alcohol use as well as school or employment status, family functioning, peer-social relationships, legal status, and psychiatric status. The main disadvantages of the ASI are its length (more than 200 items that take up to an hour to complete) and the requirement that it be administered by a trained technician.

Timeline Follow-Back

The Timeline Follow-Back (TLFB) (Sobell and Sobell 1992) is a calendar method that asks patients to reconstruct type, quantity, and frequency of substance use over a discrete period of time. The TLFB has been widely used to measure alcohol consumption and has more recently been applied to assess cigarette, cannabis, heroin, and cocaine use (Brandon et al. 1995; Hersh et al. 1999). Typically, the TLFB queries about substance use during the past month or the past 3 months, but it has also been used to assess substance use up to the past year. Usually, the assessor begins by asking about the most recent use and then proceeds with more retrospective assessment. When administering the TLFB, it is helpful to use memory-enhancing landmarks such as holidays, birthdays, and other important events.

The advantage of the TLFB is that it has been shown to be reliable and valid for the measurement of alcohol consumption (Sobell and Sobell 1992). Although fewer psychometric data exist for other substances, the TLFB has recently been shown to have fair to moderate validity for measurement of cocaine use (Hersh et al. 1999). Its disadvantages are that it may be too detailed for some clinical purposes and that it may take a long time to administer when there is extensive substance use. This method is recommended when precise estimates of use are desired, especially when a complete picture of usage is needed (e.g., determining high-risk versus low-risk days) and when a detailed comparison of pretreatment and post-treatment substance use is desired.

Drinker Inventory of Consequences

The Drinker Inventory of Consequences (DrInC), developed by Miller and colleagues (1995), is a self-administered 50-item questionnaire designed to measure adverse consequences of alcohol abuse in five areas: interpersonal, physical, social, impulsive, and intrapersonal. It is used clinically for treatment planning and for measurement of behavioral treatment outcomes in either clinical or research settings. The DrInC can measure consequences of drinking both over an individual's lifetime and during the past 3 months. Normative data are available for interpretation of results, and a brief version, the Short Index of Problems (SIP), can be used when assessment time is limited.

The advantages of the DrInC are that minimal training is required for administration, psychometric data are available, and the scale has been shown to have good reliability and validity. The disadvantage is that it inquires only about consequences of alcohol use and not other substances.

Treatment Services Review

The Treatment Services Review (TSR), developed by McLellan and colleagues (1992a), is a 5-minute, technician-administered interview that provides a quantitative measure of the number and types of services received by patients during substance abuse treatment. The TSR also inquires about self-help group attendance, an important variable in SUD treatment. The TSR was designed to be administered with the ASI; whereas the latter instrument identifies problem areas for patients with SUDs, the TSR examines the degree to which these problem areas are being addressed in treatment. The advantages of the TSR are that it is quick and comprehensive, has good psychometric properties, and appears to be appropriate for a variety of settings. However, although the TSR allows the assessor to calculate the quantity and type of services pursued, it cannot be used to evaluate the quality of these services.

World Health Organization Quality of Life Scale

The World Health Organization Quality of Life (WHOQOL) Scale, developed by the World Health Organization (1998), asks about four domains of quality of life: physical health, psychological functioning, social relationships, and environment (e.g., work, finances, and transportation). There are two versions of the WHOQOL: one consisting of 100 items, and the other consisting of 25 items. Although both scales have been found to be reliable and valid in their multiple language versions, there are limited data about their psychometric properties for patients with nonalcohol SUDs.

Biological Markers

Biological markers to detect substance use offer information regarding the extent, frequency, and impact of substance use in selected populations. Biological markers are tested through analyses of breath, urine, blood, hair, and saliva.

Five major considerations should guide the choice and scheduling of biological marker tests (Anton et al. 1995). First, the *purpose* of the test (e.g., preemployment testing) needs to be defined according to type of population studied and the setting in which testing is occurring. Second, the *window of assessment*, defined as the amount of time that the marker will remain positive after substance use, needs to be determined. Third, the assessor needs to determine *test sensitivity*, defined as the ability of a given test to detect the presence of a substance when it is truly present (i.e., a low rate of false-negative results). Fourth, it is important to determine *test specificity*, defined as the ability to detect the absence of the substance when it is truly absent (i.e., a low occurrence of false-positive results). And finally, a decision needs to be made whether to administer the test on a predetermined or a random schedule. Although random administration may increase the likelihood of detecting ongoing use and enhance the deterrent value of the testing program, random testing may not always be feasible due to resource limitations.

Breath

Breath analysis is a frequently used method to screen for recent alcohol use. Breath alcohol testing is considered to have both high sensitivity and specificity. This method is advantageous because of the immediacy of the results, the noninvasiveness of the procedure, and the relatively low cost. Moreover, little training is required to carry out this test. The disadvantage is that breath analysis has a narrow window of assessment, generally ranging from minutes to several hours after drinking (depending on the quantity consumed and the individual rate of metabolism).

Urine

Urine testing is based on the premise that metabolites of many substances of abuse are found in urine. Although this is the most frequently used test in clinical settings, it carries several disadvantages. The main disadvantage is that metabolites have different durations of detection time. Some metabolites (e.g., from cannabis) remain in urine for a long time, and a false-positive result may be obtained when testing for recent use. In contrast, other metabolites (e.g., from cocaine) are present in urine for brief time periods, and a negative result may prevent detecting use that has occurred as recently as 3 to 4 days before the test. Moreover, durations of detection time vary according to a number of other factors, including dose, frequency of administration, cutoff concentration level at which a test is considered positive, and the patient's metabolism rate (Cone 1997). Therefore, deciding when to collect urine is challenging, especially when there is an interest in detecting metabolites of multiple substances.

Some of the limitations of urine screens may be mitigated by quantitative rather than qualitative urine screens. Quantitative analysis allows one to limit the number of false-positive results that may occur due to carryover effect from frequent tests, as well as false-negative results that may occur when patients try to avoid detection of substance use by diluting their urine through consumption of other fluids (water loading). However, quantitative analysis is expensive, and it is a relatively new technology that needs further assessment. It is important to consider the susceptibility of urine tests to tampering through the use of additives, dilutions, and substitutions.

Blood

In clinical settings, direct detection of substance use through serum testing has been used primarily for detection of recent heavy substance use (e.g., in emergency room settings when an overdose is suspected). Blood analysis for alcohol is more frequently used to test for biological *consequences* of extensive drinking, because certain tissues and functions become compromised as a result of heavy alcohol use.

Frequently used markers of consequences of heavy alcohol use include increased red blood cell mean corpuscular volume (MCV), elevated levels of the glycoprotein carbohydrate-deficient transferrin (CDT), and elevated levels of the following liver enzymes: γ-glutamyltransferase (GGT), aspartate aminotransferase (AST), and alanine aminotransferase (ALT). Elevated CDT and liver enzyme levels may be indicative of serious hepatic injury that may result from heavy alcohol use (e.g., alcoholic hepatitis or cirrhosis). Increased MCV may also point to liver damage as well as to hematologic problems including certain types of anemia such as that due to vitamin B_{12} or folate deficiency.

There are advantages and disadvantages of using blood markers. Obtaining information about these markers allows the clinician to track physical health outcomes, and this information may be especially useful in clinical settings in which it can be used to enhance patients' motivation to reduce their alcohol use. However, these markers reflect tissue pathology resulting from high long-term levels of alcohol intake *or* from other disease processes. Moreover, studies show that normal levels of blood markers vary according to individual characteristics such as gender, age, body mass index, smoking, and use of caffeine and certain medications (Aubin et al. 1998; Daeppen et al. 1998). Thus, sensitivity and specificity of blood serum markers may be lower than for other biological indicators.

Hair

Testing hair for the presence of drugs is a relatively new technology that has progressed rapidly during the past decade. Although there continues to be controversy about how a drug enters hair, the most likely routes are through diffusion from blood, excretion in sweat and oily secretions, and the environment. The advantage of hair testing is that it is less invasive and less prone to decay than blood, urine, or saliva tests. Hair testing may also provide a longer duration of time in which to detect substance use than can blood or urine; in some cases substances may be detected for months after use (Cone 1997).

There are several disadvantages to hair testing, however. First, the newness of the technology limits knowledge about drug detectability, especially as it relates to dose and time relationships. Second, passive exposure to substances (especially cocaine) may result in false-positive hair test results. Third, results of hair tests may be dependent on the characteristics of the hair obtained (e.g., hair length). Fourth, there is some concern about racial bias in hair testing, even though recent studies using improved technology have not supported this concern (Hoffman 1999).

Saliva

Substances may enter saliva by passive diffusion from blood (the most important entry for most drugs), ultrafiltration (for alcohol), or active secretion. Detection time for most substances varies between 12 and 24 hours. The primary use of saliva testing is to detect very recent substance use, for example, to link drug use to behavior and performance impairment. Saliva testing is used in detection of substance use in automobile drivers, accident victims, and employees before they engage in safety-sensitive activities. The major advantage of saliva testing is that it is less invasive and less costly than urine or blood tests. The major disadvantage is the fact that saliva testing has a small window of assessment. Moreover, the technology is still somewhat new and is not widely available, and limited information exists about its validity.

Sweat

Sweat testing, a rarely utilized technology in clinical settings, has been investigated for detection of less recent substance use. A variety of substances have been found in sweat, including amphetamine, cocaine, alcohol, and methadone. The major advantage of sweat testing is that it can serve as a cumulative measure of drug use. However, routine sweat collection is difficult because of large variations in the rate of sweat production, high potential for environmental contamination, and the lack of devices suitable for collection of this type of biological fluid. To date, very limited information exists regarding its applicability.

Another important area for improvement lies in increasing training and sensitivity of service providers. In 1996, Carey et al. presented a set of guidelines for conducting assessments with patients who carry comorbid psychiatric diagnoses. The guidelines are focused on the elements that pay attention to respondent characteristics (psychiatric stability, level of intoxication or withdrawal, cognitive processes), motivation (reasons for distorting information, confidentiality assurances, other sources of information), and task variables (length of recall period, interviewer style and training, normalization of wide patterns of substance use).

When considering test sensitivity and test specificity, it is important to pay attention to the prevalence of particular substance use in the population being assessed. Specifically, a highly sensitive but not necessarily specific test is desired when prevalence of substance use is low (e.g., among employees in a work setting). In contrast, a highly specific test (even with moderate sensitivity) is preferred when prevalence of substance use is high (e.g., among individuals seeking substance abuse treatment). Taking these test characteristics into consideration may help minimize the number of people who are falsely identified.

CHALLENGES IN ASSESSING SUBSTANCE USE OUTCOMES

Adequate assessment of substance use outcomes is complicated because of a variety of factors that may limit the validity of responses. These factors include instrument disadvantages described earlier, heterogeneity of the patient population (also described earlier), and setting characteristics. Setting-related limitations have been linked to limited training and insufficient attention to substance abuse in mental health settings; these limitations may become obstacles in obtaining optimal information from patients (Lyons et al. 1997).

Furthermore, validity of patient self-reports may be compromised by factors such as not knowing or remembering the quantity of a particular substance used. This may occur when there is 1) use of multiple substances, 2) use of illicit drugs that can be modified or sold under a false name, 3) use of substances that affect memory (e.g., alcohol or benzodiazepines), or 4) presence of other disorders or psychiatric symptoms that may compromise memory (e.g., active psychosis). Moreover, the patient may be intentionally untruthful in certain contexts. For example, more valid responses may be expected in research studies in which patients expect no negative consequences from positive urine tests or self-reports of substance use. However, these contingencies may be different in treatment programs that may discharge patients for substance use, or in contexts in which information regarding substance use has real or perceived negative consequences. In such situations, certain biological markers such as urine screens assume more importance in assessing treatment outcome.

Validity of self-reports may be also affected by perceived stigma associated with a particular substance; the greater the stigma, the greater is the likelihood of suppression of valid reporting. For example, some population samples have been found to be more willing to validly report their marijuana use than the use of opioids, amphetamines, or cocaine (Gfroerer et al. 1997).

RECENT DEVELOPMENTS

Recent developments in assessment of substance abuse treatment outcomes are related to improving validity of the reports. These developments have been taking place in the areas of multimethod assessment and technology improvements.

Multimethod assessment pertains to using several instruments to measure more than one parameter of substance use. For example, el-Guebaly and colleagues (1999) developed an outcome evaluation package for use with patients who have comorbid psychiatric and SUDs. The package consists of standardized interviews and self-administered measures related to substance use, psychiatric status, and psychosocial functioning, as well as expectations and satisfaction with treatment. These authors found this to be a comprehensive tool that could be used to assess patients at initial evaluation, treatment discharge, and follow-up points.

Other approaches to multimethod assessment consist of using multiple types of measures such as self-report measures, biological markers, and collateral reports from the patient's social network. Collateral reports, known for their low cost and ease of use, are considered an important source of information in research settings and are used increasingly in clinical contexts. Recent studies suggest that the validity of collateral reports is enhanced when patients maintain close contact with their collateral informants and when the informants report high confidence in the information (Sobell et al. 1997).

Moreover, in an effort to further develop multiple indicators of substance use, significant attention has been paid to biological markers. Newer markers such as sweat have been examined (Cone 1997), and considerable research has been conducted to further investigate blood markers of alcohol use. This research has aimed to identify new markers such as hemoglobin-acetaldehyde (Laposata 1999) and to examine which markers are most sensitive and specific with respect to alcohol intake. For example, recent studies suggest that combining tests for CDT, MCV, and GGT may allow for more accurate detection of recent heavy alcohol use than can the use of each marker alone (Mundle et al. 1999).

Another important area of recent development pertains to technology improvements, such as computer-assisted self-interviewing (CASI), CASI with an audio component (audio-CASI), and interactive voice response (IVR) technology. With CASI, respondents read questions as they appear on the computer screen and enter their answers with a keyboard or some other input device. Audio-CASI consists of attaching an audio box to the computer; the respondent then follows the questions on the screen with headphones (Lessler and O'Reilly 1997). With IVR, respondents telephone in to a central location at random or predetermined intervals to report substance use (Perrine et al. 1995).

These techniques are believed to have several advantages over traditional self-reporting measures. CASI may reduce the time that it takes to complete measures, and in some cases it may improve the reporting rate because it increases privacy of the respondent. Other advantages include its ability to tailor questions based on previous responses, control inconsistent or out-of-range responses, and standardize the interview. Both the ASI and the TLFB, structured interviews that require a trained technician to administer, have recently been adapted for computer-based administration. Addition of the audio component may reduce the visual and reading burden for some respondents and has been associated with better comprehension because of limiting the external stimuli (Lessler and O'Reilly 1997). The IVR allows for more frequent, prospective reporting of substance use than is possible in treatment and research settings. Thus far, these technologies have been evaluated primarily for alcohol users; their utility for individuals who take other substances remains to be investigated.

CONCLUSION

Multiple tools are needed to adequately assess treatment outcomes for SUDs. Ease of implementation, cost, and patient matching should be considered critical variables in selecting relevant measures. Moreover, it is important to note that the overall sensitivity of an interview, a self-administered measure, or a biological marker may relate to type and severity of the SUD. The judicious use of SUD outcome measures will thus depend on knowledgeable staff trained in a variety of substance use assessments.

REFERENCES

American Psychiatric Association: Practice Guideline for Treatment of Patients with Substance Use Disorders. Washington, DC, American Psychiatric Association, 1995

Anton RF, Litten RZ, Allen JP: Biological assessment of alcohol consumption, in Assessing Alcohol Problems: A Guide for Clinicians and Researchers. Edited by Allen JP, Columbus M (NIAAA Treatment Handbook Series 4) (NIH Publ No 95-3745). Bethesda, MD, U.S. Department of Health and Human Services, 1995, pp 31–40

Aubin HJ, Laureaux C, Zerah F, et al: Joint influence of alcohol, tobacco, and coffee on biological markers of heavy drinking in alcoholics. Biol Psychiatry 44:638–643, 1998

Brandon TH, Copeland AL, Saper ZL: Programmed therapeutic messages as a smoking treatment adjunct: Reducing the impact of negative affect. Health Psychol 14:41–47, 1995

Carey KB, Cocco KM, Simons JS: Concurrent validity of clinicians' ratings of substance abuse among psychiatric outpatients. Psychiatr Serv 47(8):842–847, 1996

Cone EJ: New developments in biological measures of drug prevalence, in The Validity of Self-Reported Drug Use: Improving the Accuracy of Survey Estimates. Edited by Harrison L, Hughes A (NIDA Research Monograph 167) (NIH Publ No 97-4147). Rockville, MD, U.S. Department of Health and Human Services, 1997, pp 108–129

Daeppen JB, Smith TL, Schuckit MA: Influence of age and body mass index on gamma glutamyltransferase activity: a 15-year follow-up evaluation in a community sample. Alcohol Clin Exp Res 22:941–944, 1998

Drake RE, Mercer-McFadden C, Mueser KT, et al: Review of integrated mental health and substance abuse treatment for patients with dual disorders. Schizophr Bull 24:589–608, 1998

el-Guebaly N, Hodgins DC, Armstrong S, et al: Methodological and clinical challenges in evaluating treatment outcome of substance-related disorders and comorbidity. Can J Psychiatry 44:264–270, 1999

Gfroerer J, Lessler J, Parsley T: Studies of nonresponse and measurement error in the National Household Survey on Drug Abuse, in The Validity of Self-Reported Drug Use: Improving the Accuracy of Survey Estimates. Edited by Harrison L, Hughes A (NIDA Research Monograph 167) (NIH Publ No 97-4147). Rockville, MD, U.S. Department of Health and Human Services, 1997, pp 273–295

Hersh D, Mulgrew CL, Van Kirk J, et al: The validity of self-reported cocaine use in two groups of cocaine abusers. J Consult Clin Psychol 67:37–42, 1999

Hoffman BH: Analysis of race effects on drug-test results. J Occup Environ Med 41:612–614, 1999

Kaminer Y, Bukstein OG, Tarter RE: The Teen Addiction Severity Index: rationale and reliability. International Journal of the Addictions 26:219–226, 1991

Laposata M: Assessment of ethanol intake. Current tests and new assays on the horizon. Am J Clin Pathol 112:443–450, 1999

Lessler JT, O'Reilly JM: Mode of interview and reporting of sensitive issues: design and implementation of audio computer-assisted self-interviewing, in The Validity of Self-Reported Drug Use: Improving the Accuracy of Survey Estimates. Edited by Harrison L, Hughes A (NIDA Research Monograph 167) (NIH Publ No 97-4147). Rockville, MD, U.S. Department of Health and Human Services, 1997, pp 366–382

Lyons JS, Howard KI, O'Mahoney MT, et al: The Measurement and Management of Clinical Outcomes in Mental Health. New York, Wiley, 1997

McLellan AT, Luborsky L, O'Brien CP, et al: An improved evaluation instrument for substance abuse patients: the Addiction Severity Index. J Nerv Ment Dis 168:26–33, 1980

McLellan AT, Alterman AI, Cacciola J, et al: A new measure of substance abuse treatment: initial studies of the Treatment Services Review. J Nerv Ment Dis 180:101–110, 1992a

McLellan AT, Kushner H, Metzger D, et al: The fifth edition of the Addiction Severity Index. J Subst Abuse Treat 9:199–213, 1992b

Miller WR, Tonigan JS, Longabaugh R: The Drinker Inventory of Consequences (DrInC): An Instrument for Assessing Adverse Consequences of Alcohol Abuse. Test Manual (NIAAA Project MATCH Monograph Series, Vol 4). NIH Publ No 95-3911. Washington, DC, U.S. Government Printing Office, 1995

Mundle G, Ackermann K, Munkes J, et al: Influence of age, alcohol consumption and abstinence on the sensitivity of carbohydrate-deficient transferrin, gamma-glutamyltransferase and mean corpuscular volume. Alcohol Alcohol 34:760–766, 1999

Perrine MW, Mundt JC, Searles JS, et al: Validation of daily self-reported alcohol consumption using interactive voice response (IVR) technology. J Stud Alcohol 56:487–490, 1995

Sobell LC, Sobell MB: Timeline Follow-Back: a technique for assessing self-reported alcohol consumption, in Measuring Alcohol Consumption: Psychosocial and Biological Methods. Edited by Litten RZ, Allen J. Totowa, NJ, Humana, 1992, pp 41–72

Sobell LC, Agrawal S, Sobell MB: Factors affecting agreement between alcohol abusers' and their collaterals' reports. J Stud Alcohol 58:405–413, 1997

Tonigan SJ: Issues in alcohol outcome assessment, in Assessing Alcohol Problems: A Guide for Clinicians and Researchers. Edited by Allen JP, Columbus M (NIAAA Treatment Handbook Series 4) (NIH Publ No 95-3745). Bethesda, MD, U.S. Department of Health and Human Services, 1995, pp 143–154

World Health Organization: The World Health Organization Quality of Life Assessment (WHOQOL): development and general psychometric properties. Soc Sci Med 46:1569–1585, 1998

CHAPTER 13

Outcome Measurement in Somatoform Disorders

Manuel Santos, M.D.

Melanie Schwarz, M.D.

Asher Aladjem, M.D.

Somatoform disorders are a group of disorders that have in common the presence of physical symptoms suggestive of physical disorder that cannot be adequately or fully explained by a general medical condition or the direct effects of substances. According to DSM-IV-TR (American Psychiatric Association 2000), somatoform disorders are distinguished from factitious disorders and malingering by the fact that in somatoform disorders the production of symptoms is not willful. Somatoform disorders differ from psychiatric disorders due to medical conditions in that in the former there is no diagnosable medical condition to fully account for the physical symptoms.

The somatoform disorders identified in DSM-IV-TR are somatization disorder, undifferentiated somatoform disorder, conversion disorder, pain disorder, hypochondriasis, and body dysmorphic disorder. These disorders are often encountered in general medical settings and often benefit from psychiatric consultation. According to DSM-IV, the prevalence of somatoform disorders is surprisingly high. In addition, these patients are among the highest users of medical services. The estimated prevalence of somatization disorder is 0.2%–2% among women and 0.2% in men. Conversion disorder is estimated to be present in 0.01%–0.03% of the general population and has been reported as a focus of treatment in 1%–3% of outpatient referrals to outpatient mental health clinics. Pain disorder is estimated to occur in 10%–15% of adults in the United States. The prevalence of hypochondriasis in the general population is unknown, but the estimated prevalence in general medical practice has been reported at between 4% and 9%. There are no reliable data on the prevalence of body dysmorphic disorder.

The somatoform disorders present a diagnostic challenge for physicians, who often order elaborate workups that have frustrating, inconclusive findings. These disorders are very common reasons for psychiatric consultation, and they often present significant diagnostic dilemmas for liaison psychiatrists.

Structured tools in the area of diagnosis, treatment, and outcome can assist clinicians in gaining expertise with these groups of symptoms and can prevent unnecessary and expensive medical workups and alleviate some of the chronic suffering of these patients.

This chapter reviews the tools available (as determined by a literature search of MEDLINE from 1966 to January 2000) for outcome measures for this extremely challenging cluster of disorders. The review is by diagnosis. Some scales are used for a specific diagnosis only, whereas others could be used for more than one diagnosis.

SOMATIZATION DISORDER

Somatization disorder is characterized by recurrent, multiple somatic complaints (American Psychiatric Association 2000). It is remarkable for the absence of findings on appropriate clinical evaluation. Onset is usually before age 30. The disorder causes significant impairment in social, occupational, or other important areas of functioning and involves a combination of pain, gastrointestinal, sexual, and pseudoneurological complaints. The symptoms are not under voluntary control, nor are they intentionally produced. There is no secondary gain. Individuals with somatization disorder are often inconsistent in their complaints and seek treatment from more than one physician or site.

Symptom Checklist-90

The Symptom Checklist-90 (SCL-90) is a 90-item, self-reporting scale that measures the symptomatic behavior in psychiatric outpatients (Derogatis and Cleary 1977). The scale is divided into nine symptom subscales, including somatization. The somatization dimension measures the distress arising from perceptions of bodily dysfunction. The subscale consists of 12 questions, which the patient is asked to rank on a 5-point scale from 0 (no distress at all) to 4 (extreme distress associated with the symptom). The time limits can be flexible, but when the test is standardized the patient is asked about the symptoms for the past 7 days. The somatization subscale was found to have significant reliability and validity. The internal consistency was 0.87, the test-retest reliability was 0.82, and the interrater reliability was 0.73. Validity was found to be consistent for total scores, and the specificity and sensitivity are between 80% and 90% (Derogatis and Cleary 1977).

The primary advantage to the SCL-90 is that it is easily administered and scored. However, there are no guidelines to interpretation of the scores. Instead, scores are used to measures a patient's status over time, particularly to identify improvement after treatment. The entire questionnaire is quite long and is not specific for somatization disorder; one recommendation is to use the somatization subscale for a screening measure and for monitoring outcomes during and after treatment (Derogatis and Cleary 1977). The somatization subscale also does not clearly differentiate between somatization disorder and other somatoform disorders, particularly hypochondriasis. In fact, the SCL-90 also may be an appropriate outcome measure for hypochondriasis given its lack of specificity and its overlap with somatization disorder. Other scales reviewed as follows, such as the Whitely Index (Pilowsky 1967) and the Patient Pain Profile Scale (Willoughby et al. 1999), could be useful for outcome measurements for somatization disorder because there is significant overlap in symptoms.

CONVERSION DISORDER

The diagnosis of conversion disorder is characterized by symptoms affecting voluntary motor or sensory function that suggest (but are not fully or adequately explained by) a neurological or general medical condition. Psychological factors are believed to be involved, the hypothesis being that the production of symptoms helps the patient in alleviating unconscious psychic conflict. There are no specific measures for conversion disorder per se; however, there are instruments that can evaluate specific manifestations of conversion disorder. The Placebo Infusion Test and the Minnesota Multiphasic Personality Inventory (MMPI) are used to assess conversion disorder with seizures or convulsions (pseudoseizures, i.e., convulsions that have no neurologic or medical origins). The Glasgow-Edinburgh Throat Scale

(GETS) is used to assess globus pharyngis (the subjective feeling of choking, as if there were a foreign body occupying the trachea).

Placebo Infusion Test

The Placebo Infusion Test (PIT) consists of the deliberate use of a placebo (usually normal saline) to elicit typical seizure activity and is often used to assist in the diagnosis and treatment of suspected nonepileptic seizures. Typically, a patient is told that he or she will receive an electrolyte solution that may precipitate a seizure. The PIT is often quite effective in bringing about a typical seizure response in patients suspected of having nonepileptic seizures. In one study (Walczak et al. 1994), an infusion of normal saline induced typical seizure activity in 82% of patients with a known history of nonepileptic seizures (previously diagnosed with video electroencephalographic monitoring). In patients with a diagnosis of epileptic seizures, the same study found that 10% responded with typical seizures when given normal saline and 15% responded with atypical nonepileptic seizures.

Although the gold standard in diagnosing nonepileptic seizures remains video electroencephalographic monitoring, the use of the PIT as a routine screen for nonepileptic seizures in the clinical setting is well established (Bowman 1998). The PIT is a relatively simple and effective tool for the initial evaluation of suspected nonepileptic seizures that is inexpensive and easy to perform in most clinical settings. The use of the PIT as a measure of outcome is based on the premise that a patient will no longer respond positively once the nonepileptic seizures resolve. However, there is considerable uncertainty about the meaning of a positive or a negative response, and concerns are often raised about the ethics of using deception in the diagnosis and treatment of nonepileptic seizures.

Minnesota Multiphasic Personality Inventory

Wilkus and Dodrill (1984) used the MMPI to assess patients with epileptic and nonepileptic seizures. These researchers found that patients with nonepileptic seizures typically had a "conversion V" pattern, with raised scores on the scales for hypochondriasis and hysteria along with a less markedly elevated score on the depression scale. The MMPI is a 567-item true-false questionnaire with several subscales. These authors focused on three of the subscales: depression (57 questions), hypochondriasis (32 questions), and hysteria (60 questions). The patients with nonepileptic seizures also had elevated scores on both the psychopathic deviate (50 questions) and schizophrenia (81 questions) subscales. Using the criteria described above, Wilkus and Dodrill (1984) correctly classified between 80% and 90% of patients with nonepileptic seizures. A limitation in the use of the MMPI as an outcome measure is that it entails the cooperation of the patient in taking a test that can be both time consuming and laborious. The availability of a written test, however, is advantageous in that it allows for widespread screening.

Glasgow-Edinburgh Throat Scale

Globus pharyngis is one of the few examples of conversion disorder for which there is a readily available outcome measure. The GETS is a self-administered questionnaire that asks patients to rate the severity of their throat symptoms by answering 10 questions on an 8-point scale (in which 0 is none and 7 is unbearable) (Deary et al. 1995). Of the 10 questions, 3 stood out as being the most common complaints of patients with globus pharyngis: "feeling of something stuck in the throat"; "discomfort/irritation in the throat"; "want to swallow all the time." The reliability of the GETS was calculated to be 0.83 (Deary et al. 1995).

The availability of a simple and easily administered scale for the assessment of globus pharyngis provides a tool for clinicians who are not otolaryngologists to readily screen and identify a condition that is quite distressing to patients but is often overlooked (Deary et al. 1995). The GETS not only facilitates the initial assessment, but it also provides a means of following symptoms over time and of measuring improvement. Although there is no clear cutoff score for a positive response, patients who score high on the globus factor (i.e., the three questions that are closely correlated with globus pharyngis) should be administered the GETS serially and should be referred to the appropriate specialist.

PAIN DISORDER

The primary characteristic of pain disorder is the complaint of pain associated with significant psychological factors. These factors are judged to have an important role in the onset, severity, exacerbation, or maintenance of the pain. There is no secondary gain, as in malingering, nor is there a motivation to assume the sick role, as seen in factitious disorder.

The clinical complexity of issues involved in patients' experiences of and disabilities from chronic pain have challenged medical professionals. Chronic pain as a somatoform symptom or disorder continues to evolve as the psychiatric diagnostic nosology develops. The psychological, biological, and social aspects of chronic pain, complicated as they are, have been significantly difficult to study and measure.

Although there is no unified way to measure outcomes of interventions in the treatment of pain disorder, there are tools to measure certain aspects of the disorder.

Pain Anxiety Symptoms Scale

The Pain Anxiety Symptoms Scale (PASS) (McCracken et al. 1992) was developed to study particular aspects of pain-related fear and anxiety. The PASS is a 53-item patient-rated questionnaire in which each item is rated from 0 (never) to 5 (always.) It is divided into four subscales, fear of pain (14 items), cognitive anxiety (10 items), somatic anxiety (14 items), and escape and avoidance (15 items).

Preliminary studies appear to show adequate construct validity and concurrent validity of this instrument when studied in a variety of ways, but further studies are needed to fully establish the PASS as a reliable instrument whose subscales offer independent data (McCracken et al. 1992). The advantage of this instrument is that it is a relatively simple and straightforward questionnaire that can be easily self-administered. The limitation of the PASS is that it examines only one part of a complex issue (chronic pain). The subscales, which could provide means of identifying subgroups of patients, may not have adequate discriminate validity to do so (McCracken et al. 1992). Thus, the scale requires further testing and probably refinements. Yet it may be useful in identifying particular subgroups of chronic pain patients who score significantly higher on one or more of the subscales and are found to be responsive to treatment interventions, such as cognitive-behavioral therapy or psychopharmacotherapy, that target anxiety, cognitive distortions, or significant phobias.

Patient Pain Profile Scale

The Patient Pain Profile (P3) Scale (Willoughby et al. 1999) is a self-rated, multiple-choice scale designed to measure somatization, anxiety, and depression in patients complaining of pain. The scale consists of 44 self-reported items, which are divided in to three subscales—somatization, depression, and anxiety—and a validity index. The somatization subscale assesses the magnitude of the patient's concern about pain and health status. The P3 was found to have significant reliability (internal consistency from 0.85 to 0.91) and high test-retest reliability (r ranging from 0.98 to 0.99). Validity was also found to be significant, with correlations from 0.65 to 0.82 compared with corresponding scales of the MMPI (Willoughby et al. 1999). The somatization subscale also correlated well (0.69) with the somatization subscale of the Brief Symptom Inventory (a questionnaire derived from the SCL-90; its somatization subscale is a seven-item self-reporting scale in which the patient ranks on a 5-point scale the level of distress associated with specific symptoms) (Willoughby et al. 1999). There were also intercorrelations within the P3 subscales.

The somatization subscale of the P3 consists of 12 items, rated on a 3-point scale, that addresses the magnitude of the patient's concern with pain and his or her health status.

No cutoff score was determined; however, the authors of the scale set a score of 32 or greater as "above average." The brevity and convenience of this scale makes it ideal in a short-evaluation outpatient setting, and it may prove beneficial as a screening tool for patients with pain and to help identify additional psychiatric symptoms in this patient population. One drawback of the P3 is that there are intercorrelations within the subscales, which may indicate that the scale cannot accurately discriminate among different psychiatric symptoms that often coexist in patients presenting with pain. The scale also has no clear guidelines as to what any given score represents, although somatization disorder seems to have been somewhat arbitrarily set at a score of 32 or greater. This scale addresses several key psychological factors that are essential in the diagnosis of pain disorder—namely depression, anxiety, and somatization—and hence serves as a useful, albeit indirect, measure of outcome in pain disorder.

Although other scales are used to measure pain per se, such as visual analog scales and the McGill Pain Questionnaire, they do not specifically address pain disorder and therefore are not reviewed in this chapter.

HYPOCHONDRIASIS

In primary care, it is estimated that hypochondriasis diagnosable by accepted criteria is a relatively common disorder, with prevalence estimated at 4%–5%, and represents a population of high utilization of service. The main feature of hypochondriasis is a preoccupation with fears of having a serious disease based on a misinterpretation of one or more bodily signs or symptoms (American Psychiatric Association 2000). These patients often undergo extensive medical workups that do little to allay their fears and anxieties about being ill. These patients are often dissatisfied with their doctors and with their medical care in general, and they often resist referrals to a psychiatrist. There are several instruments that measure hypochondriasis.

Whiteley Index

The Whiteley Index (Pilowsky 1967) is a 14-item yes-no questionnaire that measures the degree of hypochondriasis. The questions address the patients' preoccupation with medical illnesses. The questions were selected by four psychiatrists to be useful in distinguishing between patients with and without hypochondriasis. The test-retest reliability was reported to be 0.81 ($P<0.001$) (Pilowsky 1967). The validity of the index was determined by correlating patients' responses with a modified scale completed by the patients' spouses. The correlation score between both questionnaires was 0.59 ($P<0.001$).

The Whiteley Index is a concise tool that can be easily administered and scored. The index can be reasonably useful in confirming clinical observations and might be useful on a larger scale as a screening tool in the primary care setting. One of the limitations of this instrument is the lack of a clear cutoff score for making a diagnosis of hypochondriasis. Furthermore, the scale's yes or no format does not allow for the measurement of degree of agreement with any question and is susceptible to both underreporting and overreporting of symptoms.

Somatosensory Amplification Scale

The Somatosensory Amplification Scale (SSAS) (Barsky et al. 1990) was devised to measure a patient's sensitivity to several bodily sensations that are experienced as uncomfortable but that are not obvious symptoms of disease. The SSAS has 10 statements that the patient is asked to rate on a 1–5 scale reflecting the degree to which each item is "characteristic of you in general." The SSAS is based on the premise that hypochondriacal patients tend to have an amplified perception of their bodily sensations. A scale that measures this may help identify these patients and also measure the degree of their hypochondriasis. The reliability of the SSAS was found to be significant, with a test-retest correlation of 0.79 ($P<0.0001$) and an internal consistency of 0.82 (Barsky et al. 1990). The validity of the scale measuring amplification was also found to be significant, with patients diagnosed with hypochondriasis (based on DSM-III-R criteria) having significantly higher scores (2.78 vs. 1.98, $P<0.001$) than did nonhypochondriacal patients. The scale correlated with a self-report inventory, the DSM-III-R diagnosis and primary care physician ratings of hypochondriasis. In addition, the SSAS was found to be more specific for hypochondriasis than for other psychiatric diagnosis, even when comorbid diagnoses were statistically controlled for (Barsky et al. 1990).

The scale, like other self-rated scales, is easily administered and may be useful as a screening tool; however, there are disadvantages. The items do not specifically target the DSM-III-R/DSM-IV criteria that the patients must be preoccupied with having a serious disease and that this preoccupation persists despite medical evaluation. Instead, it focuses primarily on the patient's misinterpretation of bodily symptoms. In addition, it is not clear if these worries cause the patient significant distress. Another difficulty with the SSAS is that there are no clear score ranges or cutoff scores to help specifically identify a hypochondriacal patient. The value of the scale lies in its ability to determine baseline scores and measure changes over time and/or after treatment.

Structured Diagnostic Interview for Hypochondriasis

The Structured Diagnostic Interview for Hypochondriasis (SDIH) (Barsky et al. 1992) first appeared in 1992 in response to the lack of other diagnostic tools useful for the somatoform disorders in general and for hypochondriasis in particular. This tool represents the first foray into a diagnostic and therapeutic area that is very difficult and often challenging. The SDIH, which was based on DSM-III-R diagnostic criteria, begins with four probe questions with yes-no responses. A negative answer to all four questions effectively rules out the diagnosis; however, even a single affirmative response prompts the interviewer to proceed with the full questionnaire of 12 questions. After the probe questions are four brief sections with 1–3 questions each, all yes-no except for the last, which concerns duration. Each section is specific to one of the DSM-III-R diagnostic criteria. This scale, developed as part of the Structured Clinical Interview for DSM-IV, was originally intended to be used as a diagnostic tool rather than to measure the outcome of treatment interventions. Because no accepted gold standard exists for examining either the diagnosis or response to treatment of hypochondriasis, the sensitivity and specificity of the SDIH have been difficult to assess. Reliability appears to be quite good, with interrater reliability on individual items ranging from 88% to 97% and overall diagnostic agreement being 96% (Barsky et al. 1992).

Because of difficulties with the diagnostic construct itself, the validity of the SDIH is a complicated issue. Multiple measures of validity (concurrent validity, external validity, divergent validity) all show that this tool is appropriate for selecting patients with the diagnosis of hypochondriasis and for excluding patients without it (Barsky et al. 1992).

The SDIH is a relatively simple, short tool that is easy to use. In addition, it was created in response to a real lack of other useful tools for this diagnostic category. Although it is short and relatively straightforward, the tool was designed to be administered by mental health professionals, with the prerequisite that the clinician have interviewing experience and some basic knowledge of psychopathology. This is because in each subsection the interviewer must judge, on the basis of the information elicited, whether or not that specific criterion has been met.

This tool addresses only the inclusion criteria of hypochondriasis and not at all the exclusionary criteria, namely panic attacks or delusional disorder. Therefore, these exclusions require either another tool or clinical diagnosis outside the realm of this instrument.

Perhaps a more significant weakness of this tool has more to do with the diagnostic construct of hypochondriasis, which in practice appears to be a dimensional rather than a categorical diagnostic entity (Barsky et al. 1992).

BODY DYSMORPHIC DISORDER

Body dysmorphic disorder (BDD) is characterized by a preoccupation with a perceived defect in appearance, in which the defect is either imagined or very slight (American Psychiatric Association 2000).

Yale-Brown Obsessive-Compulsive Scale Modified for Body Dysmorphic Disorder

The Yale-Brown Obsessive-Compulsive Scale Modified for Body Dysmorphic Disorder (BDD-YBOCS) is a 12-item semistructured, clinician-administered instrument used to assess the severity of BDD (Phillips et al. 1997). Each of the 12 items is scored from 0 (no symptoms) to 4 (extreme symptoms). Questions 1–5 assess obsessional symptoms, and questions 6–10 address compulsive symptoms. Items 11 and 12 address insight and avoidance, respectively. The interrater reliability was quite good, at 0.88 (Phillips et al. 1997). The BDD-YBOCS was positively correlated with the Clinical Global Impressions (CGI) Scale ($r=0.55$, $P=0.003$) and was negatively correlated with the Global Assessment of Function (GAF) ($r=-0.51$, $P<0.001$). To assess the scale's sensitivity to change, patients were treated with fluvoxamine and then readministered the BDD-YBOCS; an average change in BDD-YBOCS score of 50.8% was noted. The BDD-YBOCS score was also noted to correlate with global response (as measured by the CGI) of BDD symptoms to treatment ($r=0.79$, $P<0.001$). The specificity of the scale was 93% (as determined by comparison with the CGI) (Phillips et al. 1997).

In general, the BDD-YBOCS is a useful tool for the assessment of outcome in BDD, with well-established reliability and validity and high sensitivity and specificity. The widespread use of this scale would allow for the early detection of patients who could benefit from psychiatric treatment if properly diagnosed and referred. Furthermore, the scale serves as an objective measure of response to treatment that can supplement clinical assessment and subjective reports by the patient.

Brown Assessment of Beliefs Scale

The Brown Assessment of Beliefs Scale (Eisen et al. 1998) is a clinician-administered scale designed to assess delusions across three disorders: body dysmorphic disorder, obsessive-compulsive disorder, and mood disorder with psychotic features. It is a seven-item clinician-administered, semi-structured scale designed to assess delusions. The instrument first establishes the dominant belief the patient has had during the past week. The belief or delusion is evaluated with seven items, each being scored on a 5-point scale (from 0, nondelusional or least pathological, to 4, delusional or most pathological). The seven items evaluate conviction, perception of others' views of the belief, explanation of differing view, fixity of ideas, attempt to disprove the belief, insight, and idea/delusion of reference.

The scale has been found to have a significant interclass reliability of $c=0.96$ and test-retest reliability of a median of 0.95 ($P<0.01$) (Eisen et al. 1998). However, discriminant validity was not found when comparing total score on the scale with scores on other scales, particularly the BDD-YBOCS. There was significant convergent validity between the total score on the Brown Assessment of Beliefs Scale and several scales that specifically target delusions, including rating scales of unawareness of a mental disorder, conviction of delusions, fixity of beliefs, and characteristics of delusions (all with $P<0.001$). No threshold score was established for a particular diagnosis. Twenty patients with a diagnosis of body dysmorphic disorder were evaluated for delusionality. The scale's cutoff point of 18 was established to have a sensitivity of 100% and a specificity of 86% for delusions. Finally, the scale's sensitivity to change was examined by administering the scale to patients before and after treatment with sertraline. A significant decrease in the mean score ($t=5.47$, $df=37$, $P<0.001$) was found (Eisen et al. 1998).

The advantages of the scale are that it is short, requires a minimal amount of clinician time, eliminates the possibly of patient bias because it is clinician administered, and has good reliability. However, the scale lacks discriminant validity, which indicates that it is not appropriate for measuring specific diagnoses but rather is more appropriate for evaluating delusions in general. The scale may prove useful for measuring changes in delusional beliefs after treatment. However, it was examined with only a small sample size and thus needs to be further evaluated in other studies with more subjects before it can be fully established as useful.

FUTURE DIRECTIONS

The somatoform disorders are a heterogeneous group of disorders characterized by the presence of somatic complaints in the absence of demonstrable medical etiology. The diagnoses of these illnesses are complicated and often arrived at only after elaborate, expensive, and extensive medical evaluation. The ability to diagnose these disorders early would be clearly advantageous for the patient and for the overall containment of medical costs. Unfortunately, the early detection of somatoform disorders is often difficult, and there are very few tools to assist the clinician in doing so. Clearly, improvements in early diagnosis along with measurements of outcome after treatment are important. This task is made difficult, however, by the very nature of the disorders being studied. For the most part, the somatoform disorders are a heterogeneous group of disorders, each having a phenomenological cohesion that gives the impression that there is a unique pathophysiology when in fact this may not be the case. Thus, conversion disorder and somatization disorder describe myriad clinical presentations that are quite dissimilar (as evidenced by the inclusion in this chapter of both pseudoseizures and globus pharyngis as examples of conversion). Similarly, the definition of pain disorder is so broad that it encompasses a multitude of psychological factors and medical illnesses with tremendous pathophysiological diversity. This lack of diagnostic specificity limits the assessment of pain disorder. Similarly, there is a dimensional aspect inherent to the diagnosis of hypochondriasis, which renders the disorder less suitable to measurement by any given tool because what is measured lacks coherence. Body dysmorphic disorder seems to be an exception in that the BDD-YBOCS is not only reliable and valid, but easy to administer and quite useful. The reason that BDD is more amenable to outcome measurement may be that it can be conceptualized as a subset of obsessive-compulsive disorder, for which there already is a reliable and valid measure of outcome.

This chapter reviews the few instruments available to evaluate outcomes in patients with somatoform disorders, and the ones available have significant limitations and are used infrequently. Thus, although it is clear that there is a definite need for the development of more tools that are proven to be useful, reliable, valid, and easy to administer, it may be necessary to clarify the overall understanding of these enigmatic disorders before treatment outcomes can be measured in a meaningful way.

REFERENCES

American Psychiatric Association: Diagnostic and Statistical Manual of Mental Disorders, 4th Edition, Text Revision. Washington, DC, American Psychiatric Association, 2000

Barsky AJ, Wyshak G, Klerman GL: The somatosensory amplification scale and its relationship to hypochondriasis. J Psychiatr Res 24:323–334, 1990

Barsky AJ, Cleary PD, Wyshak G, et al: A structured diagnostic interview for hypochondriasis. J Nerv Ment Dis 180:20–27, 1992

Bowman ES: Pseudoseizures. Psychiatr Clin North Am 21:649–657, 1998

Deary IJ, Wilson JA, Harris MB, et al: Globus pharyngis: Development of a symptom assessment scale. J Psychosom Res 39:203–213, 1995

Derogatis LR, Cleary PA: Confirmation of the dimensional structure of the SCL-90: a study in construct validation. J Clin Psychol 33:982–989, 1977

Eisen JL, Phillips KA, Baer L, et al: The Brown Assessment of Beliefs Scale: reliability and validity. Am J Psychiatry 155:102–108, 1998

McCracken LM, Zayfert C, Gross RT: The pain anxiety symptoms scale: development and validation of a scale to measure fear of pain. Pain 50:67–73, 1992

Phillips KA, Hollander E, Rasmussen SA, et al: A severity rating scale for body dysmorphic disorder: development, reliability, and validity of a modified version of the Yale-Brown Obsessive-Compulsive Scale. Psychopharmacology Bulletin 33:17–22, 1997

Pilowsky I: Dimensions of hypochondriasis. Br J Psychiatry 113:89–93, 1967

Walczak TS, Williams DT, Berten W: Utility and reliability of placebo infusion in the evaluation of patients with seizures. Neurology 44:394–399, 1994

Wilkus RJ, Dodrill CB: Intensive EEG monitoring and psychological studies of patients with pseudoepileptic seizures. Epilepsia 25:100–107, 1984

Willoughby SG, Hailey J, Wheeler LC: Pain patient profile: a scale to measure psychological distress. Arch Phys Med Rehabil 80:1300–1302, 1999

CHAPTER 14

Outcome Measurement in Personality Disorders

J. Christopher Perry, M.P.H., M.D.
Natali H. Sanlian, M.Ps.

CHARACTERISTICS OF THE POPULATION OF PERSONALITY DISORDER

An old clinical aphorism suggests that individuals with neurotic disorders suffer because their symptoms are ego-dystonic, whereas those with personality disorders make others suffer because their symptoms are ego-syntonic. Research on personality disorders has shown this dichotomy to be mistaken in its broadest sense. In fact, many individuals with personality disorders have comorbid Axis I symptom disorders, which often bring them to seek help. The converse is also true: of those with Axis I disorders, the subpopulations with the most treatment-refractory conditions often include those with comorbid Axis II disorders. Both clinicians and researchers alike have learned that whenever treating or studying any psychiatric disorder, one ignores personality disorders at one's peril.

Personality disorders may be found in up to 10% of the adult community population; significantly higher percentages are found in clinical settings (30% or more). Certain types, such as certain cluster B types, may be found more in younger than in older adult populations, whereas others, such as clusters A and C, may be more evenly distributed. Although certain types of personality disorder are differentially related to gender (e.g., antisocial and narcissistic types predominantly occur in males; borderline and histrionic types predominantly occur in females), overall, personality disorders are distributed roughly equally between the sexes. Certain temperaments may predispose to the development of a personality disorder (e.g., impulsive, depending on the interaction of the child with environment in early development). The prevalence of personality disorders is higher in environments with poor social integration; low economic and educational conditions; and abusive, neglectful, or chaotic family situations. Nonetheless, a surprising number of cases arise even in privileged environments, which indicates that the understanding of risk factors should not be unidimensional.

PARAMETERS PERTINENT TO MEASURING THE IMPACT OF TREATMENT

In two recent reviews of outcome studies of psychotherapy in personality disorders (Perry and Bond 2000; Perry et al. 1999), several measurement distinctions were found to be meaningful: measurement perspective, measurement domain or content area, assessment time frame, and quantification of change.

Measurement Perspective

Most existing assessment methods are either self-reporting or observer-rated. Self-reporting includes questionnaires filled out by the subject to assess symptoms, personality features, and so on, as with the Symptom Checklist-90–Revised (SCL-90-R) or the Millon Clinical Multiaxial Inventory (MCMI). Observer-rated measures begin with an interview of the subject or other hard data and use the interviewer or outside rater to make the assessment, as with the Hamilton Rating Scale for Depression (HRSD) or any structured interview for Axis II. Perry et al. (1999) found that these two perspectives may produce different results in outcome, depending on treatment length and personality disorder type. In short-term treatments, with largely cluster C disorders, self-report measures may demonstrate more sizable improvement than is found when treatments are longer term, as with largely cluster B disorders. Conversely, sizable observer-rated improvements may be found in longer-term treatments of borderline personality disorder, whereas improvement on self-reporting instruments may be less.

This latter finding is consistent with the idea that as certain personality disorders improve, observable behavior may improve faster than subjective distress diminishes. This overall observation leads to a clear recommendation that outcome studies should employ assessments from both perspectives to reduce the likelihood of misrepresenting the overall degree of change.

Assessment theory also includes several other perspectives. These include objective tests of abilities (e.g., intelligence, neuropsychological tests), projective tests (such as scored data from the Rorschach or Thematic Apperception Test), and biological tests (such as psychophysiological procedures or hormonal responses to provocation tests). Most assessments using these perspectives are further from clinical phenomena than are the self-report or observer-rating assessments, more oriented toward understanding the basic mechanisms in personality and other disorders, and more experimental. As a result, they are not yet developed to the point where they can be meaningfully used as treatment outcome measures (see Chapter 25, in this volume).

Measurement Domain

The measurement domain is the traditional content area of an assessment. Perry et al. (1999) identified four overall domains relevant to the outcome of personality disorders: 1) diagnosis and diagnostic criteria, 2) symptoms and symptomatic behaviors, 3) social role functioning, and 4) core psychopathology and mechanisms. Assessment instruments can generally be categorized in one domain, although there are exceptions, such as the Global Assessment of Functioning (GAF), which spans both the symptoms/symptomatic behaviors and social role functioning domains. The ideal treatment will result in improvement in all domains, whereas improvement that is more limited, suspect, or largely due to a state change might be reflected largely in one domain, such as a decrease in self-reported distress. This observation further supports the recommendation that thorough assessment of outcome should include multiple domains.

Assessment Time Frame

Time is an integral factor in every aspect of outcome assessment and its interpretation. First is the time period covered by the assessment. For some scales, such as the SCL-90-R or the HRSD, the time frame covered is short, such as the last week. Other assessments may cover a longer time frame, such as follow-up interviews to ascertain whether a suicide attempt has been made in the past follow-up interval (such as 6 months or a year). The shorter the time period covered, the more the measure is subject to short-term state changes, whereas longer time periods tend to better represent the subject's average level.

Second is the time elapsed since the baseline assessment. Elapsed time needs to be sufficient to detect lasting change. A short-term treatment for borderline personality disorder, focusing on reduction of self-mutilation, might demonstrate an immediate decrease in self-mutilation by the end of treatment, but 1 or 2 years might be required to determine whether this improvement is durable. Thus, even impressive changes in short-term treatments are hard to interpret without sufficient follow-up.

Third, and related to the foregoing, is whether the final assessment is made at termination of treatment or at subsequent follow-up. A treatment might be quite helpful and show clear improvement at termination, and still be followed by regression to the pretreatment status quo. Only sufficient follow-up after treatment termination can differentiate between transient and durable improvements.

Fourth is whether change is measured by a follow-up or follow-along design. The former uses the common preassessment and postassessment times, perhaps including additional assessments during treatment. However, this design does not yield data about the durability of change. By contrast, the follow-along design uses multiple assessments over time, including after treatment termination, and employs statistical procedures that smooth out the state-related variability to reveal the underlying rate and amount of change. Coupling this design with a long posttreatment period of assessments produces the most stable and convincing evidence of what has changed and by how much.

Considering these points, we recommend that outcome be assessed at both termination and follow-up, preferably using multiple assessments over follow-up. The duration of follow-up should be sufficient to detect that change is stable. Because personality disorders are associated with many phenomena that occur infrequently or at irregular intervals—such as suicide attempts, self-mutilation, depressive episodes or job loss—for many disorders, 1–2 years may be a minimal length of follow-up to yield a stable estimate of change.

Quantification of Change

Whenever change is measured in a sample, comparing assessments at two points in time, the probability that the difference in scores is due to chance is expressed as its P value. However, the P value alone does not disclose certain facts that allow one to better interpret whether clinically meaningful change has occurred. These data include the severity at baseline, the magnitude of the difference between baseline (time 1) and time 2, and whether the score at time 2 is now outside of the pathological range. Studies that supply these additional data are easier to interpret and allow the reader to better determine the generalizability of the findings.

The scale of measurement determines how change is examined. Categorical measures include clinical diagnosis (e.g., definite borderline personality disorder, significant borderline personality disorder traits only, not borderline personality disorder), the proportion of a sample attaining a cutoff score on a scale, or the proportion of a sample scoring positive for a clinical item (e.g., suicide attempt in the past year). Whenever comparing assessments at two or more points in time, one usually examines the difference in proportions at each time. For instance, 45% were unemployed at baseline, whereas 25% were unemployed after 2 years. Whenever the time elapsed from baseline until an event occurs is also known, then survival analysis is a more powerful tool: for instance, comparing two treated groups on the time elapsed from beginning treatment until the patients no longer meet the criteria for the personality disorder.

Although diagnostic data are usually presented categorically, whenever dimensional (continuous) scales are available, there are several reasons for which it is desirable to present both kinds of data. First, there is an ongoing debate about whether personality disorders are better described by categorical or dimensional approaches, and therefore presenting both informs adherents of either viewpoint. Second, psychometrically, dimensional approaches have greater reliability and statistical power to detect change and have advantages in multivariate analyses.

Continuous (dimensional) measures include most clinical scales, personality measures, functioning scales, and core psychopathology measures. Many different statistical techniques can be applied to data from such measures. However, it is valuable to know the sample characteristics (such as mean, standard deviation or 95% confidence interval, range) at baseline, at treatment termination, and at follow-up. Although the amount of raw change is usually presented, there are advantages to presenting the effect size of the difference. Effect size is a measure of how meaningful is the difference between the means at baseline and at outcome. Beginning with the mean and standard deviation of the measure for the sample at baseline, this pure number reflects the number of standard deviations the measure has changed at follow-up and allows different measures to be compared (Table 14–1).

INSTRUMENTS USED IN THE ASSESSMENT OF PERSONALITY DISORDERS

The instruments discussed as follows are divided first by measurement perspective and second by measurement domain. Although there are no pub-

Table 14–1. Effect sizes for specific measures used in at least two studies

Study	Target complaints	BDI	HSRS or GAS	General symptoms	IIP	Social adjustment
Alden 1989	1.31					
Karterud et al. 1992			0.46	0.82		
Stevenson et al.1992				0.94		
Diguer et al. 1993		1.67	2.41			
Piper et al. 1993				1.17		0.64
Winston et al. 1994	2.28			0.70		0.86
Hoglend 1993			2.51			
Linehan 1994			1.36			1.07
Monroe-Blum et al. 1995				1.00		0.49
Hardy et al. 1995		1.84		1.24	1.53	
Krawitz 1997			1.66	2.33		
Barber 1997						
AVPD		1.32			0.88	
OCPD		2.21			0.41	
Wilberg et al. 1998			1.45	0.55	0.52	
Rosenthal et al. 1999					0.52	
Bateman et al. 1999		2.05		0.62	1.58	
Mean effect size	**1.80**	**1.82**	**1.64**	**1.04**	**0.91**	**0.765**
±SD	**0.48**	**0.35**	**0.76**	**0.54**	**0.53**	**0.25**

Note. AVPD=avoidant personality disorder; BDI=Beck Depression Inventory; GAS=Global Assessment of Severity; HSRS=Health–Sickness Rating Scales; IIP=Inventory of Interpersonal Problems; OCPD=obsessive-compulsive personality disorder; SD=standard deviation.

Source. Earlier versions of this table and references appeared in Perry and Bond 2000 and Perry et al. 1999.

lished outcome studies for some of the instruments (especially diagnostic instruments) discussed in this section, the instruments could be used as outcome measures with appropriate modification of the time interval assessed. Some instruments that are used in personality research have been omitted because the rationale and/or data for assessing improvement in personality disorders is not yet developed or requires further work.

Observer-Rated: Personality Diagnostic Interviews

A number of structured and semistructured interviews were devised with the advent of DSM-III and have been updated with each revision of the DSM. Although these measures are often used in studies for initial diagnoses, they also yield continuous (dimensional) scores for each personality disorder type that generally have high reliability and potential sensitivity to change. Data are presented on the latest version of these instruments whenever they are available.

Diagnostic Interview for Personality Disorders

The Diagnostic Interview for Personality Disorders (DIPD) (Zanarini et al. 1987) is a structured interview to assess DSM-III-R personality disorders. A DSM-IV version of the instrument has been modified for administration at 6-month intervals in follow-along studies. It assesses each personality disorder criterion on a month-by-month basis. It requires 2 years' duration of symptoms for items to be scored. The DIPD has 108 sets of questions, each of which elicits a DSM-IV personality disorder criterion. It takes 90 minutes to administer.

Interrater reliability was quite high for the DSM-III version, with $\kappa=0.89$ for the presence of any personality disorder and median $\kappa=0.92$ (range, 0.52–1.0) for the individual types. The 1-week retest reliability was $\kappa=0.58$ for the presence of any personality disorder type, with median $\kappa=0.68$ (range, 0.46–0.85) for the specific types. Reliability of the follow-up version has not yet been published but is reported to be high.

Initial observations using the DSM-IV versions have suggested that concordance between the baseline patient interview version and the first month of follow-up, using the follow-up version, is only moderate, characterized by a significant drop in the base rate of personality disorders. Such large changes in a short period suggest that further work is needed to separate measurement issues from true change.

International Personality Disorders Examination

The International Personality Disorders Examination (IPDE) (Loranger et al. 1994) is a structured interview for assessing DSM-III-R personality disorders. It includes 157 items grouped under the areas of work, self, interpersonal relationships, affects, reality testing, and impulse control. It has been used at centers in 11 countries with appropriate language versions. It requires 5 years' duration for items to be scored positively. The IPDE takes 90 minutes to administer. It costs $129 per kit (includes instruction manual, 25 screening questionnaires, 25 scoring booklets, and 50 answer sheets) (American Psychiatric Association 2000).

Interrater reliability of the IDPE was as follows: for 8 categorical diagnoses, median $\kappa=0.755$ (range, 0.51–0.87); for diagnosing any specific personality disorder type, $\kappa=0.70$; for the 13 dimensional scores, median correlation was 0.89 (range, 0.79–0.94). Test-retest reliability at 6 months yielded the following stability coefficients: for any specific personality disorder type, $\kappa=0.63$; for 10 categorical diagnoses, median $\kappa=0.59$ (range, 0.28–0.72); and for 13 dimensional scores, median intraclass $r=0.77$ (range, 0.68–0.92). The relationship of these changes to any specific treatment is unreported, as is the amount of improvement. Lenzenweger (1999) showed that change in personality disorder ratings using the IPDE over a 3-year period was not significantly affected by the presence of an Axis I disorder.

Findings from Pilkonis et al. (1995) showed a lower interrater reliability of an overall diagnosis of any personality disorder ($\kappa=0.55$). Compared with a criterion best-estimate diagnosis made by a panel of clinicians, the level of agreement was $\kappa=0.18$ (56% overall agreement), with good positive predictive value (0.92) but poor negative predictive value (0.41), indicating that the interview yielded a high proportion of false-negative results compared with the best-estimate diagnoses. In a sample of college students, Lenzenweger (1999) also found that the 1-year stability of the categorical diagnosis of any personality disorder was only moderate ($\kappa=0.45$), whereas the median Pearson's r for the 11 personality disorder dimensions was 0.51 (range, 0.44–0.74). Because the sample was not receiving any treatment, the degree of change over 1 year suggests that changes in IPDE diagnoses and scores may represent state changes almost as much as changes in personality disorder traits.

Structured Clinical Interview for DSM-IV Axis II Personality Disorders

The Structured Clinical Interview for DSM-IV Axis II Personality Disorders (SCID-II) consists of a self-report screening personality questionnaire of 119 true-false items, followed by a structured interview of 148 items. Each personality disorder criterion is rated on a scale of 0–3 (absent, subthreshold, threshold, or true). The SCID-II assesses 12 personality disorder types, including two in the DSM-IV appendix (passive-aggressive and depressive), plus personality disorder not otherwise specified. For an item to be scored as true, the characteristic should be present over a period of at least 5 years (excepting a few items, such as a suicide attempt). The SCID-II takes 90 minutes to administer. It costs $46 for a manual and five instruments. A computer version is also available.

Interrater reliability of the SCID-II for categorical diagnoses was as follows: for the presence of at least one personality disorder, $\kappa = 0.91$; for the 12 types, median $\kappa = 0.91$ (range, 0.48–0.98); and for dimensional scores, median intraclass $r = 0.94$ (range, 0.90–0.98) (Maffei et al. 1997). Test-retest reliability of the DSM-III-R version was determined on a large sample within a 2-week period of readministration at four sites (First et al. 1995). Results showed median $\kappa = 0.50$ (range, 0.28–0.76) for 11 specific personality disorder types. Dreessen and Arntz (1998) found similar short-term stabilities, whereas Vaglum et al. (1993) found that severe personality disorders (presence of any cluster A or B type) in day treatment were moderately stable after a mean of 2.8 years of follow-up (overall $\kappa = 0.65$).

Although the duration criterion is designed to detect traits, not sporadic events, it would make the SCID-II relatively insensitive to true change occurring over a shorter time period, such as a successful treatment of several years' duration. The high interrater reliability may have been biased upward by examining the results of the screening personality questionnaire beforehand (Maffei et al. 1997).

Structured Interview for DSM-IV Personality

The latest version of the Structured Interview for DSM-IV Personality (SIDP-IV) (Pfohl et al. 1997) is composed of 101 sets of questions divided into 10 topical sections, rather than into diagnostic sections. Each set of questions asks for examples. Each DSM-IV criterion is scored on a 4-point scale (not present, subthreshold, present, strongly present). A criterion is considered present if it has been predominantly true 50% of the time over the past 5 years. For symptoms to be scored, they must have been present for 5 years. The SIDP-IV takes 90 minutes to administer. It costs $21.95 per five instruments. A computer version is also available (American Psychiatric Association 2000).

Testing an earlier version, the SIDP-R, using DSM-III-R criteria, Pilkonis et al. (1995) obtained interrater reliability of an overall diagnosis of any personality disorder of $\kappa = 0.58$.

When the SIDP-R results were compared against a best-estimate diagnosis made by a panel of clinicians, the level of agreement was $\kappa = 0.37$ (75% overall agreement), with good positive predictive value (0.88) but poor negative predictive value (0.32), indicating that the interview yielded a high proportion of false-negative results compared with the best-estimate diagnoses (Pilkonis et al. 1995). Trull et al. (1998) examined a sample of borderline and nonborderline patients at initial evaluation and after 2 years. The stability correlation for the number of borderline personality disorder features was low ($r=0.28$), with a diagnostic agreement of $\kappa=0.03$, and with the scores generally lower after 2 years.

Observer-Rated: Symptoms and Behaviors

Global Assessment of Functioning and Health-Sickness Rating Scales

The Global Assessment of Functioning (GAF) and the Health-Sickness Rating Scales (HSRS) (Luborsky et al. 1993), from which it was derived, are global scales with anchor-point descriptions for each 10-point range. Either scale can be used to rate current functioning in the last week or the best level of functioning in the past 2 years, after any clinical interview.

Both scales mix symptoms, distress, and social role impairment and are highly correlated, usually about $r=0.90$ or above (Luborsky et al. 1993). The scales are quite popular and generally obtain reliabilities above intraclass $r=0.70$ in most studies.

Although they are very valuable for characterizing how symptomatic or impaired an individual is, they do not differentiate the contributing factors, and hence their results may fluctuate widely (for further details see Chapter 9, in this volume).

Observer-Rated: Social Role Functioning

Social Adjustment Scale

The interview schedule of the Social Adjustment Scale (SAS) (Weissman et al. 1971) assesses seven domains of social functioning, including work, student or household roles, social and leisure activities, relationships with extended family, relationship with spouse, parental functioning, and functioning in the family unit. Each area is assessed for the past 2 months on a 5-point scale anchored with descriptions from severe impairment to no impairment. A longitudinal version (LIFE-Psychosocial Functioning) (Keller et al. 1987) is also available with some modifications for tracking month-by-month changes in functioning for each social role.

The interrater reliability of the longitudinal version was median intraclass $r=0.79$ (range, 0.58–0.91) for the current month, and $r=0.77$ (range, 0.63–0.87) for the past 6 months.

In outcome studies of psychotherapy with personality disorders, the mean effect size of the combined observer-rated and self-report versions is 0.77, the smallest of all measures in Table 14–1 (for further details see Chapter 9, in this volume).

Observer-Rated: Core Psychopathology and Mechanisms

Observer-rated measures of core psychopathology and mechanisms are underrepresented in outcome studies. Based on recent presentations at meetings, measures for which findings are likely to be published soon include the Defense Mechanism Rating Scales (DMRS), the Core Conflictual Relationship Theme (CCRT), Wishes and Fears, and the Psychodynamic Conflict Rating Scales (PCRS).

Self-Report: Personality Disorder Diagnostic Assessments

Self-report diagnostic assessment instruments for personality disorder are generally intended to assess the criteria or features of the DSM-IV personality disorder types. Some instruments are designed with broader personality theory in mind in attempts to assess general personality traits in addition to traits more tied to the DSM systems. They have been used as screening instruments for selecting probable cases or noncases and as general measures of personality psychopathology. They do not generally yield categorical diagnoses that are highly comparable to interview methods.

Dimensional Assessment of Personality Pathology Basic Questionnaire

The Dimensional Assessment of Personality Pathology Basic Questionnaire (DAPP-BQ) (Livesley et al. 1989) is a 290-item questionnaire that measures 18 personality dimensions derived from an analysis of prototypical features of personality disorders. Each item is scored on a 5-point Likert-type scale.

Internal consistencies are high (range, 0.84–0.94) in a clinical sample. Similarly, retest stability figures are high over 6 weeks (range, 0.81–0.93). Clark et al. (1996) found that the average correlation with similar scales on the Schedule for Nonadaptive and Adaptive Personality (SNAP) (see later) was $r=0.53$ (range, 0.01 to 0.78).

The instrument has largely been used in cross-sectional research, such as in twin studies of the genetics of personality traits, and its change characteristics with time or treatment have yet to be reported.

Millon Clinical Multiaxial Inventory

The Millon Clinical Multiaxial Inventory (MCMI-III) (American Psychiatric Association 2000) was devised according to Millon's theory of personality to assess the DSM personality disorder types for DSM-III (MCMI-I),

DSM-III-R (MCMI-II), and DSM-IV (MCMI-III). The MCMI-II has 175 items in a true-false format divided into 13 personality disorder scales and 9 symptom scales tapping anxiety, depression, thought disorder, etc. It takes 20–30 minutes to complete. It costs $225 for a manual, 10 test booklets, 50 answer sheets, and answer keys. There is a computerized version.

Lenzenweger (1999) examined 250 college students with the MCMI-II in their freshman, sophomore, and senior years. The stability for the dimension of total personality disorder features was 0.77 after 1 year and 0.70 after 3 years, with median and ranges for 11 individual dimensions of $r=0.74$ (range, 0.63–0.78) at 1 year and $r=0.64$ (range, 0.55–0.73) at 3 years.

Comparison of the MCMI-I to other instruments yielded low correlations (Perry 1992). Millon (1992) reported that the most recent version has improved reliability and scale separation over its precursor. Lenzenweger (1999) found that the effect sizes representing naturalistic change in college students were small at 1 and 3 years (0.26 and 0.39) for a group without personality disorders but were moderate for a group with probable personality disorder (0.44 and 0.64).

Personality Diagnostic Questionnaire for DSM-IV

The Personality Diagnostic Questionnaire for DSM-IV (PDQ-4) (Hyler 1994) is a revision of early versions (PDQ, PDQ-R) to assess the 10 personality disorder types in DSM-IV, as well as 2 types in the DSM-IV appendix. The latest version has 100 true-false items, presented in random order as to personality disorder type. It takes 20–30 minutes to complete. It has been translated into several languages, and a computer version exists. The PDQ-4 can be ordered on the Internet (http://www.pdq4.com/).

An Italian version was tested on a large sample of outpatients. An average internal consistency for the 12 scales of 0.64 (range, 0.46–0.74, κ-r-20 formula) was found (Fossati et al. 1998). Using the PDQ-R, Trull et al. (1998) examined a sample of patients with and without borderline personality disorder at initial assessment and after 2 years. The stability correlation for the number of borderline personality disorder features was $r=0.54$, with a diagnostic agreement of $\kappa=0.34$, and with the scores generally lower after 2 years.

The Clinical Significance Scale was designed to minimize false diagnoses. However, more research is needed to establish this characteristic. Using the suggested cutoff scores, the PDQ-4 diagnosed a mean of 4.3 types compared with the SCID-II version 2.0, which diagnosed a mean of 1.0 types in the sample; the correlation between the respective scales was low (median $r=0.36$; range, 0.19–0.42). Agreement on the presence of any personality disorder was also low ($\kappa=0.10$). These results showed that the PDQ-4 was not a substitute for a structured diagnostic interview (Fossati et al. 1998).

Personality Assessment Inventory

The Personality Assessment Inventory (PAI) (Morey 1991) is a 344-item questionnaire devised as a general diagnostic aid and measure of psychopathology. There are 22 scales, including 11 assessing major syndromal symptoms, 2 assessing interpersonal phenomena, 5 assessing data useful for treatment consideration, and 4 assessing test validity. A 160-item short form covering the full scales only is also available. Two scales and their subscales cover personality types: Borderline Features, which includes affective instability, identity problems, negative relationships with others, and impulsive self-harm; and Antisocial Features, which includes egocentricity and poor empathy, and stimulus seeking. The two interpersonal scales reflect the two major dimensions of the circumplex model of personality: dominating and controlling versus meekly submissive, and warm and affiliative versus cold and rejecting. Items are scored on a 4-point Likert-type scale. The PAI requires up to an hour to complete. Norms are available with t scores for the general adult population and instructions for interpreting test profiles (Morey 1996).

The median internal consistency of the PAI full scales and subscales were originally reported as 0.80 and 0.70 (Morey 1991), whereas a more recent study reported a median of 0.82 for the full scales and 0.66 for subscales (Boone 1998). Median short-term stability ranged from 0.73 to 0.85 for full scales, 0.77–0.80 for subscales, and 0.60–0.90 for the personality scales, depending on sample (Morey 1991). There was good discrimination between the Borderline Features and Antisocial Features scales in clinical samples.

From the standpoint of its construction, psychometrics, and availability of population-sampled norms, the PAI is a promising instrument. However, although it is intended as a general diagnostic aid, it includes only two specific personality disorder types, thus limiting its coverage in a mixed personality disorder population. Furthermore, data are yet unreported regarding long-term change in treated samples, including state versus trait change characteristics.

Schedule for Nonadaptive and Adaptive Personality

The SNAP (Clark 1993) assesses 12 clinical traits and 3 broader temperament scales, derived from clinically identified personality disorder criteria.

The scales generally have good internal consistency, with median $\alpha = 0.81$ (range, 0.71–0.92), and good retest reliability, with median 1-week stability $r = 0.79$ (range, 0.70–0.86), in inpatients. The average interscale correlations are low, suggesting that the dimensions have good separation. Clark et al. (1996) found that the average correlation with similar scales on the SNAP was $r=0.53$ (range, 0.01–0.78), indicating good convergent validity.

The SNAP has largely been used in cross-sectional research, and its use as a change measure is yet to be reported.

Wisconsin Personality Inventory

The Wisconsin Personality Inventory (WISPI) (Klein et al. 1993) is a self-report questionnaire that assesses 240 items each on a 10-point Likert-type scale. Subjects are asked to rate themselves as usual over the past 5 years. It yields 11 scales, converted to z scores, each representing a personality disorder type based on interpersonal themes representative of 11 DSM-III-R types but formulated according to L. Benjamin's theory of the structural analysis of social behavior. The WISPI takes 60 minutes to complete. It is copyrighted and is available for free use.

The scales have high internal consistency, with median $\alpha=0.90$ (range, 0.84–0.96). Their 2-week retest reliabilities were also high, with median $r=0.88$ (range, 0.71–0.94). The stabilities were somewhat lower at 3–4 months, with median $r=0.75$ (range, 0.69–0.80); the mean scores of all but one scale were significantly lower, consistent with effects due to state changes (Barber and Morse 1994). The mean raw correlations between the WISPI and the same scales of other self-report measures were 0.39 (range, −0.26–0.79) for the MCMI-I and 0.69 (range, 0.37–0.79) for the PDQ (Klein et al. 1993); the correlations with the dimensional scores of structured interviews were somewhat lower: median $r=0.46$ (range, 0.15–0.65) for the SCID-II-R, and median $r=0.39$ (range, 0.11–0.58) for the IPDE (Barber and Morse 1994).

In a psychotherapy study of avoidant personality disorder (AVPD) and obsessive-compulsive personality disorder (OCPD), Barber et al. (1997) found that after up to 52 sessions, only 38.5% of subjects with AVPD and 15.4% of subjects with OCPD still scored above the cutoff for their respective personality disorders. Curiously, the change in personality disorder status was evident by the fourth month of treatment for OCPD. Such rapid improvement in a personality disorder type known for persistence also suggests that the instrument may be sensitive to state effects, such as distress or depression at time of seeking treatment, and thus may be susceptible to false-positive diagnoses. This is consistent with the authors' finding of a large decrease in scores on the Beck Depression Inventory with treatment for both OCPD and AVPD. On the two personality disorder dimensional scores, by treatment termination, the OCPD subjects had changed significantly, whereas the AVPD subjects showed a nonsignificant trend. Computerized scoring of the WISPI is available, because hand scoring is time consuming (American Psychiatric Association 2000).

Self-Report: Symptoms and Behaviors

Beck Depression Inventory

The Beck Depression Inventory (BDI) (Beck et al. 1961), a 21-item questionnaire, is the most commonly used measure of depressive symptoms in psychotherapy research. The original split-half reliability (Pearson's r) was 0.86, and the scale has been widely validated against clinical ratings of depression. It is used most commonly as a change measure. In studies of depressed patients, those with concurrent personality disorders generally demonstrate less change than those without personality disorders. Nonetheless, even patients with cluster C personality disorders not selected for depression may show large improvement on the BDI (Barber et al. 1997), consistent with changes in distress levels associated with treatment seeking. As demonstrated in Table 14–1, the BDI yields one of the highest mean effect sizes of all measures: 1.82 (for further details see Chapter 10, in this volume).

Symptom Checklist-90-R

The 90-item Symptom Checklist-90–Revised (SCL-90-R) (Derogatis 1983) questionnaire and its 55-item short version, the Brief Symptom Inventory (BSI), are widely used as measures of overall distress. Items are scored on a 5-point scale. Studies usually report a summary score, the Global Severity Index (GSI), because the subscales assess specific symptom dimensions that are not specific to personality disorders. The mean baseline GSI score varies widely from around 2.0 in samples of inpatients with severe personality disorders to around 1.0 in samples of outpatients with less severe cluster C disorders. Thus, as shown in Table 14–1, there is a wide range of effects sizes (0.55–2.33) (for further details see Chapter 9, in this volume).

Minnesota Multiphasic Personality Inventory

The Minnesota Multiphasic Personality Inventory (MMPI) was devised as a general self-report measure of psychopathology based on the association of each item with a particular criterion group (e.g., schizophrenia) The revised MMPI-2 has 567 true-false items, and a version for adolescents (MMPI-A) has 478. The instrument has eight basic criterion group scales (hypochondriasis, depression, hysteria, psychopathic deviance, paranoia, psychasthenia, schizophrenia, and mania), two clinical personality scales (masculinity-femininity and social introversion), and three validity scales (lie, infrequency, and correction-defensiveness), which can be used to interpret the validity or adjust the raw scores for response tendencies.

Scoring produces raw scores and t scores, which adjust the mean of each scale to 50, with a standard deviation equaling 10 points. The internal consistencies of the basic criterion group scales range from 0.34 to 0.88, and 1-week retest validity ranges from 0.58 to 0.92. There are a large number of empirically derived scales that researchers have developed over the years from the total pool of items. Norms for different demographic and clinical groups are available (Butcher et al. 1989; Greene 1991). Administration requires up to 1.5 hours, although both hand-scored and computer versions are available.

The MMPI was one of the first and most successful all-inclusive self-report assessments. However, the legacy of its origin makes it nonspecific to any of the DSM personality disorders, with the partial exception of antisocial personality disorder, which overlaps with the psychopathic deviance scale construct. Researchers have coped with this by developing new scales, drawing from the total item pool. Nevertheless, because of the time consumed in administration and scoring, the training required for interpretation, and the instrument's relative lack of application in longitudinal research on personality disorders, the MMPI-2 is not well suited for use in assessing change in personality disorders.

Self-Report: Social Role Functioning

Social Adjustment Scale-SR

A self-report questionnaire version of the Social Adjustment Scale interview schedule, the Social Adjustment Scale-SR (SAS-SR) (Weissman and Bothwell 1976) assesses overall adjustment and the same six social role areas as the parent observer-rated instrument.

In a sample of depressed outpatients, the agreement with the interviewer version was good for overall adjustment ($r=0.72$) but lower for the six role areas (median $r=0.55$; range, 0.40–0.76). In a later study of symptomatic women, a 45-item modified version (the SAS-M) correlated moderately well with the interview version on overall adjustment ($r=0.80$), whereas for the six domains the median was $r=0.74$ (range, 0.52–0.79) (Cooper et al. 1982).

Subjects rated themselves as more impaired than did the interviewer (Cooper et al 1982), which confirmed the original finding by Weissman and Bothwell (1976). Furthermore, change on the self-report version was highly correlated with changes on both observer-rated symptoms using the Psychiatric Status Examination ($r=0.54$) and self-reported mood using the Profile of Mood States ($r=0.49$), suggesting that the self-report version is susceptible to state effects. As indicated in Table 14–1, combined interview and questionnaire data from psychotherapy studies of personality disorders yielded a mean effect size of 0.77. This is the smallest effect size of all the measures shown in Table 14–1 and is also less than the improvement (effect size = 1.02) found after 8 weeks of treatment in the sample of depressed patients reported by Weissman and Bothwell (1976).

Inventory of Interpersonal Problems

The Inventory of Interpersonal Problems (IIP) (Horowitz et al. 1988) is a 127-item questionnaire that assesses interpersonal situations that the subject finds either hard to do or that he or she does too much. Each item is rated on a 5-point Likert-type scale and yields scores on six dimensions reflecting things that are hard to do (H) or that are done too much (T): H. assertive, H. submissive, H. intimate, H. sociable, T. responsible, and T. controlling. The IIP takes 20–30 minutes to complete. A 64-item version (IIP-64) was developed that represents the subject's overall score on a two-dimensional circumplex grid (Alden et al. 1990). Each of eight octants on the grid has a clinical description. The 64-item version takes 10–15 minutes to complete. A 32-item version (IIP-32) takes 5–10 minutes to complete. A complete kit includes a manual, a package of 64-item question sheets, a package of 64-item scoring sheets, and a package of 32-item question/scoring sheets. It can be obtained from the Psychological Corporation at a cost of $105.00.

The scales have good internal consistency, with a median $\alpha = 0.87$ (range, 0.82–0.93).

As indicated in Table 14–1, in psychotherapy studies of personality disorders, the mean effect size improvement on the IIP was 0.91, representing change in the mean item score after treatment. More research is needed to establish the validity of this instrument.

Self-Report: Core Psychopathology and Mechanisms

The area of self-report measures on core psychopathology and mechanisms is relatively underrepresented in outcome studies, partly because most research has focused on surface traits and functioning. However, some data on change have emerged for at least one measure. Measures for which data are likely to appear in the future include the Defense Style Questionnaire (DSQ), the Dysfunctional Attitudes Scale (DAS), and the Depressive Experiences Questionnaire (DEQ).

Defense Style Questionnaire

The original DSQ consists of 88 items, each rated on a 9-point Likert-type scale. The items were selected to reflect conscious derivatives of 29 defense mechanisms. These are arranged according to the hierarchy of defenses and are divided into four defense styles: maladaptive (e.g., acting out, passive-aggression), image-distorting (e.g., splitting, devaluation), self-sacrificing (e.g., pseudoaltruism, reaction formation), and adaptive (e.g., humor, suppression). Ten items also assess social desirability.

Because each defense is represented by only a few items, and because of problems validating the individual defenses, only the four defense styles or an overall defensive functioning score is generally used. The 6-month retest reliability of the styles ranged from 0.68 to 0.73. A shorter 36-item version has been proposed by Andrews and Pollock (1989) based on their finding of a three-factor structure (maladaptive, neurotic, and adaptive). When compared with clinical defense ratings, the DSQ defense styles correlate only modestly with their clinical counterparts (Bond et al. 1989). Both maladaptive and image-distorting styles have been associated with personality disorders, especially borderline personality disorder.

Perry and Hoglend (1998) found that the DSQ was factorially independent of Axis I and II and global functioning but overlapped with both subjective distress (SCL-90-R) and clinical ratings of defenses, whereas the clinical ratings were independent of all other measures. This is consistent with the idea that subjective distress may distort conscious reporting of defensive functioning. Furthermore, Hoglend and Perry (1998) found that baseline observer ratings of defense were better predictors of recovery of major depression after 6 months than were the DSQ or personality disorder diagnosis. An outcome study of patients treated for major depression found that the maladaptive style improved significantly after 6 months, indicating a sizable state effect (Akkerman et al. 1992); however, those continuing in treatment for up to 2 years continued to show reduction in the maladaptive style, more consistent with trait change (Akkerman et al. 1999). Overall, the DSQ clearly taps some aspects of defensive functioning, especially at both maladaptive and adaptive ends of the continuum, although with less precision or predictive ability than clinical ratings. The defense styles have more apparent validity than the individual constituent defenses, but the factor structure varies somewhat across different samples. Nonetheless, the DSQ is promising for assessing change in underlying defensive functioning in personality disorders.

DISCUSSION

A sizable body of empirical literature is being amassed on the personality disorders and other associated characteristics. However, most of this information is gathered at one point in time, without relationship to subsequent treatment, and without determination of sample characteristics at outcome. The most meaningful measures will be those that are relatively stable in naturalistic follow-up but that demonstrate much more change after treatment, especially more than a control condition. An important caveat is that whenever any two measures have been compared, only moderate to low levels of concordance between them are obtained. This has the clear implication that one cannot substitute a near-neighbor measure at follow-up for the original measure used at baseline without introducing a sizable amount of measurement error. The measures described are all candidates for acceptable outcome measures, but further work is required on many to determine their usefulness in documenting improvement.

Table 14–1 compares the within-condition effect sizes from controlled and uncontrolled treatment studies of personality disorders, arranged in descending order of magnitude. The measures included have been used in at least two studies, thus allowing the calculation of a mean and standard deviation. All means reflect moderate to large amounts of change. Perry et al. (1999) found that overall change was of similar magnitude in both controlled and uncontrolled studies, and change was larger than that observed in the few control conditions, at least for self-reporting. Target complaints and symptom measures demonstrated the most change, whereas interpersonal and social role functioning demonstrated the least. To-date change in core measures of psychopathology is largely unknown. Finally, Table 14–1 does not include some observations that are quite important in the outcome of disorders like borderline personality disorder, such as suicide attempts, self-mutilation, hospital days used, and reduction in medication use, because these are not standardized measures per se.

Looking toward future studies, we reiterate some previous recommendations (Perry and Bond 2000; Perry et al. 1999). Outcome should be assessed using both self-reporting and observer-rated methods. Assessments should include the three standard assessment domains, as well as core psychopathology and mechanisms whenever possible. These should reflect the phenomena targeted by the theoretical perspective of the treatment but may include other theoretical perspectives as well. Assessment at multiple points in time will help separate state and true trait changes. Longer-term follow-up after treatment (1 year or more) is essential to determine the durability of change. Finally, treatment process and outcome should be assessed in the same studies. Whenever therapeutic interventions are associated with responses in core mechanisms and then both with ultimate outcome, a study will provide the kind of data most likely to improve treatments. In this way, improvements in outcome assessment will facilitate the process of improving treatments.

Personality disorders continue to be one of the stepchildren of psychiatry, in terms of the scientific resources devoted to their study and improvement of their treatments. The result is that our understanding of their psychopathology often remains fixed on a superficial focus on diagnostic criteria, and assessment is left to similar diagnostic measures and off-the-shelf instruments developed for other reasons. Part of this problem has been the lack of intensive study of the personality disorders that is hypothesis driven, based on particular theories of their etiology and mechanisms. To paraphrase Kant, measurement without theory is blind. A secondary result is that the ability to assess the efficacy and effectiveness of existing or new treatments has been hampered by a focus on symptoms common to many disorders and a failure to assess core psychopathology that may be specific to the personality disorders. As the rest of medicine clearly shows, advances in assessment often precede developments in the etiology and treatment of a disorder. Keeping this in mind, the survey in this chapter demonstrates that, even with imperfect assessments, it is clear that studies demonstrate beneficial changes in personality disorders with psychotherapy.

REFERENCES

Akkerman K, Carr V, Lewin T: Changes in ego defenses with recovery from depression. J Nerv Ment Dis 180:634–638, 1992

Akkerman K, Lewin TJ, Carr VJ: Long-term changes in defense style among patients recovering from major depression. J Nerv Ment Dis 187:80–87, 1999

Alden L: Short-term structured treatment for avoidant personality disorder. J Consult Clin Psychol 57(6):756–764, 1989

Alden LE, Wigins JS, Pincus AL: Construction of circumplex scales for the Inventory of Interpersonal Problems. J Pers Assess 55:521–536, 1990

American Psychiatric Association: Handbook of Psychiatric Measures. Washington, DC, American Psychiatric Press, 2000

Andrews G, Pollock C, Stewart G: The determination of defense style by questionnaire. Arch Gen Psychiatry 46:455–460, 1989

Barber JP, Morse J: Validation of the Wisconsin Personality Disorders Inventory with the SCID-II and PDE. J Personal Disord 8:307–319, 1994

Barber JP, Morse JQ, Krakauer ID, et al: Change in obsessive-compulsive and avoidant personality disorders following time-limited supportive-expressive therapy. Psychotherapy 34:133–143, 1997

Bateman A, Fonagy P: Effectiveness of partial hospitalization in the treatment of borderline personality disorder: a randomized controlled trial. Am J Psychiatry 156(10):1563–1569, 1999

Beck AT, Ward CH, Mendelson M, et al: An inventory for measuring depression. Arch Gen Psychiatry 4:561–571, 1961

Bond M, Perry JC, Gautier M, et al: Validating the self-report of defense styles. J Personal Disord 3:101–112, 1989

Boone D: Internal consistency reliability of the Personality Assessment Inventory with psychiatric inpatients. J Clin Psychol 54:839–843, 1998

Butcher JN, Dahlstrom WG, Graham JR, et al: Minnesota Multiphasic Personality Inventory–2 (MMPI-2): Manual for Administration and Scoring. Minneapolis, University of Minnesota Press, 1989

Clark LA: Manual for the Schedule for Nonadaptive and Adaptive Personality. Minneapolis, University of Minnesota Press, 1993

Clark LA, Livesley WJ, Schroeder ML, et al: Convergence of two systems for assessing specific traits of personality disorders. Psychol Assess 8:294–303, 1996

Cooper P, Osborn M, Gath D, et al: Evaluation of a modified self-report measure of social adjustment. Br J Psychiatry 141:68–75, 1982

Derogatis LR: SCL-90-R: Administration, Scoring, Procedures Manual II. Towson, MD, Clinical Psychometric Research, 1983

Diguer L, Barber JP, Luborsky L: Three concomitants: personality disorders, psychiatric severity, and outcome of dynamic psychotherapy of major depression. Am J Psychiatry 150(8):1246–1248, 1993

Dreessen L, Arntz A: Short-interval test-retest interrater reliability of the Structured Clinical Interview for DSM-III-R Personality Disorders (SCID-II) in outpatients. J Personal Disord 12:138–148, 1998

First MB, Spitzer RL, Gibbon M, et al: The Structured Clinical Interview for DSM-III-R Personality Disorders (SCID-II). Part II: multi-site test-retest reliability study. J Personal Disord 9:92–104, 1995

Fossati A, Maffei C, Bagnato M, et al: Brief Communication: criterion validity of the Personality Diagnostic Questionnaire-4+ (PDQ-4+) in a mixed psychiatric sample. J Personal Disord 12:172–178, 1998

Greene RL: MMPI/MMPI-2: An Interpretive Manual. Boston, MA, Allyn & Bacon, 1991

Hardy GE, Barkham M, Shapiro DA, et al: Credibility and outcome of cognitive-behavioural and psychodynamic-interpersonal psychotherapy. Br J Clin Psychol 34(part 4):555–569, 1995

Hoglend P: Transference interpretations and long-term change after dynamic psychotherapy of brief to moderate length. Am J Psychother 47(4):494–507, 1993

Hoglend P, Perry JC: Defensive functioning predicts improvement in treated major depressive episodes. J Nerv Ment Dis 186:238–243, 1998

Horowitz LM, Rosenberg SE, Baer BA, et al: The Inventory of Interpersonal Problems: psychometric properties and clinical applications. J Consult Clin Psychol 56:885–892, 1988

Hyler SE: Personality Diagnostic Questionnaire C 4+ (PDQ-4+). New York, New York State Psychiatric Institute, 1994

Karterud S, Vaglum S, Friis S, et al: Day hospital therapeutic community treatment for patients with personality disorders: an empirical evaluation of the containment function. J Nerv Ment Dis 180(4):238–243, 1992

Keller M, Lavori PW, Friedman B, et al: Longitudinal Interval Follow-up Evaluation: a comprehensive method for assessing outcome in prospective longitudinal studies. Arch Gen Psychiatry 44:540–548, 1987

Klein MH, Benjamin LS, Rosenfeld R, et al: The Wisconsin Personality Disorders Inventory: development, reliability and validity. J Personal Disord 7:285–303, 1993

Krawitz R: A prospective psychotherapy outcome study. Aust N Z J Psychiatry 31(4):465–473, 1997

Lenzenweger MF: Stability and change in personality disorder features: the Longitudinal Study of Personality Disorders. Arch Gen Psychiatry 56:1009–1015, 1999

Linehan MM, Tutek DA, Heard HL, et al: Interpersonal outcome of cognitive behavioral treatment for chronically suicidal borderline patients. Am J Psychiatry 151(12):1771–1776, 1994

Livesley WJ, Jackson DN, Schroeder ML: A study of the factorial structure of personality pathology. J Personal Disord 3:292–306, 1989

Loranger AW, Sartorius N, Andreoli A, et al: The International Personality Disorder Examination (IPDE). The WHO/ADAMHA international pilot study of personality disorders. Arch Gen Psychiatry 51:215–224, 1994

Luborsky LL, Diguer L, Luborsky E, et al: Psychological health as a predictor of outcomes in dynamic and other psychotherapies. J Consult Clin Psychol 61:542–554, 1993

Maffei C, Fossati A, Agostoni I, et al: Inter-rater reliability and internal consistency of the Structured Clinical Interview for DSM-IV Axis II Personality Disorders (SCID-II), version 2.0. J Personal Disord 11:279–284, 1997

Millon T: Millon Clinical Multiaxial Inventory: I and II. Journal of Counseling and Development 70:421–426, 1992

Monroe-Blum H, Marziali E: A controlled trial of short-term group treatment for borderline personality disorder. Journal of Personality Disorders 9:190–198, 1995

Morey LC: Personality Assessment Inventory: Professional Manual. Odessa, FL, Psychological Assessment Resources, 1991

Morey LC: An Interpretive Guide to the Personality Assessment Inventory (PAI). Odessa, FL, Psychological Assessment Resources, 1996

Perry JC: Problems and considerations in the valid assessment of personality disorders. Am J Psychiatry 149:1645–1653, 1992

Perry JC, Bond M: Empirical studies of psychotherapy for personality disorders, in Psychotherapy of Personality Disorders. Edited by Gunderson JG, Gabbard GO (Review of Psychiatry Series, Oldham JM, Riba MB, series eds.). Washington, DC, American Psychiatric Press, 2000, pp 1–31

Perry JC, Hoglend P: Convergent and discriminant validity of overall defensive functioning. J Nerv Ment Dis 186:529–535 1998

Perry JC, Banon L, Ianni F: The effectiveness of psychotherapy for personality disorders. Am J Psychiatry 156:1312–1321, 1999

Pfohl B, Blum M, Zimmerman M: Structured Interview for DSM-IV Personality (SIDP-IV). Washington, DC, American Psychiatric Press, 1997

Pilkonis PA, Heape CL, Proietti JM, et al: The reliability and validity of two structured diagnostic interviews for personality disorders. Arch Gen Psychiatry 52:1025–1033, 1995

Piper WE, Rosie JS, Azim HF, et al: A randomized trial of psychiatric day treatment for patients with affective and personality disorders. Hosp Community Psychiatry 44(8):757–763, 1993

Rosenthal RN, Muran JC, Pinsker H, et al: Interpersonal change in brief supportive psychotherapy. J Psychother Pract Res 8(1):55–63, 1999

Stevenson J, Meares R: An outcome study of psychotherapy for patients with borderline personality disorder. Am J Psychiatry 149(3):358–362, 1992

Trull TJ, Useda D, Doan B-T, et al: Two-year stability of borderline personality measures. J Personal Disord 12:187–197, 1998

Vaglum P, Friis S, Karterud S, et al: Stability of the severe personality disorder diagnosis: a 2- to 5-year prospective study. J Personal Disord 7:348–353, 1993

Weissman MM, Bothwell S: Assessment of social adjustment by patient self-report. Arch Gen Psychiatry 33:1111–1115, 1976

Weissman MM, Paykel ES, Siegel R, et al: The social role performance of depressed women: a comparison with a normal sample. Am J Orthopsychiatry 41:390–405, 1971

Wilberg T, Karterud S, Urnes O, et al: Outcomes of poorly functioning patients with personality disorders in a day treatment program. Psychiatr Serv 49(11): 1462–1467, 1998

Winston A, Laikin M, Pollack J, et al: Short-term psychotherapy of personality disorders. Am J Psychiatry 151(2):190–194, 1994

Zanarini MC, Frankenburg FR, Chauncey DL, et al: The Diagnostic Interview for Personality Disorders: interrater and test-retest reliability. Compr Psychiatry 28:467–480, 1987

CHAPTER 15

Outcome Measurement in Sleep Disorders

Harry Baker, M.D.
Lloyd I. Sederer, M.D.

Sleep is a complex and reversible physiologic state of relative immobility and diminished awareness of external stimuli. Sleep exhibits highly organized cerebral activity and has many functions, including rest. Humans spend about one-third of their lives sleeping.

There are more than 80 sleep pathologies. Sleep-related symptoms are extremely common. Insomnia affects one of every three adults every year, making it possibly the most common symptom after pain. Sleep apnea is a prevalent condition that endangers the lives of about 4% of males and 2% of females. Sleep disorders also generate enormous costs to individuals and society. Sleep disorders adversely affect occupational performance and emotional well-being: they promote accidents, facilitate mood and social maladjustment, and may lead to or exacerbate medical and psychiatric disorders, thereby decreasing life expectancy and its quality. Sleep complaints are commonly voiced by psychiatric patients, because virtually all psychiatric disorders affect sleep.

The scientific study of sleep-related disorders has significantly enhanced the diagnosis and treatment of sleep pathologies. The evaluation of sleep complaints includes a medical history (including interview with the bed partner), physical evaluation, biochemical and imaging techniques, the use of questionnaires and scales, and sleep laboratory examinations. Sleep laboratories and clinics are commonly available for the evaluation of sleep states and their physiologic parameters. Polysomnography involves the electrophysiologic recording of brain electrical activity, eye movements, and muscle tone during sleep. Most of the time, polysomnography also includes air flow, respiratory effort, heart rate, oximetry, and leg movements. Other measures can be included, such as sound and video recording, esophageal pH, and penile tumescence. Polysomnography is considered the gold standard of sleep assessment, but it is expensive and cumbersome, and its results may not necessarily correlate with the patient's complaint (for example, a person might complain of unrefreshing sleep, yet have a normal sleep recording).

Another polysomnographic tool is the Multiple Sleep Latency Test (MSLT). It is a test designed to objectively measure daytime sleepiness. The MSLT measures the latency to fall asleep while lying down in a quiet and dark room. The subject is provided four to five opportunities to try to fall asleep at 2-hour intervals throughout the day. Its use has been shown to be reliable and valid in clinical and research situations. Its disadvantages are that it is a long, expensive, and labor-intensive test.

SLEEP PARAMETERS

A variety of sleep scales and questionnaires have been developed that are less expensive and easier to use than polysomnography. The most important sleep-related parameters they assess are listed below.

- *Sleep habits.* Sleep affects daytime functioning. What people do when awake affects the way they sleep. Naps, bedtime, arousal time, use of drugs (including caffeine, nicotine, and alcohol) and medication, activities before or during bedtime (exercise, watching TV, reading, sex, bath and toilet habits) and meals all influence sleep. Many sleep clinics have developed general sleep-habit questionnaires.
- *Sleep symptoms.* Because there are so many sleep disorders, some very specific—even pathognomonic—sleep symptoms, if not specifically searched for, may not be detected. Loud snoring, a cardinal symptom of sleep apnea, is not routinely questioned in psychiatric practice. Cataplexy (loss of muscle tone triggered by strong emotions) can suggest narcolepsy. A patient with sleep-related symptoms may benefit from the

administration of a comprehensive sleep questionnaire to supplement the psychiatric examination.

- *Sleep quality.* Sleep quality is a construct that physicians and patients often talk about. However, defining or objectively measuring the quality of sleep is a difficult task. Sleep quality is a function of patient perception of sleep onset, duration, perceived depth, symptoms, and level of restfulness after awakening.
- *Sleepiness.* There is a tendency to confuse tiredness or fatigue (which are related to physical fitness motivation and amount of activity) with sleepiness, which is the tendency to fall asleep. Mild sleepiness from insomnia is a symptom. More pronounced sleepiness, inducing sleepiness at inappropriate times (such as when working or driving), creates significant distress and functional impairment.
- *Specific disorders.* Specific tools have been developed to research specific disorders. For example, comprehensive questionnaires now exist for narcolepsy, sleep apnea, restless legs, and other disorders. Some tools focus on cognitive aspects (such as distortions or expectations) related to sleep that can be useful to address in treatment.

ASSESSMENT INSTRUMENTS

Although many instruments exist for the evaluation of sleep, there is no standardized or widely used questionnaire or scale for the evaluation of sleep habits and symptoms. Many sleep centers develop their own instruments according to their interests or focus. Some of the better-known instruments assess several of the areas mentioned above.

Sleep Log

The sleep log is a simple graphic registry of longitudinal data about sleep habits during a defined period of time. It is usually an 8½" × 11" or 8¾" × 14" sheet of paper with instructions and a 14-day by 24-hour grid in which each square represents 1 hour. The patient records four basic parameters of sleep: the time to bed, the estimated time(s) of sleep onset, the time(s) of awakening, and the time out of bed (Figure 15–1).

The typical symbols used in a sleep log are a downward arrow signaling getting into bed, an upward arrow signaling getting out of bed, filling in the space when the patient thinks he or she was asleep, and an empty space when the patient thinks he or she was awake.

The patient is instructed to record nighttime awakenings in the morning as best as he or she remembers, because recording them at night might keep him or her from falling asleep again. These data provide subjective

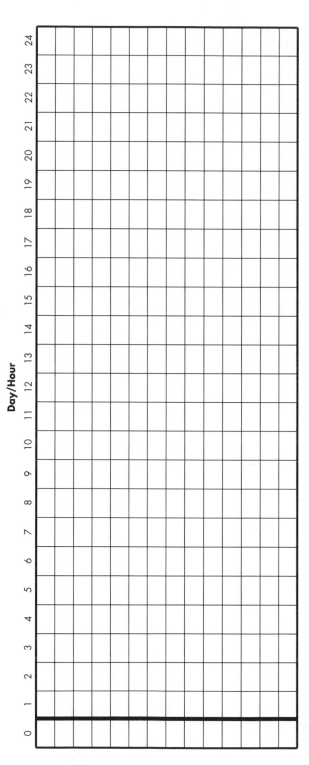

Instructions: Each morning and after each nap, please do the following:

1. Write in the first column today's date.
2. With an arrow(s) pointing down, mark the time(s) you got into bed.
3. Mark the time you think you were asleep by filling the appropriate space.
4. Leave empty when you think you were awake.
5. With an arrow(s) pointing up, mark the time(s) you got out of bed.

Figure 15–1.   Example of a sleep log.

information on sleep habits; sleep latency; number, time, and length of awakenings; final awakening time; and nap time(s).

Sleep log data can be complemented with other information of clinical interest such as exercise, sexual activity, substance use (e.g., caffeine, alcohol, nicotine, stimulants), or bath taking; specific symptoms (such as chest pain); or ratings of sleepiness or mood during waking hours. Therefore, sleep logs can vary significantly from center to center.

A sleep log can be used in patients with either insomnia or sleep-wake schedule disorders when the clinician wants to better understand sleep habits and identify any patterns that provoke symptoms. It takes 5–15 minutes to explain a sleep log to most patients. The vast majority of patients find it easy to fill out the appropriate log every day.

The sleep log can also be useful over an extended period of time. It can provide a baseline from the beginning of treatment. The graphic design can serve as a useful, educational tool to help the patient understand the relation between behaviors or habits and sleep, as well as the consequences of deviating from prescribed instructions.

The sleep log has several disadvantages. Because the patient is asked to respond (in the morning) without looking at a clock about what time he or she fell asleep, what time(s) he or she awakened during the night, and how long he or she was awake (each time) during the night, the information is highly subjective. Patients are commonly inaccurate in their reporting of the times they wake up and especially when they fall asleep. It has been demonstrated that healthy control subjects tend to overestimate, whereas insomniacs underestimate, their ability to sleep. There is also a tendency by some patients to exaggerate their symptoms. Because of its graphic nature, it is complicated to administer or score the sleep log with a computer. However, a computer program with optical recognition capabilities can be developed to process graphical information.

No studies that we know of address the psychometric properties of the sleep log. Such comparisons, when done, are usually against objective polysomnography or data obtained by a device, called an Actigraph, that records movements and has been proved to differentiate adequately between sleep and waking. However, the sleep log does provide data on the patient's perception of the problem that brought him or her to consultation, even if it is very different from objective data. The log also elicits the patient's perception of response (if any) to treatment.

In summary, the sleep log is a simple, user friendly, inexpensive, subjective tool for the evaluation and ongoing assessment of insomnia and sleep-wake schedule disorders that can be used in most clinical settings with most literate patients. It can be an educational aid in treatment. It is not yet easy to adapt the sleep log to research purposes.

Sleep Questionnaire and Assessment of Wakefulness

One of the earliest efforts to develop a sleep-oriented questionnaire was written by Miles at Stanford University in 1979. The Sleep Questionnaire and Assessment of Wakefulness (SQAW) (Miles 1982) is an 863-item questionnaire covering the following dimensions: sleep habits and symptoms, medical and psychiatric symptoms, dreaming experience, sleep history, daytime functioning, medical history, family medical and sleep history, education and occupation, and current living situation.

The SQAW is a self-report with several types of questions: Likert-type judgments, yes-no questions, check or mark items, queries of number of times or periods or amounts of time, and open-ended questions. The instrument evaluates a period covering the last 6 months. It is perhaps the most comprehensive way to evaluate sleep by self-reporting.

The target population for the SQAW is the individual patient (or control subject) for whom one wants to obtain comprehensive information on most aspects of sleep. There is no scoring manual. The measure can take up to 3 hours to complete. The SQAW has been translated into several languages (e.g., Spanish, Norwegian, French). There appear to be no studies evaluating its psychometric properties.

The SQAW has the advantage of providing an enormous amount of information, thereby helping to ensure that most sleep-related symptoms have been considered. It can be a very comprehensive resource for the development of new sleep-related questionnaires and scales.

The SQAW is not widely used because of its length, low completion rate among patients, and lack of specific focus. Although it can be presented on a computer screen, there is no program or threshold to establish pathology. However, a completed SQAW will enable the clinician to rapidly detect variances and thereby allow for careful further inquiry.

Sleep Disorders Questionnaire

In 1986, Alan Douglass and colleagues tried to simplify the SQAW. The result was the Sleep Disorders Questionnaire (SDQ) (Douglass et al. 1994). The language is easier to understand than that used in the SQAW, and the number of items was reduced to 175 questions that elicit pathognomonic symptoms of the major sleep disorders. There is a scoring manual and scoring software. Copyright release from the author is required.

SDQ questions are answered on a 1–5 scale that reflects frequency (never to always), agreement with a statement (strongly disagree to agree strongly), or quantity (e.g., numbers like sleep hours or cups of coffee per day). The SDQ queries sleep symptoms and habits over the last 6 months.

It takes between 60 and 90 minutes to complete, and patients with an eighth grade reading level can complete it. It has been used with a high degree of patient acceptability and provides satisfactory data quality. There are translations of the SDQ into several languages (e.g., Spanish, French, German).

Answers to the SDQ are coded for multivariate analysis, making it convenient to use for research. Its psychometric properties were studied by administering the SDQ to psychiatric inpatients ($n=108$) and to patients with polysomnographically confirmed diagnoses of sleep apnea ($n=158$), narcolepsy ($n=73$), and sleep periodic leg movement disorder ($n=96$). The results were compared with those of 84 control subjects. Internal consistency values measured by Cronbach's α were 0.855 for sleep apnea, 0.853 for narcolepsy, 0.800 for psychiatric inpatients, and 0.715 for periodic leg movements. Test-retest reliability (Pearson's r) values were 0.842 for sleep apnea, 0.753 for narcolepsy, 0.848 for psychiatric inpatients, and 0.817 for periodic leg movements. All correlations were highly significant ($P<0.00001$). This might mean that reducing the number of questions on the measure would still obtain a reasonable P value (e.g., $P<0.001$).

The SDQ has been well accepted. It provides adequate and reliable information on a broad range of sleep symptoms and habits.

The disadvantages of the SDQ include false-positive responses (e.g., a positive answer for a noncurrent symptom), and the fact that the psychiatric subscale is overly focused on depressive symptoms.

The SDQ is a user-friendly instrument focused on sleep symptoms. Its scales have been validated for sleep apnea, narcolepsy, sleep-related periodic leg movements, and depressive symptoms. It can be used in epidemiological studies, and there is now a computer scoring program, accessible via the Internet (http://www.sleeplabsoftware.com/sdq.html), which may prove to be a convenient tool.

Structured Interview for Sleep Disorders

There are two main classifications of sleep disorders: the International Classification of Sleep Disorders nosology (American Sleep Disorders Association 1990) and the DSM nosology (American Psychiatric Association 2000). The former is more specific and complex; the latter is simpler and clinically oriented, although it has been criticized for not considering physical disorders associated with sleep disturbance. The DSM classification lends itself to the development of structured clinical interviews.

In 1993, Schramm and colleagues developed an instrument for epidemiologic studies of the sleep disorders considered in Axes I and II of DSM-III-R. They called this instrument the Structured Interview for Sleep Disorders according to DSM-III-R (SIS-D). The SIS-D has three parts: 1) a brief, semistructured questionnaire for demographic, general health, drug, physical, and psychiatric history; 2) a structured interview for specific sleep symptoms; and 3) a summary score sheet to be completed by the rater after the interview.

The authors of the SIS-D recommend that it be used by experienced psychiatric interviewers with specific training in the instrument. Axis I diagnoses are coded as current (in the last 4 weeks) or lifetime, whereas Axis III sleep disorders can be evaluated only as current (and must be confirmed by polysomnography). The average time to administer the scale is 20–30 minutes, because interviewers can skip irrelevant sections.

Psychometric analysis of the SIS-D has high to excellent agreement among interviewers; Cohen's κ values are generally in the 0.80–0.90 range. Test-retest reliability is very high, ranging from 97% to 100%, with a mean κ of 0.77.

Adequate concordance was found with the SIS-D diagnoses and polysomnographic results. SIS-D concordance was highest for insomnia and lowest for dyssomnia not otherwise specified and sleep-wake schedule disorders (although the sample size was quite low).

SIS-D is a useful instrument for psychiatric research. Because it is in a format similar to the widely used Structured Clinical Interview for DSM-IV, it can also be used as a screening instrument in clinical practice, where it can be completed in 20–30 minutes.

The disadvantages of the SIS-D include the fact that it requires an advanced level of experience and training to administer properly. SIS-D is less specific on various nosologic entities because it is based on DSM-III-R instead of the International Classification of Sleep Disorders, the classification commonly used by most sleep disorders specialists. There is still not much experience in its use, and there is inadequate research experience because most research done in the area is by sleep specialists rather than general psychiatrists.

Sleep-Wake Activity Inventory

Rosenthal and colleagues in 1993 published the Sleep-Wake Activity Inventory (SWAI). The inventory was derived from existing psychiatric and sleep self-report scales.

The SWAI is answered using a Likert-type frequency scale ranging from 1 (always) to 9 (never). There are 59 questions that reflect six factors: excessive daytime sleepiness (EDS), psychic distress, social desirability, energy level, ability to relax, and sleep. The main focus of the questionnaire is excessive daytime sleepiness experienced by the subject over the last 7 days. The SWAI is simple to answer and takes about 15 minutes.

In a study of 421 individuals with sleep complaints and 133 without sleep complaints, Cronbach's coefficients for the six factors noted above were 0.89 for EDS, 0.72 for psychic distress, 0.76 for social desirability, 0.71 for energy level, 0.69 for ability to relax, and 0.69 for sleep. The items within each scale are moderately correlated (range, 0.4–0.5). In the same study, a subgroup of 20 sleep apnea patients answered the SWAI before and after successful treatment. Only two of the subscales changed significantly; therefore, the inclusion of the other four factors is questionable.

The main advantage of the SWAI is that it is validated by a comparison with the MSLT. The EDS subscale produced an r value of 0.386 ($P<0.001$) in a regression analysis for variables contributing to EDS measured by the MSLT. Analysis of the subscales showed that it is a valid and reliable questionnaire. However, it remains to be determined if social desirability or ability to relax are useful clinical correlations with EDS.

Stanford Sleepiness Scale

One of the earliest scales to measure sleepiness was the Stanford Sleepiness Scale (SSS) developed by Hoddes and associates (1973). The SSS was constructed to measure sleepiness during the day or night. It consists of seven statements sensitive to discrete changes in sleepiness. These range from 1 (feeling active and vital; wide awake) to 7 (almost in reverie, sleep onset soon, lost struggle to remain awake). The SSS is a quick (2–5 minutes), inexpensive, and easy-to-use tool that provides a numerical measure of the tendency to fall asleep at a defined moment. It does not provide information on sleepiness over a period of time. The SSS does not have a high individual consistency, because some people do not offer an accurate evaluation of their actual tendency to fall asleep at any moment. The SSS also has not been well studied. Its results are not significantly correlated with sleep latency as measured by the MSLT.

Epworth Sleepiness Scale

The author of the Epworth Sleepiness Scale (ESS) (Johns 1991) noted that sleepy people fall asleep inadvertently in activities with low levels of stimulation (like watching television), even if they do not want or intend to sleep. On the other hand, some people without excessive sleepiness choose (to combat boredom, kill time, or to socially withdraw) to sleep during the day. Therefore, frequency or length of sleep during daytime may not distinguish pathological sleepiness from voluntary daytime sleep. To distinguish both instances, the ESS asks subjects to rate, in recent everyday life, on a scale from 0 (never) to 3 (high), the chances they would fall asleep in eight different situations. These include situations where normal persons would likely fall asleep (such as lying down in the afternoon) and situations where only very sleepy persons would doze off (such as talking to someone, or in a car stopped for a few minutes in traffic).

The ESS can distinguish patients with sleep apnea and sleep disorders and snorers from control subjects without sleep disorders ($F=50.00$; $df=6,173$; $P<0.0001$). Insomniacs have significantly lower scores than do control subjects ($P<0.01$). The ESS can even differentiate patients with severe sleep apnea from those with moderate sleep apnea ($P<0.001$). It has been proved that the ESS is sensitive to changes in sleep apnea due to treatment. The ESS can distinguish snorers from patients with sleep apnea of different severity and provides a cutoff point for identifying persons with a significant sleep disorder. The ESS provides clinically relevant sleepiness levels, whereby 10 is a level for concern and 16 is a problem (scale from 0 to 24). Low scores on the ESS in patients with insomnia are consistent with a low sleep propensity, even when they are able to relax.

The authors have demonstrated that there is a good correlation between scores on the ESS and on the MSLT ($r=-0.514$; $N=27$; $P<0.01$; linear regression $SL=3.353$; this was -0.091 in the ESS score). However, the notion that the ESS correlates significantly with daytime sleep latency as measured by the MSLT has recently been challenged (Chervin and Aldrich 1999). An advantage of the ESS is that it differentiates tiredness from sleepiness. The ESS does not ask how many times the patient has actually fallen asleep at inappropriate times, only the likelihood of this happening, which controls for motivation. The ESS is probably the most widely used sleepiness scale in sleep centers. It is inexpensive to administer, and most patients can answer it in a few minutes.

Disadvantages of the ESS include that it is a subjective and simple tool that assumes that the likelihood of falling asleep is the mirror of EDS.

Pittsburgh Sleep Quality Index

The Pittsburgh Sleep Quality Index (PSQI) was published in 1989 by Buysee and associates. The authors view sleep quality as a concept that includes sleep duration, sleep latency, number of arousals, and depth and "restfulness" of sleep.

The PSQI assesses sleep quality over a continuous period of the previous month to avoid night-to-night natural variations. There are 19 self-rated questions answered on a 0–3 scale, in which the higher number represents greater severity. The 19 questions are grouped into seven components: subjective sleep quality, sleep latency, sleep duration, habitual sleep efficiency, sleep disturbance, use of sleeping medication, and daytime dysfunction. These components are summed to yield a global sleep quality score (from 0 to 21). The PSQI also includes 5 questions rated by the bed partner that are not tabulated in the scoring. The PSQI requires around 10 minutes to complete and is easy to score.

The PSQI was initially studied in 52 healthy control subjects, 34 poor sleepers with major depression, and 62 patients with specific sleep disorders. Internal consistency was reliable (Cronbach's $\alpha=0.83$). Scores for individuals who completed the PSQI on two separate occasions showed no differences, except for depressed patients who had undergone treatment. Overall test-retest reliability was 0.85 ($P<0.001$). PSQI validity scores differed between subject groups ($P<0.001$), demonstrating that the PSQI can discriminate patients from control subjects. Results were consistent with polysomnographic data.

The PSQI provides a simple quantitative method with different components as well as a global score that correlates with severity. Direct comparisons can be made of the same patient across time, as well as among groups. A PSQI global score of 5 or higher is indicative of poor sleep quality. The PSQI does not provide valid or reliable clinical diagnoses.

The PSQI can be used as a simple screening measure for the identification of poor sleepers in both clinical and epidemiologic research settings. It can be used to prompt clinicians to investigate sleep-related symptoms, and it provides a measure of the effectiveness of individual treatment. It is simple and quick to use.

Dysfunctional Beliefs and Attitudes About Sleep Scale

Clinical experience indicates that faulty cognitions, in the form of unrealistic expectations, dysfunctional beliefs, catastrophic consequences, and unstable and external attributions, are prevalent and causal factors in insomnia mediated by emotional arousal.

Charles Morin studied the influence of faulty cognitions in insomnia. In 1994, he published the Dysfunctional Beliefs and Attitudes About Sleep (DBAS) scale (Morin 1994). The DBAS is a self-report instrument that consists of 30 items drawn both from clinical practice and a theoretical conceptualization of insomnia. Subjects rate their level of agreement in a 100-mm visual analog scale anchored at each end by "strongly agree" and "strongly disagree." There are five clusters: misconceptions, misattributions or amplification of consequences, unrealistic expectations, control and predictability of sleep, and faulty beliefs about sleep-promoting practices.

The DBAS has fine internal consistency (Cronbach's $\alpha=0.8$). One disadvantage is that the DBAS does not provide a numeric end result that can be translated into a clear cutoff point. Another problem is that a patient can have one strong faulty cognition that is of clinical relevance, whereas a healthy person who functions well can have several mild faulty cognitions and have a higher global score.

The DBAS can be used in the course of insomnia treatment. Patients are asked to monitor and report their sleep and insomnia cognitions. The DBAS is sensitive to change with cognitive-behavioral therapy.

The DBAS needs further research and development. It has a positive potential to become an interesting and useful clinical and research tool. An improvement would be to have the aforementioned cutoff point for pathology, both in single questions and in a global score.

Summary

The objective measurements provided by sleep laboratories in the form of the polysomnogram and the MSLT remain today's gold standard, even if these measures are cumbersome, expensive, and not available everywhere. Despite some interesting accomplishments, there are still too few well-researched assessment instruments. Many people are developing their own scales, and these efforts might eventually produce some useful instruments. For example, an important tool can be a semistructured interview that provides clinical diagnosis according to the International Classification of Sleep Disorders.

CONCLUSION

The field of clinical sleep problems continues to expand. Most studies in this field measure outcomes in physiologic variables (blood pressure, oximetry, use of continuous positive airway pressure, mortality rate) mostly in relation to patients with obstructive sleep apnea. With the exception of sleep laboratory studies, there is no widely used and well-standardized and accepted instrument in use by most sleep researchers and psychiatrists, which may be viewed as a disadvantage or an open field for opportunity.

REFERENCES

American Psychiatric Association: Diagnostic and Statistical Manual of Mental Disorders, 4th Edition, Text Revision. Washington, DC, American Psychiatric Association, 2000

American Sleep Disorders Association Diagnostic Classification Steering Committee: International Classification of Sleep Disorders: Diagnostic and Coding Manual. Rochester, MN, American Sleep Disorders Association, 1990

Buysee DJ, Reynolds CF, Monk TH, et al: The Pittsburgh Sleep Quality Index: a new instrument for psychiatric practice and research. Psychiatry Res 28:193–213, 1989

Chervin RD, Aldrich MS: The Epworth Sleepiness Scale may not reflect objective measures of sleepiness or sleep apnea. Neurology 52:1–7, 1999

Douglass AB, Bornstein R, Nino-Murcia G, et al: The Sleep Disorders Questionnaire I: creation and multivariate structure of SDQ. Sleep 172(29):160–167, 1994

Hoddes E, Zarcone V, Smythe H, et al: Quantification of sleepiness: a new approach. Psychophysiology 10(4):431–436, 1973

Johns MW: A new method for measuring daytime sleepiness: the Epworth Sleepiness Scale. Sleep 14(6):540–545, 1991

Miles L: A sleep questionnaire, in Sleeping and Waking Disorders. Indications and Techniques. Edited by Guilleminault C. Menlo Park, CA, Addisson-Wesley, 1982

Morin CM: Dysfunctional Beliefs and Attitudes About Sleep (DBAS). Behavior Therapist 2:163–164, 1994

Rosenthal L, Roehrs TA, Roth T: The Sleep-Wake Activity Inventory: a self-report measure of daytime sleepiness. Biol Psychiatry 34:810–820, 1993

Schramm E, Hohagen F, Grasshoff U, et al: Test-retest reliability and validity of the Structured Interview for Sleep Disorders according to DSM-III-R. Am J Psychiatry 150:867–872, 1993

16

Outcome Measurement in Sexual Disorders

Laura Berman, L.C.S.W., Ph.D.

Jennifer Berman, M.D.

Mary Christina Zierak, B.A., M.A.

Ciara Marley, B.A., M.A.

Sexuality is a basic part of general health and wellness as well as quality of life for both men and women. Yet in the most recent national survey addressing this topic, the National Health and Social Life Survey (Laumann et al. 1999), it was found that 43% of women and 31% of men have complaints about their sexual functioning. In recent years, science has made major advances toward understanding the neurovascular mechanisms of sexual response in men and women. Furthermore, the potential for drug therapy to treat certain types of sexual complaints is tremendous. However, most experts agree that sexual dysfunction is a multicausal and multidimensional problem combining biological, intrapsychic, and interpersonal determinants. For many people, sexual dysfunction is physically disconcerting, emotionally distressing, and socially disruptive.

According to DSM-IV-TR (American Psychiatric Association 2000), sexual dysfunctions are characterized by disturbance in desire as well as psychophysiologic changes. Categories of sexual dysfunction include sexual desire disorders, sexual arousal disorders, orgasmic disorders, sexual pain disorders, sexual dysfunction due to a general medical condition, substance-induced sexual dysfunction, and sexual dysfunction not otherwise specified. A sexual dysfunction is characterized by a disturbance in the processes that characterize the sexual response cycle (desire, excitement, orgasm, and resolution) or by pain associated with sexual activity.

However, with recent attention paid to the evaluation and treatment of female sexual dysfunction, greater focus is being placed on the difference between men and women and the importance of taking a multidimensional approach to treatment and treatment evaluation. The Consensus Development Panel on Female Sexual Dysfunction was convened in 1998 by the Sexual Function Health Council of the American Foundation for Urologic Disease (AFUD) to evaluate and revise existing definitions and classifications of female sexual dysfunction. The resulting consensus panel built on the existing framework of DSM-IV-TR. The consensus panel recommended adoption of a new diagnostic and classification system for female sexual dysfunction based on physiologic as well as psychological pathologies and a "personal distress" criterion for most of the diagnostic criterion. In particular, definitions of sexual arousal disorder and hypoactive sexual desire disorder were developed, and a new category of noncoital sexual pain diagnosis was devised (Basson et al. 2000). This is an important issue to consider in terms of outcome measures; however, no "personal distress" scales currently exist.

DSM-IV-TR SEXUAL DYSFUNCTION DISORDERS

Each of the diagnoses listed below are to be subtyped as follows: 1) lifelong or acquired; 2) generalized or situational; and 3) organic, psychogenic, mixed, or unknown etiologic origin. Subtyping is based on the best evidence from the medical history, laboratory tests, and physical examination.

Sexual Desire Disorders

Hypoactive sexual desire disorder is the persistent or recurrent deficiency (or absence) of fantasies, thoughts, and/or desire for or receptivity to sexual activity, which causes personal distress (American Psychiatric Association 2000; Basson et al. 2000).

Sexual aversion disorder is the persistent or recurrent aversion to and active avoidance of sexual contact with a sexual partner, which causes personal distress. The individual reports anxiety, fear, or disgust when confronted by a sexual opportunity with a partner. The intensity of the individual reaction with exposure to the aversive stimulus ranges from moderate anxiety to extreme psychological distress (American Psychiatric Association 2000; Basson et al. 2000).

Sexual Arousal Disorders

Female sexual arousal disorder is the persistent or recurrent inability to attain or to maintain sufficient sexual excitement, causing personal distress. It may be expressed as a lack of subjective excitement or of genital (lubrication/swelling) or other somatic responses (American Psychiatric Association 2000; Basson et al. 2000).

Male erectile disorder is a persistent or recurrent inability to attain or to maintain until completion of the sexual activity an adequate erection, which causes personal distress. There are different patterns or erectile dysfunction; some men report the inability to obtain any erection from the outset of a sexual experience. Others complain of losing tumescence once an adequate erection has been achieved (American Psychiatric Association 2000).

Orgasmic Disorders

Female orgasmic disorder is a persistent or recurrent delay in or absence of orgasm following a normal sexual excitement phase. Women exhibit wide variability in the type and intensity of stimulation that triggers orgasm. The diagnosis includes consideration of the woman's age and sexual experience and the adequacy of sexual stimulation she receives. The disturbance must cause marked distress or interpersonal difficulty to be diagnosed (American Psychiatric Association 2000; Basson et al. 2000).

Male orgasmic disorder is a persistent or recurrent delay in or absence of orgasm following a normal sexual excitement phase. The diagnosis takes into consideration the person's age and whether the stimulation is adequate in focus, intensity, and duration. The disturbance must cause marked distress or interpersonal difficulty to be diagnosed (American Psychiatric Association 2000).

Premature ejaculation is the persistent or recurrent onset of orgasm and ejaculation with minimal sexual stimulation, which causes personal distress. The diagnosis includes consideration of age, novelty of the sexual partner or situation, and recent frequency of sexual activity (American Psychiatric Association 2000).

Sexual Pain Disorders

Dyspareunia is genital pain that occurs with sexual activity. It is most commonly experienced during intercourse, although it may also occur before or after coitus. The symptoms may range from mild discomfort to sharp pain, and the disturbance causes marked personal distress. Vaginismus or lack of lubrication alone does not cause the disturbance (American Psychiatric Association 2000; Basson et al. 2000).

Vaginismus is the recurrent or persistent involuntary contraction of the perineal muscles surrounding the outer third of the vagina when vaginal penetration is attempted, which causes personal distress. In some women, even the anticipation of vaginal insertion may result in muscle spasm. The contraction may range from mild (inducing some tightness and discomfort) to severe (preventing penetration) (American Psychiatric Association 2000; Basson et al. 2000).

Noncoital sexual pain disorder is recurrent or persistent genital pain induced by noncoital sexual stimulation (American Psychiatric Association 2000; Basson et al. 2000).

Other categories of sexual dysfunction include sexual dysfunction due to a general medical condition, substance-induced sexual dysfunction, and sexual dysfunction not otherwise specified. The category of sexual disorders also contains the paraphilias, which include exhibitionism, fetishism, frotteurism, pedophilia, sexual masochism, sexual sadism, voyeurism, and transvestic fetishism. Also related are the gender identity disorders (American Psychiatric Association 2000).

DSM-IV-TR GENDER IDENTITY DISORDERS

Gender identity disorder is the presence of strong and persistent cross-gender identification, which is the desire to be of the other sex. Adults with gender identity disorder are preoccupied with their wish to live as a member of the opposite sex. This preoccupation may be manifested in a desire to adopt the social role and/or appearance of the other sex through hormonal manipulation or surgery (American Psychiatric Association 2000).

Distress or disability in individuals with gender identity disorder is manifested differently across the life cycle. In children, distress is manifested by the unhappiness with the assigned sex. In adults, preoccupations with cross-gender desire often interfere with work, school, and relationships.

OUTCOME MEASUREMENTS

Valid and reliable outcome measures in the area of sexuality are greatly limited. There is a need for more research and updated instruments to address all the sexual issues and concerns addressed in DSM-IV-TR. All of the measurements described below can be used as outcome measures to determine the effectiveness of an intervention on components of male and female sexuality.

Measures of Global Sexual Function

Sexual History Form

The Single Summary Score for Nowinski and LoPiccolo's Sexual History Form (SHF) (Creti et al. 1987, 1988) is a widely used self-report sexual history measure on sexual behavior and function for men and women. The questionnaire evaluates the frequency of sexual activity; sexual function relating to desire, arousal, orgasm, and pain; and overall sexual satisfaction. The SHF is frequently used in sex therapy clinics, in clinical studies, and in longitudinal assessments of the impact of chronic illness on sexuality. The format is multiple choice, and the measure is scored on an item-by-item basis.

Global sexual functioning scores have good temporal stability, with reliability coefficients ranging from 0.92 to 0.98 (Creti et al. 1988; Libman et al. 1989). Internal consistency was established for male and female sexual functioning scores. The Cronbach's α coefficient had a high of 0.65 for male global functioning and 0.85 for female global functioning (Creti et al. 1988).

Data on this instrument indicate that it can differentiate sexually well-functioning from poorly functioning individuals and is sensitive to changes with therapy (Creti et al. 1987). Furthermore, the measure is sensitive to age differences in sexual function and is related to other sexual functioning measures, including sexual self-efficacy, sexual satisfaction, sexual repertoire, and sexual drive (Creti and Libman 1989; Creti et al. 1987; Libman et al. 1989).

The SHF is a 46-item measure that takes approximately 15 minutes to complete. It focuses on function as well as effects associated with function (e.g., reactions when lovemaking does not go well). This provides opportunities for outcome measurements in coping strategies as well as function following treatment. It would be useful, however, to determine the effectiveness of this measure in longitudinal studies. No validity or reliability scores are established in this context.

Derogatis Sexual Functioning Inventory

The Derogatis Sexual Functioning Inventory (DSFI) (Derogatis and Melisaratos 1979) measures constructs of sexual functioning (e.g., body image, sexual satisfaction) as well as basic signs of general well-being (e.g., effects psychological distress). This self-report inventory considers the quality of current sexual functioning of an individual.

The DSFI is composed of 10 dimensions that are judged to replace fundamental components of sexual behavior. Of the 10 subtests in the DSFI, two of them, psychological symptoms and affects, are themselves complete, multidimensional tests.

Reliability coefficients range from 0.60 to 0.97, and test-retest coefficients across a 14-day interval range from the high 0.70s to the low 0.90s (Derogatis and Melisaratos 1979).

The DSFI has been established as being highly sensitive to naturally occurring and disease-induced interference with sexual functioning, as well as to positive treatment effects (Derogatis 1980).

The DSFI is composed of 26 items and takes 15–20 minutes to complete. It is a comprehensive measure that considers sexual information (e.g., knowledge), experiences, drive, attitudes, psychological distress, affect, gender identity, fantasy, body image, and sexual satisfaction. It does not include any information on relationship stability or satisfaction, and the literature associated with it is dated. Further data are needed on the clinical application of this instrument.

Sexual Interaction Inventory

The Sexual Interaction Inventory (SII) (LoPiccolo and Steger 1974) is a self-report measure for differentiating between "dysfunctional" and "nondysfunctional" couples and for the diagnosis of sexual dysfunction. The SII measures the current nature of a couple's sexual relationship with respect to satisfaction and level of functioning.

Reliability was established, with test-retest reliability coefficients ranging from 0.53 to 0.90 on the 11 scales and with all the correlations significant ($P<0.05$) (LoPiccolo and Steger 1974). The Cronbach's α for each scale ranged between 0.79 and 0.93, indicating good internal consistency. Validity was not as established in this measure, because although almost all scales had correlations that were significant ($P<0.05$ or better), the absolute magnitude of these correlations was low.

The SII consists of 102 items and takes an average of 15–30 minutes to complete. It includes illustrations of sexual activity (except intercourse) and asks the couple to provide information about 17 different sexual behaviors. The inventory collects information about several parameters: current sexual frequency; desired sexual frequency; current level of sexual satisfaction; estimate of partner's current level of sexual satisfaction; desired level of satisfaction in "ideal" self; and desired level of satisfaction in an "ideal" partner. It is especially useful for determining perceptual accuracy in terms of partner expectations and reactions. More recent literature applying this measure is needed.

Measures of Male Sexual Functioning

Erectile Dysfunction Inventory of Treatment Satisfaction

The Erectile Dysfunction Inventory of Treatment Satisfaction (EDITS) (Althof et al. 1999) was developed to assess satisfaction with medical treatments for erectile dysfunction. Two versions of the EDITS are available, one measuring patient treatment satisfaction and the other measuring partner satisfaction. The patient and partner EDITS are brief, psychometrically sound questionnaires that include subjective assessments about the effectiveness of treatment, side effects, ease or use, naturalness, and impact on significant others.

Test-retest reliability for the summary score was 0.98 for the patient version and 0.83 for the partner version. The high test-retest reliability suggests that the measurement of treatment satisfaction is not being influenced by error due to fluctuations in such matters as a respondent's mood, level of fatigue, or recent sexual experience.

Content validity was assessed, as was construct validity, for individual items. The validity coefficient, a Spearman's rank-order correlation coefficient, was calculated by correlating the target person's response with his or her partner's responses to the similar item. The correlation was positive and significant ($P < 0.05$) (Althof et al. 1999).

The EDITS is very brief (five items) and intervention specific. It would be useful in medical or clinical settings to determine the effectiveness of concrete interventions such as drug therapy.

Brief Male Sexual Function Inventory for Urology

The Brief Male Sexual Function Inventory for Urology (BMSFI) is a brief questionnaire to measure male sexual function and may be useful in practice and research. An initial set of questions was refined and reduced through cognitive testing and two serial validation studies. In both studies, men were recruited from a sexual dysfunction clinic and a general medicine practice to complete the instrument. This instrument addresses four domains: sexual drive (two items), erection (three items), ejaculation (two items), perceptions of problems in each area (three items), and overall satisfaction (one item). This inventory is a self-administered report designed to avoid issues of interview bias that can be problematic in outcome research.

Gender Identity and Erotic Preferences in Males

Gender Identity and Erotic Preferences in Males is a test packet that encompasses seven scales assessing erotic preference, erotic anomalies, and gender identity. These scales include the Feminine Gender Identity Scale

for Males (FGIS), the Androphilia Scale, the Gynephilia Scale, the Heterosexual Experience Scale, the Fetishism Scale, the Masochism Scale, and the
Sadism Scale. Part A of the FGIS was constructed from items endorsed
by adult gynephiles and nontranssexual androphiles. Parts B and C of the
FGIS were constructed from items endorsed by transsexuals and nontranssexual homosexuals.

The α reliability coefficients are as follows: FGIS part A, 0.93; FGIS
parts B and C, 0.89; Androphilia, 0.93; Gynephilia, 0.85; Heterosexual
Experience, 0.82; Fetishism, 0.91; Masochism, 0.83; and Sadism, 0.87
(Blanchard 1985; Blanchard and Freund 1983; Freund et al. 1982).

The evidence for the construct validity of the FGIS is the demonstration of reliable group differences among heterosexual, nontranssexual
homosexual, and transsexual homosexual males (Freund et al. 1982). There
was also good agreement between clinicians' assessment of erotic partner
preference (heterosexual vs. homosexual) and assessment by means of the
Androphilia and Gynephilia scales.

Each scale in this packet has only one response option and takes at
most 15 minutes to complete. This is a comprehensive packet with many
scales and subscales that could be useful in outcome measurement in this
area. One limitation is that test-retest reliabilities have never been established.

Measures of Female Sexual Functioning

McCoy Female Sexuality Questionnaire

The McCoy Female Sexuality Questionnaire (MFSQ) (McCoy and Matyas
1996) assesses a woman's general level of interest in sexual activities at the
time of evaluation. It is used to monitor changes in sexual functioning or as
a diagnostic tool. Some of the questions explore enjoyment, arousal, interest, and satisfaction with a partner and feelings of attractiveness. Some of
the questions focus on heterosexual coitus, including frequency, enjoyment, orgasm and pleasure, lubrication, and the incidence of decreased satisfaction as a result of a partner's erectile difficulty. Three optional sections
address masturbation, sexual activity without coitus, and heterosexual anal
intercourse.

McCoy and Matyas (1996) reported an internal consistency α of 0.77.
Test-retest correlations (α) following a 2-week time interval for individual
items ranged from 0.69 to 0.95, with an average test-retest correlation of
0.83.

The MFSQ has been utilized in clinical and nonclinical samples of
menopausal-age women. Significant within-subject differences have been
established, as have connections between interest before and after men-

strual cycles as well as in relation to estradiol levels and oral contraceptive use (McCoy 1990; McCoy and Davidson 1985; McCoy and Matyas 1996).

The MFSQ consists of 19 questions; 18 are answered on a 7-point scale ranging from very low or absent to extremely high. The final question deals with the overall frequency of heterosexual coitus during the preceding 4 weeks. The questionnaire should take 15–30 minutes to complete. This is an easy-to-use, brief questionnaire that is designed as an outcome measure and covers both function and affect associated with the experience in terms of pleasure and enjoyment experienced.

Brief Index of Sexual Functioning for Women

The Brief Index of Sexual Functioning for Women (BISF-W) (Rosen et al. 1993) was developed to provide a brief, standardized self-report measure of overall sexual function (i.e., sexual interest, activity, desire, arousal, orgasm, satisfaction, and preference) in women. The questions were formulated to target three major aspects of women's sexual functioning: factor 1, sexual desire; factor 2, sexual activity; and factor 3, sexual satisfaction.

The internal consistency measured by Cronbach's α ranged from 0.39 for factor 1 to 0.83 for factor 2. The test-retest reliability of factor scores, calculated by means of Pearson correlation coefficient at baseline and at the 1-month retest interval, ranged from 0.68 to 0.78.

Concurrent validity was assessed by means of comparison of specific factor scores corresponding to the DSFI. Correlations between the BISF-W and the DSFI subscales were positive, ranging from 0.59 to 0.69. Body image was significantly correlated with the DSFI body image scale ($r=0.62$; $P<0.001$) (Rosen et al. 1993).

The BISF-W is a 22-item questionnaire that takes about 10–15 minutes to complete. It has been one of the most widely used measures for global assessment of sexual functioning in recent years. It is a useful measurement to use in longer-term work where global functioning may shift. However, the arousal questions could be more female specific in terms of genital sensation and swelling/engorgement.

Female Sexual Arousal Index

The Female Sexual Arousal Index (FSAI) is a self-report measure focusing on female sexual arousal. The time context is centered on the past month, and questions concern sexual desire, general sexual arousal, vaginal lubrication, genital sensation, orgasm, pain, and sexual satisfaction; some questions concern satisfaction with sexual technique of the partner and satisfaction.

Validity and reliability were established through a multiphase process starting with the establishment of face validity and group analysis. The second phase included factor analysis, discriminate validity, and test-retest reliability in a population consisting of 250 age-matched women, half of whom had a diagnosis of female sexual dysfunction (Rosen et al. 2000).

This measure is the newest of the female sexual dysfunction assessments and is unique in that it addresses quantity and quality of sexual function. For instance, ability to achieve and maintain levels of arousal are assessed, as are perceptions of satisfaction with those levels. This is a useful measure for assessment of female global sexual dysfunction as well as for evaluation of treatment effectiveness.

Measures of Sexual Self-Concept

Multidimensional Sexual Self-Concept Questionnaire

The Multidimensional Sexual Self-Concept Questionnaire (MSSCQ) (Snell 1995) is a self-report measure that examines 20 psychological aspects of human sexuality: sexual anxiety, sexual self-efficacy, sexual consciousness, motivation to avoid risky sex, chance/luck sexual control, sexual preoccupation, sexual assertiveness, sexual optimism, sexual problem self-blame, sexual monitoring, sexual motivation, sexual problem management, sexual esteem, sexual satisfaction, power–other sexual control, sexual self-schemata, fear of sex, sexual problem prevention, sexual depression, and internal sexual control.

The internal consistency of the MSSCQ was determined using the Cronbach α coefficients. The α values for all subjects on the 20 subscales ranged from 0.84 to 0.94. Evidence for the validity of the MSSCQ comes from a recent research investigation (Snell 1995), which found a relationship between the MSSCQ and men's and women's contraceptive use and gender differences.

The MSSCQ consists of 100 items that are answered based on how characteristic each statement is of the respondent. The items can be treated as individual difference measures of the constructs or as dependent variables when examining predictive correlates of these concepts. This is a comprehensive measure of sexual self-concept that would be useful when determining effective treatment outcomes.

Sexual Self-Efficacy Scale for Erectile Functioning

The Sexual Self-Efficacy Scale for Erectile Functioning (SSES-E; Libman et al. 1985) measures the cognitive dimension of erectile functioning and adjustment in men with a focus on beliefs about sexual and erectile competence in a variety of sexual situations.

Libman et al. (1985) evaluated the reliability of the SSES-E. They calculated α coefficients of 0.92 for a group of dysfunctional men and 0.94 for their female partners' ratings of their male partners; α values for the control group were 0.92 for the men and 0.86 for their female partners. Test-retest reliability was $\alpha=0.98$ for males and $\alpha=0.97$ for females.

The concurrent validity estimates were found by correlating the dysfunctional men's SSES-E scores and selected items on the SHF (Nowinski and LoPiccolo 1979). These correlations ranged from $\alpha = 0.47$ to $\alpha = 0.68$ for items related to quality of erections and feelings of sexual arousal. Results of a known-groups validity study demonstrated that dysfunctional men and their partners score lower on the SSES-E than do functional men and their partners (Libman et al. 1985). Dysfunctional and functional men were able to be classified with 88% accuracy based on SSES-E scores.

This 25-item measure evaluates confidence in sexual activity using a 10-point interval scale ranging from 10 to 100. Higher scores in the scale indicate greater confidence in the man's erectile function. It can be used in the clinical assessment of sexual dysfunction, as a treatment outcome measure for sex therapy, or in the evaluation of how confidence changes in relation to biological events.

Sexual Self-Efficacy Scale for Female Functioning

The Sexual Self-Efficacy Scale for Female Functioning (SSES-F) measures perceived competence in the behavioral, cognitive, and affective dimensions of a woman's sexual response. This scale is based on the self-efficacy theory, which holds that expectations about how well one can perform in a given situation can significantly influence behavior in that situation. The scale focuses on the sexual response dimensions of interest, desire, arousal, and orgasm.

Internal consistency evaluation in a nonclinical sample of women yielded a Cronbach's α of 0.93. Test-retest correlations for the total scores indicated good stability over time ($r=0.83$; $P<0.001$) (Bailes et al. 1989). The overall strength score of the SSES-F correlated strongly with other measures of sexual functioning, such as the SHF and the SII, and with marital satisfaction. The overall strength scores were significantly lower for women with sexual dysfunction than for women who reported no sexual dysfunction.

Women rate their confidence levels on a 37-item scale, which takes 10–15 minutes to complete. The evaluation and alteration of self-efficacy expectations in treatment are important in the cognitive-behavioral treatment of a number of psychosexual problems. This is one of the few sexual self-efficacy scales that exist for women.

Relationship Measures

Index of Sexual Satisfaction

The Index of Sexual Satisfaction (ISS) is designed to consider the degree of dissatisfaction in the sexual component of a dyadic relationship. Questions focus on elements of sexual enjoyment, excitement, libido, and sensitivity.

Cronbach's α was 0.92, and standard error of the mean was 4.24 (Hudson et al. 1981). Test-retest reliability was not established. The known-groups validity coefficient was 0.76 as determined by the correlation between four status (troubled vs. untroubled criterion) groups and the ISS scores.

The ISS contains 25 items, some of which are worded negatively to partially offset the potential for response set bias. Scores range from 0 to 100, with higher scores indicating a greater degree of sexual discord in a relationship. The questionnaire takes 5–7 minutes to complete. Full evidence of reliability and validity is still needed on this measure. However, this is a brief questionnaire that would be useful as an indication of red flags in a sexual relationship and potential resolution of those issues following treatment.

Sexual Interaction System Scale

The Sexual Interaction System Scale (SISS) is a self-report instrument designed to measure the quality of a heterosexual couple's sexual interaction, including specific sexual dysfunctions. Each partner's perception is measured by five factors, and the total couple's score is formed by the addition of each individual's score. These five factors, which are believed to interact in sexual encounters, are sexual functioning, attitudinal set, nonsexual interaction, interaction coordination, and postsexual interaction. This statement-response scale focuses on the interactions taking place during a couple's actual sexual interaction.

Internal consistency, as analyzed by the five SISS factors, resulted in a Cronbach's α of 0.90 (Woody and D'Souza 1994). The t tests showed significant difference between the sexual dysfunction group and the nonclinical group ($t=7.14$; $P<0.001$). Validity was also supported by a Pearson's correlation coefficient ($r=0.80$; $P<0.001$) between the SISS couple's score and the couple's score on a criterion question dealing with sexual satisfaction.

This 48-statement scale is filled out by partners independently, preferably on the same day, and takes approximately 10 minutes to complete. This is a good outcome measure to use to determine the effectiveness of couples' sexual therapy on general function, satisfaction, and attitudes toward the sexual relationship.

Sexual Relationship Scale

The Sexual Relationship Scale (SRS) is an objective self-report scale designed to measure communal and exchange approaches to sexual relationships. The communal approach is feeling responsible for the partner's needs, whereas the exchange approach is feeling no responsibility for the partner's needs.

Internal consistency was determined using Cronbach's α coefficients. The results were 0.77 for men, 0.79 for women, and 0.78 for both together. Validity for women, factor I, consisted of sexual communion items (eigenvalue, 4.81; variance, 20%), and factor II contained sexual exchange items (eigenvalue, 2.98; variance, 12%). Men reported significantly higher scores than did women on the sexual exchange subscale, but no difference was found for the sexual exchange scale (Hughes and Snell 1990).

The SRS is a 24-item Likert-type response scale that takes 10–15 minutes to complete. The scale is useful to determine the effectiveness of treatment for addressing chronic dispositional differences in the type of approach two partners take to their sexual relations as well as the way in which the treatment has changed the couple's sense of and attitude toward connection.

CONCLUSION

Sexuality is a basic part of the general health, wellness, and quality of life for both men and women. With the media attention paid to sexual dysfunction as well as the pharmaceutical options that have been made available, more and more individuals will be presenting for evaluation and treatment of sexual dysfunction. For mental health care providers, the challenge will be to adequately assess men and women who are appropriate candidates for medication. The measurements to assess sexual function presented here will be one useful method of identifying individuals with sexual dysfunction and of evaluating the effectiveness of treatment.

However, no medication will effectively resolve sexual dysfunction that is rooted in psychopathology, emotional stresses, or relational conflicts. It will therefore be crucial that mental health professionals and prescribing physicians adequately assess not only the presence of sexual function complaints but also their emotional or relational sources. This will be a significant challenge facing mental health professionals treating sexual dysfunction for the next millennium.

REFERENCES

Althof SE, Corty EW, Levine SB, et al: EDITS: the development of questionnaires for evaluating satisfaction with treatments for erectile dysfunction. Urology 53:793–799, 1999

American Psychiatric Association: Diagnostic and Statistical Manual of Mental Disorders, 4th Edition, Text Revision. Washington, DC, American Psychiatric Association, 2000

Bailes S, Creti, L, Fitchen C, et al: The SSES-F: a multidimensional measure of sexual self-efficacy for women. Poster presented at the annual convention of the American Psychological Association, New Orleans, LA, August 1989

Basson R, Berman J, Burnett A, et al: Report of the International Consensus Development Conference on Female Sexual Dysfunction: definitions and classifications. J Urol 163:888–893, 2000

Blanchard R: Research methods for the typological study of gender disorders in males, in Gender Dysphoria: Development, Research, Management. Edited by Steiner BW. New York, Plenum, 1985, pp 227–257

Blanchard R, Freund K: Measuring masculine gender identity in females. J Consult Clin Psychol 51:205–214, 1983

Creti L, Libman E: Cognition and sexual expression in the aging. J Sex Marital Ther 15:83–101, 1989

Creti L, Fitchen CS, Libman E, et al: A global score for the "Sexual History Form" and its effectiveness. Paper presented at the 21st annual convention of the Association for Advancement of Behavior Therapy, Boston, MA, November 1987

Creti L, Fitchten CS, Amsel R, et al: Female sexual functioning: a global score for Nowinski and LoPiccolo's Sexual History Form. Paper presented at the annual convention of the Canadian Psychological Association, Montreal, QC, Canada, June 1988 [Abstracted in Canadian Psychology 29 (2a), Abstract 164, 1988]

Derogatis LR: Psychological assessment of psychosexual functioning, in The Psychiatric Clinics of North America Symposium on Sexuality. Edited by Meyer JK. Philadelphia, PA, Saunders, 1980, pp 113–131

Derogatis LR, Melisaratos N: The DSFI: a multidimensional measure of sexual functioning. J Sex Marital Ther 5:244–281, 1979

Freund K, Scher H, Chan S, et al: Experimental analysis of pedophilia. Behav Res Ther 20:105–112, 1982

Hudson WW, Harrison DF, Crosscup PC: A short-form scale to measure sexual discord in dyadic relationships. Journal of Sex Research 17:157–174, 1981

Hughes T, Snell WE: Communal and exchange approaches to sexual relations. Annals of Sex Research 3:149–163, 1990

Laumann E, Paik A, Rosen R: Sexual dysfunction in the United States: prevalence and predictors. JAMA 281:537–544, 1999

Libman E, Rothenberg I, Fitchen CS, et al: The SSES-E: a measure of sexual self-efficacy in erectile functioning. J Sex Marital Ther 11:233–244, 1985

Libman E, Fitchen CS, Rothenberg P, et al: Transurethral prostatectomy: differential effects of age category and presurgery sexual functioning on post-prostatectomy sexual adjustment. J Behav Med 12:469–485, 1989

LoPiccolo J, Steger JC: The Sexual Interaction Inventory: a new instrument for assessment of sexual dysfunction. Arch Sex Behav 3:585–595, 1974

McCoy NL: Estrogen levels in relation to self-reported symptoms and sexuality in perimenopausal women. Ann N Y Acad Sci 592:450–452, 1990

McCoy NL, Davidson JM: A longitudinal study of the effects of menopause on sexuality. Maturitas 7:203–210, 1985

McCoy NL, Matyas JR: Oral contraceptives and sexuality in university women. Arch Sex Behav 25:73–90, 1996

Nowinski JK, LoPiccolo J: Assessing sexual behavior in couples. J Sex Marital Ther 5:225–243, 1979

Rosen RC, Taylor JF, Leiblum SR, et al: Prevalence of sexual dysfunction in women: results of a survey study of 329 women in an outpatient gynecological clinic. J Sex Marital Ther 19:171–188, 1993

Rosen R, Brown C, Heiman J, et al: The Female Sexual Function Index (FSFI): a multidimensional self-report instrument for the assessment of female sexual function. J Sex Marital Ther 26(2):191–208, 2000

Snell WE: The Extended Multidimensional Sexuality Questionnaire: measuring psychological tendencies associated with human sexuality. Paper presented at the annual meeting of the Southwestern Psychological Association, Houston, TX, April 1995

Woody JD, D'Souza, HJ: The Sexual Interaction System Scale: a new inventory for assessing sexual dysfunction and sexual distress. J Sex Marital Ther 20:210–228, 1994

Outcome Measurement in Eating Disorders

Drew A. Anderson, Ph.D.
Donald A. Williamson, Ph.D.

Eating disorders have become a significant problem over the past 30 years. Two eating disorders, anorexia nervosa and bulimia nervosa, are recognized in DSM-IV-TR (American Psychiatric Association 2000). Although binge-eating disorder is not yet recognized as an independent diagnosis, criteria for it are provided in DSM-IV-TR for further study.

This chapter describes the research literature on methods for evaluating treatment outcome with eating disorders. In recent years, many assessment methods have been developed and tested in psychometric studies. Most of these procedures were developed for measuring the symptoms of eating disorders or some feature of eating disorders, for example, cognition associated with eating disorders or concerns about body size and shape. Few assessment methods have been developed specifically for the purpose of evaluating outcome of therapy with eating disorders. This chapter focuses on these methods. For each method, studies of the reliability and validity of the procedure are summarized and the utility of the method for measuring treatment outcome is addressed.

CHARACTERISTICS OF EATING DISORDERS

Anorexia Nervosa

The essential characteristics of anorexia nervosa are a refusal to maintain a minimally normal body weight, an intense fear of gaining weight, significant disturbance in the perception of the shape or size of the body, and in the case of postmenarchal females, amenorrhea (American Psychiatric Association 2000). There are two subtypes of anorexia nervosa: individuals with restricting type anorexia nervosa do not regularly engage in binge eating or purging behavior, whereas those with binge-eating/purging type anorexia nervosa do regularly engage in those behaviors.

Anorexia nervosa affects primarily females, with onset typically occurring in adolescence or early adulthood. Approximately 0.5%–1.0% of females in this age range meet full criteria for anorexia nervosa, and many more will meet subthreshold criteria for the disorder (American Psychiatric Association 2000). Anorexia nervosa is associated with high rates of comorbid psychiatric disorders, particularly mood, anxiety, and substance use disorders (American Psychiatric Association 2000), and it has the highest mortality rate of all the psychiatric disorders (Sullivan 1995).

Bulimia Nervosa

The essential characteristics of bulimia nervosa are binge eating and inappropriate compensatory methods to prevent weight gain, along with excessive influence of shape and weight on self-evaluation. Individuals with purging type bulimia nervosa regularly use self-induced vomiting or misuse of laxatives, diuretics, or enemas as compensatory methods. Individuals with nonpurging type bulimia nervosa do not regularly engage in self-induced vomiting or misuse laxatives, diuretics, or enemas but do regularly use other inappropriate compensatory methods such as strict dieting and/or excessive exercise (American Psychiatric Association 2000). Like anorexia nervosa, bulimia nervosa affects primarily females, with onset typically occurring in adolescence or early adulthood. Approximately 1%–3% of females in this age range meet criteria for bulimia nervosa (American Psychiatric Association 2000). Bulimia nervosa is associated with high rates of comorbid psychiatric disorders, particularly mood, anxiety, and substance use disorders (American Psychiatric Association 2000).

Binge-Eating Disorder

In recent years, interest has begun to focus on individuals who report problems with binge eating but do not use compensatory methods to control their weight. This pattern of behavior has been termed binge-eating disorder. Although the American Psychiatric Association Task Force on Eating Disorders believed that there was insufficient information on the disorder to warrant its inclusion as a separate diagnosis (American Psychiatric Association 2000), binge-eating disorder is currently provided as a specific example of eating disorder not otherwise specified and is a criteria set provided for further study. Binge-eating disorder is defined by episodes of binge eating without regular use of compensatory behaviors. Individuals with binge-eating disorder must have marked distress regarding binge eating. Because of the number of calories ingested during binge episodes, persons with binge-eating disorder are typically overweight or obese (American Psychiatric Association 2000). Binge-eating disorder is associated with elevated levels of comorbid psychopathology compared with obese non-binge-eaters, but lower levels of psychopathology compared with persons with bulimia nervosa (Spitzer et al. 1993).

IMPORTANT PARAMETERS OF THE EATING DISORDERS

Factor analytical studies have found that the central features of anorexia nervosa and bulimia nervosa are 1) negative affect, 2) dietary restraint, 3) bulimic behavior, and 4) body image disturbance (Williamson et al. 1996). Fairburn and colleagues have developed a cognitive-behavioral model of the maintenance of bulimia nervosa that informs their successful treatment approach (Fairburn 1997). According to this model, five factors underlie the maintenance of bulimia nervosa: 1) low self-esteem, 2) extreme concerns with body shape and weight, 3) dietary restriction, 4) binge eating, and 5) purgative behavior. A similar model is thought to operate in anorexia nervosa as well (Fairburn 1997).

Much less research has been done to identify the core symptoms of binge-eating disorder beyond the symptoms episodes that are described in DSM-IV-TR (i.e., binge eating and distress following binge episodes). Extreme concerns with shape and weight may not be present in persons with binge-eating disorder to the same degree as in those with anorexia nervosa and bulimia nervosa.

EATING DISORDERS: DISCRETE CATEGORIES OR POINTS ON A CONTINUUM?

There has been considerable debate over whether mental illness is best conceptualized as a set of categorically discrete disorders or a series of dimensional attributes on which individuals can vary in degree but not in kind. The categorical approach is generally taken in DSM-IV-TR, although the limitations of such approach and the strengths of a dimensional system are acknowledged (American Psychiatric Association 2000, p. xxxii). In the field of eating disorders, this debate has taken the form of two questions: 1) is the eating behavior seen in individuals with eating disorders qualitatively different from normal eating, or does it represent extreme points on a continuum of eating behavior; and 2) are the eating disorders qualitatively different from each other, or do they represent different points on a continuum of eating behavior?

Research on the first question has found that behavior related to eating disorders appears to be qualitatively different from eating by persons without eating disorders. Laboratory studies of eating behavior have shown strikingly different patterns of eating between patients with eating disorders and control subjects (e.g., Cooke et al. 1997; Hadigan et al. 1989). In addition, qualitative differences between persons with and without eating disorders were found in an investigation of the latent structure of eating disorder symptoms (D.A. Williamson et al., unpublished observations, 2000).

Research on the second question has yielded mixed results. It is not yet clear if the diagnoses of eating disorders in DSM-IV-TR themselves represent quantitatively or qualitatively different syndromes; evidence from a recent taxometric study of eating disorder symptoms suggests that some features of eating disorders are dimensional, whereas others are categorical (D.A. Williamson et al., unpublished observations, 2000).

Although the categorical/dimensional debate is of enormous theoretical and diagnostic importance for the eating disorders, at the present time it is less vital when discussing the assessment of treatment outcome. Several of the assessment instruments reviewed as follows have been shown to discriminate between individuals with eating disorders and those without eating disorders as well as distinguishing specific eating disorder diagnoses (as they are currently defined) from each other.

AVAILABLE MEASURES

General Problems in Measuring Outcome

Many individuals with eating disorders, particularly anorexia nervosa and bulimia nervosa, hide their disorder. Most individuals with bulimia nervosa, for example, will binge eat and purge only when alone. The eating disorders are also associated with high levels of deception and resistance to treatment. On the other hand, most measures of eating disorders symptoms have high face validity, which make them vulnerable to dissimulation ("faking good"). Because of this, it can be difficult to obtain accurate information of the severity and nature of eating disorder symptoms. Interviewing family members or using test meals (see the following) can provide more objective information concerning eating disorder symptoms.

There are particular problems associated with evaluating binge eating. According to DSM-IV-TR, a binge episode must involve eating an amount of food that is definitely larger than most people would consider normal under the circumstances and must be accompanied by sense of lack of control over eating during the episode. However, individuals with bulimia nervosa have been found to significantly overestimate the caloric intake of a meal (Hadigan et al. 1992), and individuals who binge eat are more likely to define a meal as an overeating episode in comparison to individuals who do not have frequent binges (Williamson et al. 1991). There is also evidence that persons who binge eat rely more on feelings of loss of control rather than the amount of food eaten to define an eating episode as a binge (Beglin and Fairburn 1992). Although some researchers have argued that the objective size of a binge episode is not important (e.g., Pratt et al. 1998), current DSM-IV-TR criteria require that a large amount of food be eaten. Thus, there is evidence that self-reporting of binge episodes may be an overestimation of the actual frequency of their occurrence.

It is important to assess all critical symptom domains associated with the eating disorders. Unless gains are observed in all symptom domains, treatment cannot be viewed as successful, and relapse is more likely. In particular, Fairburn and colleagues suggest that anorexia nervosa and bulimia nervosa are driven by extreme concerns with body weight and shape, and treatment success is likely to be short-lived unless these concerns are successfully addressed (Fairburn 1997). Unfortunately, there is no clear consensus in the eating disorders literature on which measures should be used to measure outcome (Williamson et al. 1996). This chapter provides some guidelines for measuring outcome in the treatment of eating disorders.

Interview Methods

Eating Disorders Examination

The Eating Disorders Examination (EDE) (Fairburn and Cooper 1993) is a semistructured interview designed to assess a broad range of the specific psychopathology of anorexia nervosa and bulimia nervosa and their variants. The EDE is an investigator-based interview, in which the interviewer is trained so that he or she understands the concepts being assessed and can rate the severity of symptoms based on these concepts. Thus the investigator, not the subject, rates the severity of symptoms on the EDE. This distinction is particularly important in the eating disorders because there is a great deal of variability in how laypersons and professionals define key terms such as *binge* (see above).

The EDE focuses exclusively on behavior and attitudes in the 4 weeks (28 days) preceding the interview. Each item consists of one or more obligatory probe questions that must be asked. The interviewer may supplement these probes with questions of his or her own, depending on the subject's responses. Items are scored on 7-point Likert-type scales of either severity or frequency, depending on the question. Guidelines are provided to assist in rating the subject's responses. The EDE has four subscales: restraint, eating concern, shape concern, and weight concern.

The EDE uses a unique classification system to assess overeating. It categorizes overeating episodes on the bases of amount and feelings of control. Thus, a particular overeating episode could be classified as one of four types of episodes. Only episodes that include ingestion of an objectively large amount of food with accompanying feeling of loss of control meet full DSM-IV-TR criteria for a binge episode. Thus, the EDE classification system makes it easier for professionals to document actual binge episodes. It also allows professionals to document changes in eating patterns. For example, a patient in treatment might still report frequent loss of control during eating episodes, but the amount of food consumed during these episodes may have decreased significantly. Alternatively, a patient might report continued consumption of large amounts of food but may feel more in control of eating. The EDE allows professionals to distinguish between these patterns, which otherwise might be subsumed by patients under the general description of binge eating.

The subscales of the EDE have been found to have good internal consistency (generally above 0.90) and interrater reliability (0.68 or better; see Fairburn and Cooper 1993 for a detailed review of reliability). The EDE can discriminate between patients with eating disorders and control subject without eating disorders, as well as between patients with eating disorders and highly restrained eaters (Fairburn and Cooper 1993), and EDE subscale scores are sensitive to change (Fairburn and Cooper 1993)

The primary strengths of the EDE lie in its investigator-based format, which overcomes many of the problems inherent in self-reporting of eating disorders symptoms, as well as its format for rating eating episodes. The EDE also has very good psychometric properties, and it assesses the core features of the eating disorders. Because of these strengths, the EDE has been called the method of choice for assessing the specific psychopathology of the eating disorders (Fairburn and Beglin 1994), and it is used widely in research. However, the utility of the EDE in a clinical setting is somewhat limited. Interviewers must be thoroughly trained to use the EDE, which can take 30 minutes to an hour to administer (Fairburn and Cooper 1993; Williamson et al. 1995). These training and time issues render it generally impractical for clinical use. As a consequence, a questionnaire version of the EDE has been developed (see the following).

Self-Report Inventories

Eating Disorders Examination–Questionnaire Version

The Eating Disorders Examination–Questionnaire Version (EDE-Q) (Fairburn and Beglin 1994) is a 35-item self-report inventory developed from the EDE interview (see above). The EDE-Q was designed to be a simple measure that would take less than 15 minutes to complete yet still assess the main behavioral features of the eating disorders. The EDE-Q retains the initial item probes and 7-point Likert-type scale scoring format of the EDE interview format, and it generates the three key EDE subscales (restraint, shape concern, and weight concern). However, detailed guidelines for making ratings and definitions of key terms such as *binge* were eliminated to make it simple and easy to complete.

The subscales of the EDE-Q have very good internal consistency and test-retest reliability, but items measuring the occurrence and frequency of the key behavioral features of eating disorders have somewhat lower stability (Luce and Crowther 1999). Studies of the concurrent validity of the EDE-Q have found that although agreement between the EDE-Q and EDE is strong for behaviors that do not pose problems of definition, such as purging, correlations between the two measures are low when assessing more complex constructs, particularly binge eating (Fairburn and Beglin 1994; Wilfley et al. 1997). Although scores on the subscales of the EDE-Q and EDE are highly correlated, subjects consistently report higher levels of disturbance on the EDE-Q versus the EDE (Fairburn and Beglin 1994; Wilfley et al. 1997).

The EDE-Q has some advantages over the EDE, from which it was developed. The EDE-Q is brief and does not require a trained interviewer to administer. Subscales of the EDE-Q also demonstrate good reliability and validity. However, the EDE-Q may be poor at assessing symptoms as eating disorder pathology increases and at evaluating some of the more abstract constructs associated with eating disorders.

Multifactorial Assessment of Eating Disorder Symptoms

The Multifactorial Assessment of Eating Disorder Symptoms test (MAEDS) (Anderson et al. 1999) is a 56-item self-report measure designed to measure six symptom clusters thought to be important for treatment outcome of the eating disorders: depression, binge eating, purgative behavior, fear of fatness, restrictive eating, and avoidance of forbidden foods. It is relatively brief, requiring no more than 10 minutes for most people to complete it. Items on the MAEDS are scored on a 7-point Likert-style format with response choices ranging from "always" to "never." Separate subscale scores are calculated, allowing for detailed analysis of the six symptom clusters.

The reliability of the MAEDS subscales is good, with coefficient α scores ranging from 0.80 to 0.92 and test-retest reliability scores ranging from 0.89 to 0.99 (Anderson et al. 1999). The MAEDS has adequate convergent and divergent validity (Anderson et al. 1999), and a recent study found support for its criterion-related validity (Martin et al. 2000). Norms are available for college-age women.

Because the MAEDS was designed specifically to be used as a treatment outcome measure, it assesses domains relevant for treatment outcome, yet it is brief and easy to administer. Its multifactorial design allows for a detailed analysis of symptom domains. The primary disadvantage of the MAEDS is that it is a self-report questionnaire that is subject to the biases of simulation and dissimulation. We have not found this type of bias to be a substantial obstacle to the use of the MAEDS as a measure of treatment outcome in clinical and research settings, however. The MAEDS is also a new measure, and it has been used in only two outcome studies to date. In both of these studies, the subscales of the MAEDS were found to be sensitive to change. Thus, the MAEDS is a promising new addition to the eating disorders field.

Eating Attitudes Test

The Eating Attitudes Test (EAT) (Garner and Garfinkel 1979) is a 40-item self-report inventory designed to assess behaviors and attitudes associated with anorexia nervosa. Factor analysis of the EAT yielded a 26-item version (EAT-26) (Garner et al. 1982) that was highly correlated with the original EAT ($r=0.98$). Children's, adapted language, and non-English versions of the EAT have also been developed (Williamson et al. 1995).

Items on the EAT and EAT-26 are scored on a 6-point Likert-type scale. Only the three most extreme, "anorexic-like" responses on any given item are scored; the response most indicative of anorexia nervosa receives a score of 3, the response slightly less extreme receives a score of 2, and the response slightly less extreme than that receives a score of 1.

Much of the research on the psychometric properties of the EAT has been conducted using the original 40-item version of the measure. The EAT has been found to have high internal consistency (coefficient α scores of 0.79 for anorexia nervosa and 0.94 for combined anorexia nervosa and nonclinical control subjects [Williamson et al. 1995]) and internal reliability ($r=0.84$ [Williamson et al. 1995]). Scores on the EAT are moderately correlated with scores on other self-report inventories of eating disorder symptoms. Scores on the EAT appear to be sensitive to changes in anorexia nervosa symptoms after successful treatment (Williamson et al. 1995). Norms are available for individuals diagnosed with anorexia nervosa, bulimia nervosa, and binge-eating disorder, as well as obese control subjects, female control subjects, and male control subjects (Williamson et al. 1995). A cutoff score of 30 on the EAT and 20 on the EAT-26 have been suggested to identify persons with attitudes and behavior of eating disorders (Garner et al. 1982).

Although it was originally developed to assess persons with anorexia nervosa only, the EAT is useful in assessing persons with other eating disorders. For example, the EAT has been shown to differentiate persons with anorexia nervosa, bulimia nervosa, and binge-eating disorder from control subjects without eating disorders; however, it has not been shown to differentiate persons with anorexia nervosa from those with bulimia nervosa (Williamson et al. 1995).

The EAT is the most commonly used self-report inventory in the eating disorder literature (Williamson et al. 1996). It takes less than 10 minutes to complete, is easy to score, and has alternative versions for young or non-English-speaking patients. The EAT also has good reliability and validity, and norms are available. However, because the EAT renders only an omnibus total score, it does not provide details on which particular symptoms are changing during treatment. Thus, the EAT might be best used as a screening device to assess for the presence of eating disorder symptoms. Because it is brief, easily scored, and sensitive to change, the EAT might also be given regularly during treatment to provide a rough index of treatment progress.

Behavioral Measures

Self-Monitoring

Self-monitoring can provide a wealth of useful information for diagnosis and measurement of treatment outcome. In clinical practice, self-monitoring may be the only practical way to obtain information such as temporal eating patterns, type and amounts of food eaten, frequency and topography of binge episodes and purgative behavior, and mood before and after the meal. The data from self-monitoring forms can easily be quantified to provide an index of baseline symptoms. Self-monitoring can be used throughout treatment to monitor change in symptoms.

Although self-monitoring can provide a great deal of data, patients must be trained to self-monitor accurately. For example, self-monitoring data are more likely to be accurate if they are recorded immediately following a meal, rather than later that night or the next day. Self-monitoring is also vulnerable to dissimulation, particularly by patients who deny having eating problems.

Test Meals

Direct measurement of eating behavior during test meals can be a very useful method for objectively assessing dietary restraint and treatment progress, particularly for individuals who minimize or deny the extent of their eating disorder. For example, patients might be asked to eat a standard multi-item test meal (including both safe and forbidden foods) before beginning treatment to establish a baseline, and then asked to consume the same meal periodically throughout treatment to measure progress.

There are numerous advantages to using test meals. It is possible to measure total calories eaten as well as the proportion of each food consumed, which provides an objective index of dietary restraint. An increase in consumption, particularly for forbidden foods, serves as an index of improvement. Perhaps most importantly, test meals are less vulnerable to dissimulation than are other assessment measures.

There are some cautions to using test meals, however. There is often a great deal of resistance to test meals, particularly by patients who deny having eating problems. Often patients will report that they have just eaten or that they do not eat a particular (usually forbidden) food that is part of a test meal. Patients should also be supervised for at least 30 minutes after a test meal to prevent purging. The practical issues surrounding test meals (e.g., preparing food, providing supervision after the meal) may make them difficult to implement in clinical practice.

Other Measures

Weight and Body Mass Index

Many outcome studies include change in weight or body mass index (BMI) (weight in kilograms divided by the square of height in meters) as an outcome variable. For patients with anorexia nervosa, weight gain is the primary goal in the early stages of treatment. Conversely, for patients with binge-eating disorder, weight loss is usually a goal of treatment. Patients with bulimia nervosa are typically of normal weight or slightly overweight, but they fear weight gain. By measuring weight or BMI, professionals can demonstrate to those patients that they can normalize their eating patterns without gaining weight.

FUTURE DIRECTIONS

Over the past 10 years, considerable progress has been made in the development of measures for evaluating treatment outcome for eating disorders. The EDE has become the gold standard in research studies of eating disorders. The MAEDS and the EDE-Q are much more convenient self-report inventories that could be more widely used in the future. Research on the correlation of these questionnaire measures with the EDE interview method is needed so that it can be assessed whether the improvement in time efficiency with the questionnaires is justified in terms of validity of assessment.

Only the MAEDS measures psychological disturbances other than eating disorder symptoms. The MAEDS includes a scale that measures depression. Given the common finding that patients diagnosed with eating disorders are also diagnosed with personality disorders, there is a need to establish a cost-efficient method for assessing the severity of personality disturbances associated with eating disorders.

SUMMARY AND RECOMMENDATIONS

At this time, we recommend four main strategies for evaluating treatment outcome with eating disorders: 1) using a structured interview, 2) using a self-report inventory, 3) using BMI or change in body weight, and 4) using test meals.

There is no question that the EDE is the most widely respected method for evaluating treatment outcome with eating disorders. As a structured interview, the EDE has been refined in a series of psychometric studies and has been found to be sensitive to change in a number of controlled trials. The primary disadvantages of the EDE are that it is time consuming to administer and that it requires special training to administer properly. Because of these limitations, the EDE may be relegated to the status of a research tool that is used by clinical researchers, but not by mainstream clinicians who must deal with the time constraints of clinical practice and the demands of managed care, to evaluate behavior change as economically as possible.

The primary alternatives to the EDE or other structured interview are self-report inventories. The self-report inventory most appropriate for use as an outcome measure is the MAEDS. This self-report inventory was designed specifically to measure treatment outcome for eating disorders. The subscales of the MAEDS were developed to be relatively comprehensive (e.g., measuring the symptoms of depression as well as the symptoms of anorexia nervosa and bulimia nervosa). Alternatively, the EDE-Q provides some of the same information as the EDE but in a much more time-efficient manner. It has many of the same advantages (e.g., brevity, ease of administration and scoring) and disadvantages (e.g., susceptibility to dissimulation, lack of description of critical terms) as the MAEDS. Therefore, for the mainstream clinician who manages patients with eating disorders, the MAEDS or EDE-Q may be good alternatives to the EDE. Other self-report inventories (e.g., EAT, BULIT-R) have been used in controlled trials, but none were designed for use as an outcome measure and thus are not well adapted for this purpose.

The measurement of BMI or some other form of body weight that is controlled for height of the person is a crucial variable that should always be included in the evaluation of treatment outcome with eating disorders. For true cases of anorexia nervosa, increased body weight must be considered to be *the* primary outcome variable during the first few months of treatment. For bulimia nervosa, weight maintenance during treatment is the most common goal, but some patients need to gain weight and others need to lose weight. For binge-eating disorder, most patients need to lose substantial amounts of weight. Unfortunately, some of the more established treatments for binge-eating disorder (e.g., cognitive-behavioral therapy to reduce binge eating) have not typically yielded significant changes in body weight.

Lastly, for clinicians with available resources, test meals provide significant information while not being susceptible to dissimulation. Test meals need not be elaborate, multi-item affairs; a simple candy bar or bag of potato chips can serve the same purpose.

REFERENCES

American Psychiatric Association: Diagnostic and Statistical Manual of Mental Disorders, 4th Edition, Text Revision. Washington, DC, American Psychiatric Association, 2000

Anderson DA, Williamson DA, Duchmann EG, et al: Development and validation of a multifactorial treatment outcome measure for eating disorders. Assessment 6:7–20, 1999

Beglin SJ, Fairburn CG: What is meant by the term "binge"? Am J Psychiatry 149: 123–124, 1992

Cooke EA, Guss JL, Kissileff HR, et al: Patterns of food selection during binges in women with binge eating disorder. Int J Eat Disord 22:187–193, 1997

Fairburn CG: Eating disorders, in The Science and Practice of Cognitive Behaviour Therapy. Edited by Clark DM, Fairburn CG. Oxford, Oxford University Press, 1997, pp 209–242

Fairburn CG, Beglin SJ: Assessment of eating disorders: Interview or self-report questionnaire? Int J Eat Disord 16:363–370, 1994

Fairburn CG, Cooper Z: The eating disorder examination, in Binge Eating: Nature, Assessment, and Treatment, 12th Edition. Edited by Fairburn CG, Wilson GT. New York, Guilford, 1993, pp 317–360

Garner DM, Garfinkel PE: The Eating Attitudes Test: an index of the symptoms of anorexia nervosa. Psychol Med 9:273–279, 1979

Garner DM, Olmsted MP, Bohr Y, et al: The Eating Attitudes Test: psychometric features and clinical correlates. Psychol Med 12:871–878, 1982

Hadigan CM, Kissileff HR, Walsh BT: Patterns of food selection during meals in women with bulimia. Am J Clin Nutr 50:759–766, 1989

Hadigan CM, LaChaussee JL, Walsh BT, et al: 24-hour dietary recall in patients with bulimia nervosa. Int J Eat Disord 12:107–111, 1992

Luce KH, Crowther JH: The reliability of the Eating Disorder Examination—Self-Report Questionnaire Version (EDE-Q). Int J Eat Disord 25:349–351, 1999

Martin CK, Williamson DA, Thaw JM: Criterion validity of the multiaxial assessment of eating disorders symptoms. Int J Eat Disord 28:303–310, 2000

Pratt EM, Niego SH, Agras WS: Does the size of a binge matter? Int J Eat Disord 24:307–312, 1998

Spitzer RL, Yanovski S, Wadden T, et al: Binge eating disorder: its further validation in a multisite study. Int J Eat Disord 13:137–153, 1993

Sullivan PF: Mortality in anorexia nervosa. Am J Psychiatry 152:1073–1074, 1995

Wilfley DE, Schwartz MB, Spurrell EB, et al: Assessing the specific psychopathology of binge eating disorder patients: interview or self-report? Behav Res Ther 35:1151–1159, 1997

Williamson DA, Gleaves DH, Lawson OJ: Biased perception of overeating in bulimia nervosa and compulsive binge eaters. Journal of Psychopathology and Behavioral Assessment 13:257–268, 1991

Williamson DA, Anderson DA, Jackman LP, et al: Assessment of eating disordered thoughts, feelings, and behaviors, in Handbook of Assessment Methods for Eating Behaviors and Weight-Related Problems. Edited by Allison DB. Newbury Park, CA, Sage, 1995, pp 347–386

Williamson DA, Anderson DA, Gleaves DG: Anorexia and bulimia: structured interview methodologies and psychological assessment, in Body Image, Eating Disorders, and Obesity: An Integrative Guide for Assessment and Treatment. Edited by Thompson K. Washington, DC, American Psychological Association, 1996, pp 205–223

CHAPTER 18

Patient Satisfaction and Perceptions of Care

Susan V. Eisen, Ph.D.

Patient satisfaction with services is widely recognized as an important component of outcome (Donabedian 1980). Potential purposes of assessing consumer satisfaction include improving adherence to treatment recommendations, achieving optimal utilization of appropriate services, improving the quality of mental health services, and improving clinical outcome (Kalman 1983). This chapter briefly reviews earlier efforts to assess patient satisfaction and recent attempts to refine the understanding of the concept and measurement of patient satisfaction. It then describes an instrument designed to improve on earlier instruments, reports results obtained with the instrument in an inpatient psychiatric facility, how results are used internally for quality improvement purposes, and how results may be used on a national level.

BACKGROUND

Assessment of consumer satisfaction with mental health services was widespread as early as the 1970s. Many different methodologies and instruments were developed to measure satisfaction with services (Lebow 1982). Qualitative methods included focus groups, content analysis of letters written by patients and their families, and personal interviews (Edgman-Levitan and Cleary 1996; Eisen and Grob 1979). Quantitative assessments often involved customized instruments developed at each site to address unique characteristics of particular programs or clients. Methods of data collection have included self-report surveys completed by current or former patients in person or by mail and structured interviews administered in person or by telephone. Although some standardized satisfaction surveys exist, research in the field has been limited by inadequate study design, inadequate instruments, and lack of reliability or validity information for the existing instruments (Ruggeri 1994).

Two developments have shifted the focus of recent work in the field of assessing consumer satisfaction. First, national efforts to evaluate and compare services provided in different facilities or systems of care have created a need to use standardized instruments. There is pressure for facilities to give up customized instruments in exchange for standardized questionnaires that allow comparison across facilities. Several national organizations have become involved in these efforts. The National Committee for Quality Assurance (NCQA) has developed the Health Employment Data and Information Set (HEDIS 3.0), the most widely used health care report card system to compare quality of care across health plans (National Committee for Quality Assurance 1997). HEDIS 3.0 incorporates the Consumer Assessment of Health Plans Study (CAHPS) consumer survey to collect and report information from health plan enrollees about their experiences with medical services and with their insurance plans (Crofton et al. 1999). The Foundation for Accountability (FACCT) has developed quality measures for specific medical conditions, including depression (Skolnick 1997). The American Managed Behavioral Healthcare Association (AMBHA) developed Performance Measures for Managed Behavioral Healthcare Programs (PERMS), a set of 16 indicators measuring access to care, consumer satisfaction, and quality of care (Ross 1997).

The Mental Health Statistics Improvement Program (MHSIP) developed a consumer-oriented mental health report card to assess the quality of mental health treatment provided within statewide public mental health systems (Center for Mental Health Services 1996). All of these efforts focus on assessing consumer perceptions of health care quality for large systems of care or for health/behavioral health insurance plans.

At the individual facility level, the Joint Commission on Accreditation of Healthcare Organizations (JCAHO) ORYX initiative requires accredited hospitals to assess their performance using indicators and instruments within approved performance measurement systems (Joint Commission on

Accreditation of Healthcare Organizations 1997). This is the first national effort to promote standardized performance indicators at the facility level. JCAHO has approved more than 50 performance measurement systems that are applicable to behavioral health, each with multiple indicators. The approval of multiple systems and indicators allows providers great flexibility in meeting accreditation requirements. However, the need to select among JCAHO-approved indicators should help to decrease the number of indicators in use. To further decrease the number of indicators in use, JCAHO will be selecting core indicators that facilities may be required to use. Patient satisfaction is one of four performance categories identified by the ORYX initiative. Facility-specific performance data must be sent to JCAHO with the goal of creating national performance benchmarks for different types of facilities.

The second shift in thinking about patient satisfaction involves the conceptualization and methods of measurement. The concept of consumer satisfaction is becoming more refined, moving away from the global, abstract idea of *satisfaction* to more concrete, well-defined indicators of quality of care. Ware et al. (1983) distinguish between reports about care and ratings of care. Reports ask factual questions such as, "Were you given information about the benefits and risks of medication you received?" Reports may also ask for the frequency with which particular events occurred, for example, "How often did you have to wait more than 15 minutes past your appointment time?" Response options might include never, sometimes, usually, or always. Ratings ask respondents to evaluate an aspect of care, for example, "How would you rate the amount of information you received about medications you received?" Response options might include poor, fair, good, very good, and excellent.

A number of instruments have been developed to assess consumer evaluations of mental health care. However, most were designed to assess outpatient services. As a result, they include some items that do not apply to inpatient services and exclude areas that are important to inpatient care. The Client Satisfaction Questionnaire (CSQ-8) is an 8-item general satisfaction survey with high internal consistency and reliability (Attkisson and Greenfield 1996). The brevity and simplicity of the instrument make it feasible to implement with minimal burden on staff and clients. However, because the items do not focus on particular aspects of treatment, it may be difficult to use results for quality improvement purposes. The 30-item Service Satisfaction Scale provides specific information that can guide quality improvement efforts, but it was designed to evaluate outpatient services (Attkisson and Greenfield 1996). The 40-item MHSIP consumer survey was designed with a consumer orientation and geared toward the values and goals of the public mental health system (Teague et al. 1997). It does not focus on care received within a particular setting. The Consumer Assessment of Behavioral Health Services (CABHS) was designed to assess consumer perceptions of outpatient services and insurance plans covering those services. It includes all services received within a 12-month period and does not focus on care received at a particular facility (Eisen et al. 1999).

THE PERCEPTIONS OF CARE SURVEY

The intentions of the designers of the Perceptions of Care (PoC; S.V. Eisen et al., unpublished observations, 2002) survey were to develop a survey that would 1) address the important domains of quality best assessed by consumers; 2) assess care received within a particular facility; 3) apply across diverse inpatient programs to allow for comparisons among programs and against national benchmarks; 4) meet accreditation and payer requirements; 5) be useful for guiding internal quality improvement efforts; and 6) be feasible to implement in inpatient settings at minimal cost and burden to consumers and clinicians.

Development of the Survey: Design Principles

Many factors went into the process of developing the PoC survey. Most important, much of the earlier work that had been done in developing consumer surveys for both medical and behavioral health care was taken into consideration. Important conceptual and instrument development work helped identify the important domains to cover as well as the format of the survey (Cleary et al 1991; Davies and Ware 1988; Edgman-Levitan and Cleary 1996; Eisen et al. 1999; Fowler 1995; Hays et al. 1999; Rubin 1990; Rubin et al. 1990). A review of the literature suggested a number of important factors to consider in constructing the survey. For example, Edgman-Levitan and Cleary (1996) reported that outpatients' concerns about care are different from those of inpatients. Among the dimensions of care identified as salient to inpatients were respect for patients' values and needs, information, communication, education, coordination and continuity of care, involvement of family, and transition to the community. Many of these are similar to the interpersonal aspects of care identified by Donabedian (1980) and noted by Davies and Ware (1988) as aspects of care best evaluated by consumers.

The format of the survey was another important consideration. Many surveys use the same response options for every item. For example, the MHSIP survey is in the form of statements with a 5-point disagree–agree rating scale. The Patient Judgments of Hospital Quality questionnaire asks respondents to rate aspects of their care on a 5-point scale from excellent to poor. Each of these formats has advantages and disadvantages. Phrasing items as statements can allow for simple wording, resulting in items that are easily understood by a wide range of respondents whose education and socioeconomic status may vary. Using the same rating scale for every item simplifies aggregation of items into domains, each of which can then be measured on the same continuum. However, particular response options do not always fit questions equally well, especially questions that ask for reports of events. For example, a question asking if an individual received information about the benefits and risks of medication is most directly answered "yes" or "no." Dichotomous response options best fit this type of question. However, items with yes or no answers result in a very limited range of responses, often with little variance. The reduced variance of such items limits the potential for obtaining high reliability and validity estimates, possibly diminishing the psychometric strength of the measure.

Agree–disagree response options have other disadvantages. If someone is neutral or disagrees with an item, appropriate interpretation of the response may be unclear. For example, if an individual indicates that he is neutral in response to the statement, "I liked the services that I received," it could mean that he did not care either way about the services, or that he liked some but not all of the services received. The information is not specific enough to be useful for quality improvement purposes. Agree–disagree response options are also thought to be particularly vulnerable to an acquiescence response set, in which people tend to agree with whatever statement appears. Less educated respondents have been found to be particularly likely to exhibit this response set (Fowler 1995).

Other survey concern issues addressed in the literature include reading level, ease of translation into foreign languages, and comparability of a survey across different modes of administration (e.g., mail vs. telephone) (Fowler et al. 1999; Weidmer et al. 1999). Particular response options may be especially difficult to translate accurately, which suggests that numerical rating scales may offer greater comparability of translated items than do categorical response options.

Both content and item construction principles were taken into consideration in constructing items for the PoC survey. For example, it was important to state items as clearly and specifically as possible to enhance the likelihood that respondents would understand and interpret the items consistently. This was important, because research on consumer comprehension of quality care indicators has suggested that many survey items are not well understood (Jewett and Hibbard 1996). Negatively worded items (e.g., "Some of the services I received were not helpful") can be particularly confusing (Ganju et al.1998). Double-barreled questions, which combine two or more ideas into one question, are also problematic because of the difficulty of interpreting unfavorable evaluations. For example, the question "What is your overall feeling about office procedures (scheduling, forms, tests, etc.)?" includes three different kinds of office procedures. If someone is dissatisfied with office procedures it is unclear which of these procedures is problematic.

The PoC survey attempts to balance the advantages and disadvantages of specific item formats and response options by using a combination of reports and ratings, with response options tailored to fit the particular question. Principles of good survey design and item construction were employed in an effort to produce the best instrument possible for evaluating consumer perceptions of inpatient psychiatric care. The work began by reviewing many of the existing measures of consumer satisfaction for inpatient and outpatient medical and psychiatric care. From these, items judged to be relevant and appropriate for inpatient psychiatric care were extracted. Some items designed to assess medical care were adapted for inpatient psychiatric programs. Based on earlier work on patient satisfaction, items unique to inpatient mental health care were added (Eisen and Grob 1979, 1982; Eisen et al. 1999). A pilot questionnaire containing 40 items was tested on a sample of 71 patients. Items that were redundant (correlated 0.80 or higher with others items) or that did not add to the scale's reliability were eliminated, resulting in an 18-item scale.

Consumer input was also obtained before finalizing the PoC survey. Former psychiatric inpatients were asked to review a draft of the PoC survey and to rate the importance of each item in evaluating the quality of care. In addition, consumers were asked to provide feedback regarding 1) length of the survey, 2) how they interpreted each item on the survey, 3) wording of each question, 4) appropriate response options for each question, and 5) format of the survey. The input obtained from consumers was invaluable in creating questions judged to be important to the assessment of quality that were easily and consistently understood by respondents.

Description of the Survey

The PoC survey is a 20-item self-report instrument designed to assess consumer perceptions of the inpatient psychiatric hospital experience (Appendix B). The first 18 items are structured questions with forced-choice response options. Ten questions are rated on a 4-point frequency scale (never, sometimes, usually, always) to assess how often particular events occurred. Eight questions offer yes-or-no response options. In addition, two open-ended questions believed to provide useful feedback to clinical and administrative staff (but not intended for cross-program comparisons) are included. One question asks respondents to identify staff members who they feel deserve special recognition. The other asks respondents to add anything about their care that they felt was important but was omitted from the questionnaire. Responses to these questions provide qualitative information that can be useful for internal quality improvement purposes. At McLean Hospital, where the PoC was developed, both quantitative and qualitative results of the PoC survey are reported to the clinical and administrative staffs of each program. The inpatient PoC was modified slightly to create outpatient and partial-hospital versions. Results reported in this chapter pertain only to responses obtained from inpatients.

Administration of the Survey

Patients are asked by nursing staff to complete the survey the day before they are to be discharged. To enhance confidentiality, no name appears on the PoC forms, which are identified only by a unique identification number. Nursing staff members provide a preaddressed envelope in which the patient puts the completed form. These forms are sent directly to the Department of Mental Health Services for analysis.

Results reported here were obtained from 622 patients discharged in 1998 from the adult inpatient services at McLean Hospital in Belmont, Massachusetts, a private, not-for-profit psychiatric hospital affiliated with the Partners Healthcare System and Harvard Medical School. Sample characteristics are presented in Table 18–1. The majority were female, between 25 and 44 years old. Both public (Medicare and Medicaid) and private insurance plans were represented, as were the major diagnostic categories. Seventy-two percent of patients were hospitalized for 14 days or less. Multiple diagnoses were common, with 76% of patients having more than one psychiatric or medical diagnosis.

Response distributions for the 18 forced-choice PoC survey items are presented in Table 18–2. In general, responses indicated favorable perceptions of care, although clear distinctions occurred between items. For example, 90%–94% of patients reported receiving information about rules and policies of the program and about their rights as a patient. Also, 81%–87% of patients reported receiving information about how to reduce the chances of a relapse, benefits and risks of their medication, and plans for continued treatment after discharge. Fewer than 80% of patients reported being told about self-help or support groups, or whom to contact in case of a problem or emergency after discharge. Items for which frequency of occurrence was assessed (4, 5, 7–11) tended to focus on interaction between patients and staff. These items were all perceived quite favorably, with "usually" or "always" responses occurring for 78%–91% of respondents. Eighty per-

Table 18–1.   Demographic and clinical characteristics

Characteristic	N	%
Age		
14–17	16	2.6
18–24	78	12.5
25–34	164	26.4
35–44	204	32.8
45–54	105	16.9
55–64	43	6.9
65+	12	1.9
Sex		
Male	273	43.9
Female	349	56.1
Payer		
Medicare	168	27.0
Medicaid	97	15.6
Commercial nonmanaged	152	24.4
Commercial managed	194	31.2
Other	11	1.8
Primary Axis I diagnosis		
Schizophrenia/schizoaffective disorder	124	20.4
Bipolar disorder	109	18.0
Major/minor depression	163	26.8
Substance abuse disorder	161	26.5
Anxiety/dissociative disorder	31	5.1
Other disorder	19	3.1
Comorbid diagnosis		
Medical	249	40.0
Personality disorder	110	17.7
Substance abuse	170	27.3
Other	200	32.2
Comorbidity index		
0 (no comorbid diagnosis)	151	24.3
1	253	40.7
2	178	28.6
3	40	6.4
4	0	0
Length of stay		
0–7 days	265	42.6
8–14 days	184	29.6
15–21 days	77	12.4
22–30 days	43	6.9
31–60 days	35	5.6
61+ days	18	2.9

Table 18–1. Demographic and clinical characteristics *(continued)*

Characteristic	N	%
Program		
Psychotic disorders	144	23.3
Mood/anxiety disorders	119	19.3
Dual diagnosis/substance abuse	161	26.1
Short-term	193	31.3

cent reported that they were helped quite a bit or a great deal by the care received. On a 0–10 scale asking for an overall rating of care received in the hospital, 70% rated their care at 8 or higher.

Using PoC Information for Internal Quality Improvement

The McLean Hospital continuous quality improvement program has established an 80% threshold for favorable responses on each PoC item. Any item that is not favorably reported by at least 80% of respondents is targeted for quality improvement. In 1996, analysis of patients' responses to the PoC survey indicated that 25% of respondents reported that they did not receive information about patients' rights or information about rules and policies of the program (McLean Hospital 1999). Consequently, a quality improvement task force was organized to address this issue. The task force first identified the sources of the problem. Inpatient staff orientation manuals and procedures were not up to date, and the process for distributing the information to patients needed improvement. To address these problems, the task force first updated the written materials, then developed a process to ensure that the materials were distributed to all patients who arrived at the Clinical Evaluation Center (the admissions area of the hospital). A reevaluation of PoC responses indicated that in the first half of 1998, 86% of patients reported that they received information about patients' rights and 91% reported that they received information about rules and policies of the program. Thus, distribution of information to incoming patients improved after the intervention.

Using PoC Information for External Quality Assessment Purposes

One of the goals of standardizing quality indicators is to enable comparison of programs. Several national efforts to assess the quality of medical care have released comparative data for both hospitals and health plans. A recent analysis of HEDIS data supplied by managed care organizations

Table 18–2. Frequency distributions of responses to Perceptions of Care survey items

Item	Yes		No		I am not taking any medication / Unsure	
	N	%	N	%	N	%
1. Did the staff give you information about the rules and policies of the program?	579	94	39	6		
2. Did the staff give you information about your rights as a patient?	557	90	60	10		
14. Did the staff tell you about self-help or support groups?	464	77	138	23		
15. Did the staff give you information about how to reduce the chances of a relapse?	488	81	116	19		
					I am not taking any medication	
3. Did the staff tell you about the benefits and risks of the medication(s) you are taking?[a]	478	82	105	18	27	4
					Unsure	
12. Did the staff review with you plans for your continued treatment after you leave the hospital?	526	87	34	6	41	7
13. Were you told whom to contact in case you have a problem or emergency after you leave the hospital?	402	67	127	21	72	12
18. Would you recommend this facility to someone else who needed mental health or substance abuse treatment?	465	81	40	7	71	12

Table 18–2. Frequency distributions of responses to Perceptions of Care survey items (continued)

Item	Never N	Never %	Sometimes N	Sometimes %	Usually N	Usually %	Always N	Always %
4. Did the staff explain things in a way you could understand?	8	1	80	13	207	33	322	52
5. Were you involved as much as you wanted in decisions about your treatment?	23	4	109	18	185	30	293	48
7. Did the staff listen carefully to you?	9	2	72	12	230	37	304	49
8. Did the staff who treated you work well together as a team?	10	2	55	9	210	34	338	55
9. Did the staff spend enough time with you?	16	3	91	15	227	37	282	46
10. Did the staff treat you with respect and dignity?	7	1	51	8	187	30	376	61
11. Did the staff give you reassurance and support?	14	2	81	13	190	31	327	53

Item	More than I wanted N	More than I wanted %	Less than I wanted N	Less than I wanted %	About the right amount N	About the right amount %	No involvement, which is what I wanted N	No involvement, which is what I wanted %
6. How much did the staff involve your family in your treatment?	33	5	53	9	341	55	190	31

Item	Not at all N	Not at all %	Somewhat N	Somewhat %	Quite a bit N	Quite a bit %	A great deal N	A great deal %
16. How much were you helped by the care you received?	22	4	101	17	247	41	233	39

Item	1	2	3	4	5	6	7	8	9	10
17. Using any number from 1 to 10, what is your overall rating of care received in the hospital?	1%	2%	1%	2%	5%	5%	13%	27%	18%	25%

[a] Adjusted percentages based on number of patients taking medication.

nationwide was used to report rates of preventive health interventions among investor-owned and not-for-profit health care plans. The results, indicating that investor-owned health maintenance organizations delivered lower quality of care than did not-for-profit plans, were reported both in the professional literature and in local newspapers (Himmelstein et al. 1999). Thus, quality information was made available to the general public. The CAHPS project currently reports information about health care quality from the consumer's perspective that is helpful to consumers in choosing among health plans (McGee et al. 1999). In 1998, the Washington State Health Care Authority, in collaboration with the CAHPS project and the Picker Institute, distributed a report to state employees showing how 16 health plans were rated by state employees who used each plan. In 1998, in both Michigan and Massachusetts, statewide reports were made available to consumers, comparing consumer evaluations of medical, surgical, and maternity care provided by specific hospitals within each state (Veroff et al. 1998).

Such data are not yet publicly available for behavioral health providers, but they will be in the near future. The JCAHO ORYX initiative requires accredited hospitals to systematically assess their performance using a select number of indicators and instruments within approved performance measurement systems (Joint Commission on Accreditation of Healthcare Organizations 1997). Accredited facilities are required to collect data and submit them to an approved performance measurement system which, in turn, is required to produce quarterly site-specific reports, create aggregate benchmarks compiled from all sites submitting data, and transmit site-specific data and the benchmarks to JCAHO. In so doing, performance measurement systems will be able to compare results among sites using the same indicators.

Patient satisfaction is one of four performance categories identified by the ORYX initiative. The inpatient PoC survey includes four JCAHO-approved performance indicators from which accredited facilities may select. Although multisite benchmarks are not yet available for the PoC, the instrument was used to compare four different inpatient programs within McLean Hospital. The comparison reported here is for illustrative purposes to determine whether the PoC survey is sensitive enough to detect differences among programs. Because all of the programs are within the same facility, differences may not be as dramatic as they might be if different facilities were compared.

Two indicators were selected for interprogram comparisons: overall rating of care received and perceived involvement in treatment decisions. Four inpatient programs were compared: the psychotic disorders program, the dissociative disorders and trauma program, the dual diagnosis (substance abuse/mental illness) program, and the generic adult program. Results indicated that there were no statistically significant differences among programs in overall rating of care. Mean ratings for each program ranged from 7.71 to 7.97. However, there was a statistically significant difference among programs in patients' perceived involvement in treatment decisions. Patients in the mood and anxiety disorders program reported that they were more often involved in decisions about their treatment than were patients in the other three programs. Table 18–3 presents the mean ratings for patients from each program on these two PoC indicators. To determine whether these program differences could be accounted for by demographic differences among patients treated in the three programs, a multiple regression analysis was performed controlling for patients' age and sex and number of days hospitalized. Program differences remained statistically significant, suggesting that perceived involvement in treatment was greater in the mood and anxiety disorders program irrespective of patients' age, sex, or length of stay. Results should be interpreted cautiously, because it is possible that other patient characteristics may have influenced the results. However, the results suggest that PoC indicators are sensitive enough to detect differences among programs.

Implications

Although differences were found among programs on a particular PoC indicator, the PoC survey itself does not suggest why these differences occurred. Reporting such information to clinical and administrative leaders may be the first step in efforts to improve quality of care. It is up to the organization staff and leadership to analyze the structures and processes of care provided within the program to identify the program attributes that are likely to be responsible for favorable and unfavorable perceptions. Once those factors are identified it should be possible to disseminate that information for use by other programs.

MAXIMIZING USEFULNESS OF PERFORMANCE INFORMATION

To maximize the usefulness of information obtained on performance indicators (such as the PoC survey), feedback to clinical and administrative staffs is necessary. Feedback can take a number of forms and can be presented in a variety of ways. At McLean Hospital, quarterly report cards for the hospital as a whole, and separately for each program, are prepared and distributed. Part of the report card presents, in graphical form, the percentage of

Table 18–3. Program differences in overall rating of care and perceived involvement in treatment decisions

Program	Overall rating of care[a]			Involvement in treatment decisions[b]		
	Mean	F	P	Mean	F	P
Mood/anxiety disorders (n=119)	7.71	0.383	NS	3.48	4.43	<0.005
Psychotic disorders (n=143)	7.87			3.17		
Dual diagnosis (n=149)	7.97			3.21		
Short-term program (n=194)	7.93			3.13		

[a]Ratings ranged from 0, worst possible care, to 10, best possible care.
[b]Ratings: 1, never; 2, sometimes; 3, usually; 4, always.
Note: NS=not significant.

patients responding favorably to each PoC item. Staff members can quickly see which areas meet the 80% acceptability threshold and which do not.

Use of performance information for external quality assessment purposes also requires systematic reporting mechanisms. The health care quality information described previously has been presented in a variety of report formats. The CAHPS research team has especially focused on developing report formats that provide the most useful information in ways that are easily understood by both purchasers and consumers of care. Feedback from experts, focus groups, and cognitive testing were used to create a variety of report formats that include bar charts, stars (one, two, or three stars indicating below average, average, or above-average performance), and arrows (down, up, or horizontal for below average, above average, or average). Control charts are another increasingly popular format for comparing site-specific performance to a benchmark (Green 1999). A control chart presents a line graph plotted around a benchmark score with indicators for one, two, or three standard deviations around the benchmark. The line can indicate site-specific scores for each site, allowing for visual presentation of whether a specific site's score on a performance indicator falls significantly above or below the benchmark.

FUTURE DIRECTIONS

The behavioral health services field is just beginning to address issues of outcome and quality at all levels of clinical care. Much work remains to be done. With respect to the PoC survey, future efforts will be directed at developing and validating composite indices reflecting particular domains of quality. For example, four PoC indicators have been approved by JCAHO to meet ORYX requirements for inpatient (24-hour) behavioral health facilities: 1) communication with and information received from providers; 2) interpersonal interaction between clinicians and patients; 3) continuity and coordination of care; and 4) global evaluation of care. Efforts will focus on creating scoring algorithms for these domains, determining whether these domains are distinguishable from each other, and assessing their reliability and validity.

As an increasing number of facilities agree to use standardized quality indicators, it will be possible to develop benchmarks for performance comparisons. It is recognized that interpretation of comparative data can be complicated and misleading, and that risk adjustment will be necessary for appropriate interpretation of results. The purpose of risk adjustment is to take into account factors that influence performance that could lead to erroneous inferences about effectiveness or quality of care (Iezzoni 1997).

Providers and facilities want to be assured that if their outcome results are being compared to a benchmark or standard, the benchmark is derived from comparable facilities and patients. Commonly named factors that might be used for risk adjustment include demographic or clinical characteristics of patients (age, gender, race, education, socioeconomic status, diagnosis, chronicity, level of impairment). However, perceptions of quality of care can also be adjusted for facility characteristics (type of program, level of care, region, urban vs. rural setting, etc.). Iezzoni (1997) presents a comprehensive analysis of the many issues pertaining to risk adjustment, including factors to adjust for, deciding the unit of analysis (patients, providers, hospitals, health plans), and multivariate statistical methods used for risk adjustment.

With appropriate data analytic and risk adjustment methods, behavioral health care report cards are likely to become available (Dickey 1996). What remains to be seen is the form these report cards will take and to whom they will be distributed. Currently, site-specific behavioral health care report cards are routinely distributed to clinical and administrative staffs of particular facilities, and perhaps to purchasers or accrediting organizations. They have not been distributed to consumers. However, several report cards for general medical and surgical care have been made available to the general public through the local press and other media. Report cards for consumers and the general public will be part of the future of the delivery of behavioral health care.

REFERENCES

Attkisson CC, Greenfield TK: The Client Satisfaction Questionnaire–8 and the Service Satisfaction Questionnaire–30, in Outcomes Assessment in Clinical Practice. Edited by Sederer LI, Dickey B. Baltimore, MD, Williams & Wilkins, 1996, pp 120–127

Center for Mental Health Services: The MHSIP Consumer-Oriented Mental Health Report Card. The Final Report of the Mental Health Statistics Improvement Program (MHSIP) Task Force on a Consumer-Oriented Mental Health Report Card. Washington, DC, 1996

Cleary PD, Edgman-Levitan S, Roberts M, et al: Patients evaluate their hospital care: a national survey. Health Affairs (Millwood) 10:254–267, 1991

Crofton C, Lubalin JS, Darby C: Consumer assessments of health plans study (CAHPS). Foreword. Med Care 37 (3 suppl):MS1–MS9, 1999

Davies AR, Ware JE: Involving consumers in quality assessment. Health Aff (Milllwood) 7:33–48, 1988

Dickey B: The development of report cards for mental health care, in Outcomes Assessment in Clinical Practice. Edited by Sederer LI, Dickey B. Baltimore, MD, Williams & Wilkins, 1996, pp 156–160

Donabedian A: The Definition of Quality and Approaches to Its Assessment. Ann Arbor, MI, Health Administration Press, 1980

Edgman-Levitan S, Cleary PD: What information do consumers want and need? Health Aff (Millwood) 15:42–56, 1996

Eisen SV, Grob MC: Assessing consumer satisfaction from letters to the hospital. Hospital and Community Psychiatry 30:344–347, 1979

Eisen SV, Grob MC: Measuring discharged patients' satisfaction with hospital care at a private psychiatric hospital. Hospital and Community Psychiatry 33:227–228, 1982

Eisen SV, Shaul JA, Clarridge BR, et al: Development of a consumer survey for behavioral health services. Psychiatr Serv 50:793–798, 1999

Fowler FJ: Improving Survey Questions: Design and Evaluation (Applied Social Research Methods Series, Vol 38). Thousand Oaks, CA, Sage, 1995

Fowler FJ, Gallagher PM, Nederend S: Comparing telephone and mail responses to the CAHPS survey instrument. Consumer Assessment of Health Plans Study. Med Care 37(3 suppl):MS41–MS49, 1999

Ganju V, Wackwitz J, Trabin T: The mental health statistical improvement program (MHSIP) consumer survey. Unpublished report submitted for consideration by the Committee on Performance Measurement, National Committee for Quality Assurance, February 20, 1998

Green RS: The application of statistical process control to manage global client outcomes in behavioral healthcare. Evaluation and Program Planning 22:199–210, 1999

Hays RD, Shaul JA, Williams VSL, et al: Psychometric properties of the CAHPS 1.0 survey measures. Consumer Assessment of Health Plans Study. Med Care 37 (3 suppl):MS22–MS31, 1999

Himmelstein DU, Woolhandler S, Hellander I, et al: Quality of care in investor-owned vs not-for-profit HMOs. JAMA 282(2):159–164, 1999

Iezzoni LI (ed): Risk Adjustment for Measuring Healthcare Outcomes, 2nd Edition. Chicago, IL, Health Administration Press, 1997

Jewett JJ, Hibbard JH: Comprehension of quality care indicators: differences among privately insured, publicly insured, and uninsured. Health Care Financing Review 18:75–94, 1996

Joint Commission on Accreditation of Healthcare Organizations: ORYX Outcomes: The Next Evolution in Accreditation. Oakbrook Terrace, IL, Joint Commission on Accreditation of Healthcare Organizations, 1997

Kalman TP: An overview of patient satisfaction with psychiatric treatment Hospital and Community Psychiatry 34:48–54, 1983

Lebow J: Consumer satisfaction with mental health treatment. Psychol Bull 91:244–259, 1982

McGee J, Kanouse DE, Sofaer S, et al: Making survey results easy to report to consumers: how reporting needs guided survey design in CAHPS. Med Care 37 (3 suppl):MS32–MS40, 1999

McLean Hospital: McLean 1998 PoC Results (McLean Reports Clinical Quality Initiatives for Improving Patient Care Vol 6). Belmont, MA, McLean Hospital, 1999

National Committee for Quality Assurance: HEDIS 3.0 Volume 2, Technical Specifications. Washington, DC, National Committee for Quality Assurance, 1997

Ross EC: Managed behavioral health care premises, accountable systems of care, and AMBHA's PERMS. Evaluation Review 21:318–321, 1997

Rubin HR: Patient evaluations of hospital care: a review of the literature. Med Care 28 (9 suppl):S3–S9, 1990

Rubin HR, Ware JE, Nelson EC, et al: The Patient Judgments of Hospital Quality (PJHQ) questionnaire. Med Care 28 (9 suppl):S17–S18, 1990

Ruggeri M: Patients' and relatives' satisfaction with psychiatric services: the state of the art of its measurement. Soc Psychiatry Psychiatr Epidemiol 29:212–227, 1994

Skolnick AA: A FACCT-filled agenda for public information. JAMA 278:1558, 1997

Teague GB, Ganju V, Hornik JA, et al: The MHSIP mental health report card. A consumer-oriented approach to monitoring the quality of mental health plans. Evaluation Review 21:330–341, 1997

Veroff DR, Gallagher PM, Wilson V, et al: Effective reports for health care quality data: lessons from a CAHPS demonstration in Washington state. Int J Qual Health Care 10:555–560, 1998

Ware JE, Snyder MK, Wright WR, et al: Defining and measuring patient satisfaction with medical care. Evaluation and Program Planning 6:247–263, 1983

Weidmer B, Brown J, Garcia L: Translating the CAHPS 1.0 survey into Spanish. Consumer Assessment of Health Plans Study. Med Care 37 (3 suppl):MS89–MS96, 1999

PART
III

Challenges and Opportunities

CHAPTER 19

Implementation of Outcome Assessment in Systems of Mental Health Care

Manuel Trujillo, M.D.

Concerns with outcomes of clinical care are as old as medical practice. Over centuries, the observations of clinicians, who typically had very few effective interventions at their disposal, defined a range of outcomes for specific disorders related to the natural course of diseases. As medical practice became more effective, a need for more precise measurements of recovery grew.

Standardized measurements of patient baseline and posttreatment characteristics made their public debut in the 1950s, hand in hand with the expansion of clinical trials for many new and effective psychotropic medi-

I wish to thank the clinical staff at Bellevue Hospital Center for their commitment to the outcomes project. Special thanks to Hector Varas, M.D., and Susan Kleinrock for leading the Quality Improvement Program.

cations. Specially designed psychometric instruments allowed early psychopharmacologists to track the changes achieved by the use of newly introduced psychotropic medications and allowed for comparisons among patients' outcomes. By the 1990s, the escalating costs of health care prompted payers to demand increased accountability through valid and reliable quantitative assessments of the results of medical and psychiatric care. This demand prompted a rapid development of the relatively new field of outcome measurement: a development additionally enhanced by the requirements of managed care organizations for provider and system performance. Whatever the source of the pressure, both individual practitioners and systems of psychiatric care will likely have to account for the outcomes of their efforts as routinely as they now submit to the process of regulation by agencies such as the Joint Commission on Accreditation of Healthcare Organizations (JCAHO), the Health Care Financing Administration (HCFA), and state and local health and mental health authorities.

The field of outcome assessment is rapidly becoming vast. It is growing to capture data from diverse treatment settings and systems of care, such as departments of psychiatry, integrated care networks, and health plans. Ideally, outcome measurement will be expanded to track the effects of treatment interventions at the community level and at the level of targeted specific subpopulations or risk groups. The global output of larger systems of care (countywide or statewide) and quantitative performance measures of new mental health policies will increasingly be assessed as new measurement technologies are introduced, tested, and expanded.

At present, despite the dramatic growth in community-based psychiatric services that has occurred since World War II, a large majority of community-sampled psychiatric disorders remain untreated (Andrews 1999; Regier et al. 1993). Because of problems with gaining access to appropriate care, maintaining continuity, or obtaining effective treatments, the expanding mental health system has so far been unable to reduce either the prevalence of psychiatric disorders or the burden of disability caused by them. Few—if any—national or statewide mental health systems have systematically tracked two important measures of their effectiveness: reductions in community prevalence and alleviation of personal, familial, and social burden. Both sets of measures are key if mental health systems are to demonstrate their effectiveness to the public health. A conceptualization of a comprehensive matrix of measurements is depicted in Table 19–1.

In this chapter, a case study and experimental methodologies are used to discuss the issues surrounding implementation of outcome measurement in a relatively large system of care. A case study of an academic department of psychiatry of a large urban medical center is used to provide examples of 1) using outcome assessment to improve clinical programs and practices

Table 19–1. Levels and scope of measurements

1. Individual patient care	a. Symptom reduction b. Functional improvement c. Quality of life d. Adverse events e. Patient satisfaction and perception of care f. Family and community burden g. Service utilization h. Cost
2. Facilities and integrated systems (inpatient and outpatient programs)	Individual patient outcomes as in category 1, plus: a. Readmission rate b. Participation in ambulatory care (as evidenced by detection, engagement, and retention in treatment) c. Relapse prevention
3. Health care plans	Selected measures from categories 1 and 2 plus: a. Measures of access b. Measures of continuity of care c. Global population-based improvement in functioning d. Impact on population health status
4. Community level	a. Treated and untreated prevalence b. Access, utilization, and continuity of treatment c. Changes in Disability-Adjusted Life Years (DALYS)

and to track the impact of program changes (Waxman 1996); 2) the use of outcome measurement to improve clinical management of specific disorders to meet predefined standards of care; and 3) the use of patient satisfaction measurement to support or modify program activities and clinician styles. This case study covers the different levels of care, including inpatient, partial hospitalization, and outpatient services.

MEASURING OUTCOMES OF SYSTEMS OF CARE

Each stakeholder in a system of care—including administrators, providers, persons receiving treatment and their families, and society at large—holds a different set of preferences regarding clinical, functional, social, occupational, quality of life, or legal outcomes. Before an outcome measurement program is implemented, it is important to determine the audience or recipient of such measures and understand their preferences.

In 1995, for example, the New York State Office of Mental Health (Carpinello et al. 1998) conducted a mail survey to canvass opinions concerning outcomes from different mental health system stakeholders. The majority of respondents chose *wellness* (as manifested by increased independence and higher self-esteem) and improved social roles performance and living skills acquisition as preferred individual-level outcomes. The correction of system deficiencies was the preferred system-level outcome, and the elimination of stigma was the most valued social-level outcome.

In this survey, recipients chose independence and increased self-esteem as preferred outcomes, whereas clinicians and family members focused on reduction of symptoms and symptom management skills. Administrators of a system of care attempting to respond to multiple stakeholders would be wise to demonstrate performance along these diverse preference sets.

In general, systems of care participate in outcome measurement as a result of any combination of the following forces: regulatory pressures, (e.g., JCAHO and National Committee for Quality Assurance [NCQA] accreditation), internally driven quality improvement initiatives, contractual demands, and marketing and public relations efforts. Each illustrates a different piece of the outcomes pie.

Because any large practice or program may produce a virtually infinite number of measurable outcomes, this potential universe must be reduced on the basis of a careful strategic plan that takes into account the most relevant factors influencing outcome and proposes a manageable package of measures that will yield meaningful data.

There are an increasing number of measurement instruments and methods, each of which imposes a different burden of cost, time, and training. The decision to utilize a particular measure or group of measures will be dependent on the setting of care, the population served (categorized by demographics, diagnosis, comorbidities, etc.), the specific goals of the program, and regulatory requirements.

This chapter includes selected material from a case study that illustrates the selection, utilization, and results of outcome measures and performance indicators in an urban academic medical center that services a very broad array of patients. Reviewed as follows are the available measurement instruments, the selection process, and how quantitative outcomes were used to achieve better clinical and system performance.

INPATIENT CARE OUTCOMES

The great majority of inpatient programs treats patients with acute severe psychiatric disorders who are in imminent danger to self or others; who are so disorganized that they cannot safely perform basic self-care functions; or who, being highly symptomatic and dysfunctional, have been unable to function in a less restrictive level of care.

Adequate inpatient treatment for a defined diagnostic condition should maintain safety, reduce symptoms and disability, reduce the risk of relapse after discharge, and promote continuity of care, with as few adverse effects as possible.

Table 19–2 presents a matrix of functions and suggested measurements for possible implementation in inpatient settings.

In addition to monitoring the outcome of inpatients' core functions, an outcome program may have additional functions as follows:

1. Monitor clinician performance to guide it toward an optimum. Feedback to clinicians can also guide their performance to meet specified standards of care.
2. Track program performance in relation to benchmarks. Performance benchmarks may be obtained from the following sources:

   • Results of randomized clinical trials (gold standard of efficacy)
   • Practice guidelines, algorithms, and clinical consensus recommendations
   • Results of demonstration projects, evaluations of sample cohorts, analyses of treated samples, and expert opinions

Through a case illustration, this section demonstrates the methods used to measure the progress of patient outcome in an inpatient program as national practice recommendations were progressively incorporated into a clinical setting.

> The Department of Psychiatry at New York University/Bellevue Hospital Center is one of the oldest and largest general hospital psychiatric facilities in the United States. The department currently operates 319 inpatient beds distributed among the emergency, child and adolescent, substance abuse, forensic, and geriatric psychiatry divisions. The department also operates three day programs and two long-term residential treatment settings. Its ambulatory division provides over 120,000 outpatient visits per year, covering the spectrum of individual, group, and family therapies. Bellevue's psychiatric program serves a multiethnic, multicultural population that comes from diverse socioeconomic backgrounds. The typical patient has a severe psychiatric disorder that is often complicated by significant medical and substance abuse comorbidities and psychosocial stressors. In addition to the severity of their clinical conditions, many patients are severely and disproportionately affected by adverse socioeconomic situations such as poverty, homelessness, unemployment, and ethnic and/or linguistic minority status and acculturation problems. These factors are all known to have negative effects on the onset, course, and outcome of psychiatric disorders.

Table 19–2. Functions and suggested measurements for inpatient settings

Function	Outcome	Measurement methods
Maintain safety	Suicide/attempted suicide Injuries/assault Falls Restraint and seclusion	Tracking and trending
Reduce symptoms	Decreased psychotic symptoms Decreased depressive or manic symptoms	BPRS, SANS, SAPS, PANSS, SCL-90-R, SADS, SAS II[a]
Minimize adverse effects	Minimize expected side effects Monitor unexpected adverse effects and drug interactions	AIMS, Simpson Angus Scale, ESRS, Barnes Akathisia Scale;[a] Tracking and trending
Reduce disability	Activities of daily living (ADL) and other functions	GAF, BASIS-32, NOSIE,[a] and Katz ADL Scale
Reduce risk of relapse	Readmission rate (within 15 days or 30 days)	Tracking and trending
Promote continuity of care	Percentage of discharged patients with set aftercare appointments Percentage of discharged patients who kept aftercare appointments	Tracking and trending
Patient perceptions of care	Percentage satisfaction with care	PoC, CSQ-8, SSS-30[c]

[a]Abbreviations: BPRS=Brief Psychiatric Rating Scale; SANS=Scale for the Assessment of Negative Symptoms; SAPS=Scale for the Assessment of Positive Symptoms; PANSS=Positive and Negative Syndrome Scale; SCL-90-R=Symptom Checklist-90-Revised; SADS=Schedule of Affective Disorders and Schizophrenia; SAS II=Social Adjustment Scale II; AIMS=Abnormal Involuntary Movement Scale; ESRS=Extrapyramidal Symptom Rating Scale; GAF=Global Assessment of Functioning Scale; BASIS-32=Behavior and Symptom Identification Scale; NOSIE=Nurses' Observation Scale for Inpatient Evaluation. For a more detailed review of some of these instruments, please refer to Chapter 9, in this volume.

[b]Abbreviations: BDI-II=Beck Depression Inventory–II; HRSD=Hamilton Rating Scale for Depression; YMRS=Young Mania Rating Scale; IDS=Inventory for Depressive Symptomatology. For a more detailed review of some of these instruments, please refer to Chapter 10, in this volume.

[c]Abbreviations: PoC=Perceptions of Care survey; CSQ-8=Client Satisfaction Questionnaire–8; SSS-30=Service Satisfaction Survey–30. For a more detailed review of some of these instruments, please refer to Chapter 18, in this volume.

Part 1: Improving Inpatient Outcomes

In 1992, the quality improvement program in the department of psychiatry selected the 30-day readmission rate as an outcome measure and decided to track and compare it with other urban public psychiatry programs after the introduction of specific programmatic interventions. The choice of the 30-day readmission rate was based on the concept that the best output of inpatient care today is the "production" of safe discharges to a less restrictive level of care. This measure has been extensively evaluated (Lyons et al. 1997; Swett 1995; Thomas et al. 1996) in studies that have yielded significant insight about the optimum inpatient treatment of acute psychosis, such as the role of negative or deficit symptoms in the prediction of early readmissions and the importance of ensuring adequate posthospital psychosocial support. Another readmission measure (15-day) has been selected by the JCAHO (through the ORYX system, which is an initiative to integrate performance measures into the accreditation process) as a national benchmark for behavioral health care organizations, which will permit future cross-institutional comparisons. Readmission rates also have demonstrated sensitivity and responsiveness to clinical interventions such as psychoeducation (Conte et al. 1996) and intensive case management (Patterson and Lee 1998), making it possible for systems treating large numbers of psychotic patients to measure and achieve better outcomes by the systematic application of these services.

The Global Assessment of Functioning (GAF) (American Psychiatric Association 2000) is another outcome measure commonly used by inpatient units. Typically inpatients are admitted with GAF scores of 10–35 and are discharged with scores of 25–55. Even though the GAF is scored and collected by clinicians on a regular basis for every patient at points of entry, the decision was made to use the 30-day readmission rate as the main inpatient clinical indicator. Although the GAF is included in DSM-IV-TR as an Axis V diagnosis, its interrater reliability ranged from 0.61 to 0.91 depending on the level of training (Jones et al. 1995). This variability was judged to interfere with the accurate tracking of outcome in response to the policy changes implemented in the department. At baseline (1992), Bellevue's 30-day readmission rate stood at 9%, slightly higher than the 8.3% recorded for the reference group (Figure 19–1).

As noted previously, the 30-day readmission rate was selected as a key outcome measure for the introduction of a series of quality improvement initiatives in the management of severe psychosis. Psychoses represented 65%–75% of admission diagnoses. The new program for optimum inpatient management of psychotic disorders involved three sequential steps. The steps, derived from the research literature on the treatment of psycho-

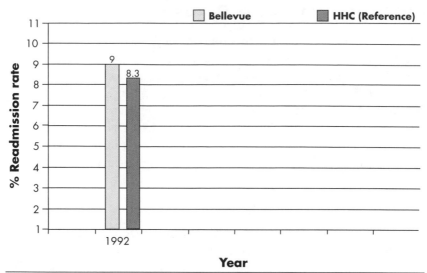

Figure 19–1.   Baseline readmission rates, Bellevue Hospital and reference facility (Health and Hospitals Corporation Benchmark [HHC]).

sis, at first drew heavily on the emerging clinical trials literature addressing the optimum psychopharmacology of psychosis and later on the recommendations of the Schizophrenia Patient Outcomes Research Team (PORT) (Lehman et. al 1998), as highlighted in Table 19–3.

Table 19–3.   Recommended steps for treatment of psychosis

1. State-of-the-art psychopharmacology
2. Patient/family psychoeducation
3. Intensive aftercare through case management and assertive community treatment (ACT)

Implementing the Continuous Quality Improvement Program

Step 1: improved psychopharmacology.   The program first aimed at optimization of psychopharmacologic management of psychosis according to empirically derived recommendations. Key components of this program are summarized in Table 19–4.

The program for the psychopharmacologic management of psychosis was introduced to the medical and clinical staffs through a variety of educational endeavors, including seminars, grand rounds, psychopharmacology conferences, and clinical case conferences. Its implementation was monitored using case-by-case review performed by an expert psychopharmacologist. The medical records of every patient admitted were reviewed

Table 19–4.   Recommendations for psychopharmacologic management
of psychosis

Evidence-based selection of agent
Identification and treatment of comorbidities such as anxiety, depression, and
  substance abuse
Age, gender, and ethnic considerations (Trujillo 2000)

by the psychopharmacologist along with the treating physician before the
patient's treatment plan was developed; the psychopharmacologist suggested medication options congruent with expert recommendations.
Although these recommendations were not binding, they were very frequently observed.

By 1995, this intervention was associated with a reduction in the 30-day
readmission rate by a statistically significant 5.05% versus the reference
group rate of 6.7% (two-tailed test, $P<0.05$) (Figure 19–2).

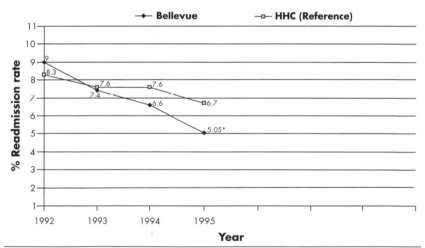

Figure 19–2.   Annual readmission rates after implementation of a psychopharmacology quality improvement program in the psychiatry department (1992–
1995), Bellevue Hospital and reference facility (Health and Hospitals Corporation
Benchmark [HHC]).

Step 2: psychoeducation.   The second step involved an increased emphasis on patient and family psychoeducation through quality improvement activity in the nursing department.

The work of McFarlane, Falloon, Leff, and others on psychoeducation
has established effectiveness in reducing relapses, possibly improving function and lowering treatment costs (Falloon et al. 1996; Leff et al. 1985;

McFarlane et al. 1995). On inpatient units, patient and family education was introduced by the nursing department as a part of milieu therapy activities, both on a one-to-one basis and in groups of 8–10 patients. Group content included awareness of diagnosis and symptoms, the different elements of treatment, medications, management of frequent side effects, and stress management. Identification and management of early signs of relapse and crisis intervention were also included. The impact of these psychoeducational efforts was assessed by a specially designed questionnaire, which rated psychoeducational status at baseline and before discharge on parameters such as patient awareness of diagnosis, symptoms, medications, and side effects. This quality initiative demonstrated a significant decrease in lack of awareness of diagnosis and symptoms from 85% at baseline to 25% at discharge. Despite the increase in the number of available measurement instruments, systems of care that have an interest in developing an outcome measurement program will, at times, need to develop their own instruments to capture the impact of interventions for which validated instruments may not be readily available. In this case, the nursing staff developed a questionnaire to assess patients' baseline and discharge knowledge using principles derived from the Juran process of quality improvement (Juran 1989).

This psychoeducational effort was associated with a second statistically significant reduction of the 30-day readmission rate to 3.51% compared with a reference rate of 4.84% (two-tailed paired samples t-tests; $t+4.3$ $[af=5]$; $P<0.01$) (Figure 19–3).

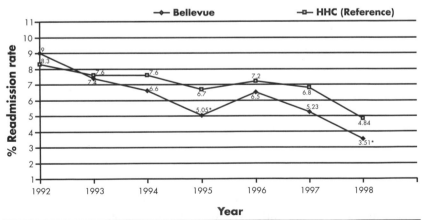

Figure 19–3. Annual readmission rates after implementation of a psychoeducation quality improvement program in the nursing department (1995–1998), Bellevue Hospital and reference facility (Health and Hospitals Corporation Benchmark [HHC]).
[*]Statistically significant at the 0.005 level.

Although the 30-day readmission rate of the reference group had also undergone a large decrease during this time period, the differences between the rate at Bellevue and the rate of the reference group remained strongly significant. All hospitals in the region were experiencing pressures to reduce their readmission rates during that period, particularly since the introduction of the JCAHO ORYX indicator in 1994. The combination of optimized psychopharmacology and psychoeducation may have enhanced such efforts at Bellevue.

Step 3: intensive aftercare. The third step involved increasing the utilization of intensive case management and assertive community treatment (Juran 1989). These services were introduced into the department as a component of the Outpatient Commitment Program, a pilot program supported by the New York State legislature to test the viability of adding an outpatient commitment statute to the state's mental hygiene laws. The use of intensive case management and assertive community treatment in the higher-risk cohort of psychotic patients was associated with a reduction in the 30-day readmission rate to 2.31% versus the 4.27% achieved by the reference group (Figure 19–4).

This multiphasic quality improvement initiative demonstrates the value of using outcome measures to track the results of program changes over extended periods of time. As large systems of care adapt their clinical practices to the requirements of evidence-based medicine, they will need to select measures that are sensitive to change over time and that are robust enough to reflect long-term program changes.

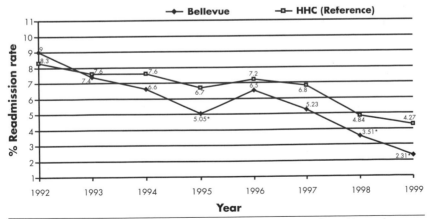

Figure 19–4. Annual readmission rates after implementation of intensive case management and assertive community treatment (1998–1999), Bellevue Hospital and reference facility (Health and Hospitals Corporation Benchmark [HHC]).
*Statistically significant at the 0.005 level.

AMBULATORY CARE OUTCOMES

Partial Hospitals

Partial hospitals are an essential component in a system of mental health care. They are used as an alternative to inpatient care for patients who are highly symptomatic and/or disorganized but who either do not meet the risk criteria for inpatient care or do not have a support system in place that can contain and support them. Optimum outcomes of partial programs revolve around further stabilizing acute symptoms and developing or strengthening self-care and social skills functions to permit the patient to maintain safety and promote recovery at a lesser level of care. Typically, patients are admitted to these programs with GAF scores between 25 and 40 and are discharged with scores of 50–60, depending on the quality of their outpatient treatment options and the availability of psychosocial supports.

Table 19–5 presents the matrix of functions and measurements that can be used to assess the outcomes of patients treated at partial hospital programs.

Table 19–5. Recommended functions and measurements for outcome assessment of patients in partial hospital programs

Function	Outcome	Measurement method
Maintain safety	Suicide attempts Violent episodes	Tracking and trending
Reduce disability	ADL and other functions Social skills and work readiness	GAF, BASIS-32, NOSIE, Katz ADL, Work Readiness Questionnaire
Reduce risk of relapse	Readmission rate (within 15 days or 30 days) and inpatient days	Tracking and trending
Promote continuity of care	Percentage of discharged patients to alternate levels of care Percentage of appointments kept	Tracking and trending
Patient perceptions of care	Percentage satisfaction with care	PoC, CSQ-8, SSS-30
Resource utilization	Planned length of stay	Tracking and trending

Note. ADL=activities of daily living; GAF=Global Assessment of Functioning; BASIS-32=Behavior and Symptom Identification Scale; NOSIE=Nurses' Observation Scale for Inpatient Evaluation; PoC=Perceptions of Care survey; CSQ-8=Client Satisfaction Questionnaire–8; SSS-30=Service Satisfaction Survey–30.

Outpatient Clinics

Outpatient facilities, within or linked to large systems of care, treat a great diversity of patients at different levels of disability and with varying intensity of treatment. Therefore, outcomes need to be controlled for differences in diagnosis, comorbidity, prognosis, and sociodemographic characteristics. A key decision in the selection of measures is the purpose of the outcome measurement system. Outpatient measurements can be performed for the following reasons:

- To improve the effectiveness of clinicians by aiding in diagnosis, standardizing the monitoring of adverse effects, and assessing complex comorbidities.
- To track physician and clinician performance with a specific patient population in relation to an internal or external reference group ("provider profiling").
- To assess program performance against known benchmarks. Do program practices conform to recommendations of national or specialty guidelines? If clinically meaningful variances are detected, they can be the forms of quality improvement initiatives through the use of process of care measures (for more details please see Chapter 3, in this volume).
- To improve the outcome of treatments applied to specific patient populations, who may fall out of acceptable ranges due to clinical, demographic, or other reasons. As an example, patients of certain linguistic or ethnic minorities have higher dropout rates when treated with individual psychodynamic therapies (McFarlane 1997).

Table 19–6 presents the matrix of functions and measurements at the outpatient level.

Part 2: Improving Depression Outcomes

In part 2 of the case study, the treatment outcomes of a specific population of patients (those with depressive disorder) are used to improve clinicians' performance.

Affective disorders in general, and depressive disorders in particular, constitute a large and growing component of the global burden of disease. These disorders carry significant mortality and morbidity, including greatly impaired functioning. Together with anxiety disorders, depression represents the greatest threat to the mental health of the human population. Depression and anxiety are extensively represented in primary care settings, private practices, and outpatient mental health services. Anti-

Table 19–6.   Recommended functions and measurements for outcome assessment of outpatients

Function	Outcome	Measurement method
Reduce symptoms	Decrease symptoms of depression, anxiety, psychosis, etc.	Specific disorder-related outcome instruments (see respective chapters)
Reduce disability	ADL and other functions Social skills and work readiness	GAF, BASIS-32, Katz ADL, Work Readiness Questionnaire
Promote independence and improvement of quality of life	Quality-of-life measures	Quality of Life Inventory (QOLI) and Quality of Life Scale (QLS)
Promote continuity of care	Percentage of appointments kept	Tracking and trending
Patient perceptions of care	Percentage satisfaction with care	PoC, CSQ-8, SSS-30

Note.   ADL=activities of daily living; GAF=Global Assessment of Functioning; BASIS-32=Behavior and Symptom Identification Scale; PoC=Perceptions of Care survey; CSQ-8=Client Satisfaction Questionnaire–8; SSS-30=Service Satisfaction Survey–30.

depressant medications and specific psychotherapies for depression (such as interpersonal and cognitive psychotherapies) offer remarkable efficacy in the treatment of depression. However, treatments studied under carefully controlled conditions have not resulted in comparable effectiveness when applied under field conditions (Eisen and Grob 1992).

Problems with access, medical and substance abuse comorbidities, and premature treatment terminations contribute to less than optimum treatment results under natural treatment conditions. Klein et al. (2000) reported a recovery rate of 52% at 5 years in a study of the treatment of dysthymic patients under naturalistic conditions. These results fall within the range of outcomes obtained in pharmacotherapy, psychotherapy, or mixed controlled studies (50% response to active treatment vs. 32% response to placebo for major depression; 59% vs. 37% response for dysthymia). The cohort observed in this study spent approximately 70% of the follow-up period fully meeting criteria for a mood disorder (Bluestone and Vela 1982).

Outpatient visits for depressive disorders represent slightly over 50% of ambulatory care visits at Bellevue. In 1998, a quality improvement initiative to assess and improve depression treatment outcomes was designed. Patients entering treatment in the ambulatory psychiatry programs would complete the Beck Depression Inventory–II (BDI-II) as a part of their initial screening. The BDI-II was selected because of its widespread use in outcome studies destined to assess symptom change over time, ease of administration (self-report), sensitivity to severe depression, and ability to detect significant change during psychotherapy and drug therapy. Outcome evaluators working in other settings also have at their disposal other instruments to assess the outcome of depression: the Hamilton Rating Scale for Depression (HRSD or Ham-D), the Inventory for Depressive Symptomatology (IDS) (with both a self-report and clinician-administered forms), and the Montgomery-Asberg Depression Rating Scale (MADRS).

Evaluators working in other settings or with other patient populations should select instruments in relation to their sensitivity to essential characteristics of their patients, such as relative homogeneity of their sample, severity of depression at baseline, and presence of comorbidities, as well as availability of time, financial resources, and trained rates. For example, few depression scales provide good coverage of psychotic symptoms in depression. The HRSD includes indirect references to psychosis in the severity anchors. The IDS, which queries about atypical symptoms, may be useful to clinicians or settings with significant numbers of patients with atypical depression. The IDS is also keyed to DSM-IV-TR criteria and tracks outcomes of individual DSM-IV-TR symptoms (American Psychiatric Association 2000). (For a more detailed review, please refer to Chapter 10, in this volume.)

Reviewers used an evaluation form based on the written algorithm. The form inquired about parameters such as percentage of missed appointments, patient adherence to medication regimens, active identification of existing comorbidities, and clinician adherence to optimum prescribing protocols. Table 19–7 compares the initial average BDI-II score for three cohorts of patients.

Table 19–7 demonstrates that each cohort achieved lower BDI-II scores earlier in the treatment, perhaps indicating more rapid improvement.

Table 19–7.   Average scores on the Beck Depression Inventory–II for outpatients with depressive disorder

Cohort	Initial month	3 months	6 months	9 months average
1	32.8	23.4	18.7	16.7
2	31.4	20.3	16.7	NA
3	28.1	18.7	NA	NA

Note.   Cohort 1 represents the eligible patients who entered treatment between 11/30/98 and 3/1/99; Cohort 2 entered treatment between 3/1/99 and 5/31/99; Cohort 3 entered treatment between 6/1/99 and 8/30/99. NA=not available.

In addition to evaluation of the improvement in average scores, the percentages of patients in each cohort that had complete response, partial response, or no response for each period of analysis were calculated. Table 19–8 presents the response in each cohort according to the month of analysis.

As shown in Table 19–8, there was a sizable improvement in the percentage of patients showing a complete response at 3 months, an effect that may be due to the feedback given to the treating clinicians as the initiative unfolded.

Results from the 3-month, 6-month, and 9-month chart reviews revealed the following most commonly noted reasons for suboptimal treatment response: complicating life stressors (55% of all charts surveyed); complicating second diagnosis (31%); complicating medical diagnosis (29%); appointment noncompliance (20%); medication refusal (17%); and substance use (15%).

The most common life stressors cited as causes of nonresponse to treatment were serious medical illnesses (30%); unemployment/financial problems (13%); and family conflict (20%). The most common secondary diagnoses associated with nonresponse to treatment were alcohol/polysubstance abuse (20%); personality disorders (8%); and other comorbid mental disorders (20%).

Table 19–8.   Outpatient response to treatment for depressive disorder

Response	3 months (%)	6 months (%)	9 months (%)
Cohort 1 (N=46)			
Complete	16.7	30.6	36.1
Partial	44.9	44.4	46.1
None	38.9	25.0	17.8
Cohort 2 (N=36)			
Complete	20.2	38.4	NA
Partial	47.5	32.3	NA
None	32.3	29.3	NA
Cohort 3 (N=58)			
Complete	30.5	NA	NA
Partial	34.8	NA	NA
None	34.8	NA	NA

Note.   Cohort 1 represents the eligible patients who entered treatment between 11/30/98 and 3/1/99; Cohort 2 entered treatment between 3/1/99 and 5/31/99; Cohort 3 entered treatment between 6/1/99 and 8/30/99. NA=not available.

Overall, it was found that patient and illness factors, rather than staff and institutional factors, accounted for poorer outcomes. Patient factors were five times more likely to be cited as contributing to poor outcomes than were staff factors. Improper medication dosing (e.g., low dosing), the only notable staff factor, was noted in 17% of the reviews and was addressed through staff educational activities. As of this writing, the impact of these activities in clinicians' practices is being evaluated.

Lessons From the Depression Outcome Project

The findings of the program to improve patient outcomes in depression are summarized below:

- In the Bellevue population, treatment-refractory primary depression was seldom the major reason for poorer outcomes. Other factors—such as accompanying psychosocial stressors, comorbid drug and alcohol use, and patient noncompliance with medication regimens or treatment recommendations—were much more likely to be the associated factors.
- The 3-month effectiveness rates have been above 64%, and the 6-month effectiveness rates have been above 72%. These are comparable to results obtained in randomized clinical trials for the treatment of depression and are better than those obtained in most naturalistic studies.
- Improper dosing of medication is the only staff factor that has been noted consistently in the chart reviews.
- Feedback to clinicians using data gathered from selected chart reviews may improve outcome at 3 months and beyond.
- The process of outcome evaluation, supplemented by other reviews (with results fed back to the treating clinician), may be valuable in improving treatment outcome in difficult-to-treat disorders. Improvements may be obtained by identifying comorbidities and additional factors specific to a particular treatment setting or population of patients, which can focus quality improvement efforts.

Patient Satisfaction Guiding Program Changes

The measurement of patient and family satisfaction with treatment has become an established practice in systems of care, making it perhaps the most frequently used measure of quality. First used commonly as a public relations tool by private proprietary psychiatric facilities in the 1980s, patient satisfaction surveys have become more respectable. They are an important response to the increasingly visible and active role of consumers in health care.

Evidence has accumulated about the correlation between patient satisfaction and clinical outcomes (Klein et al. 2000). Originally designed to assess primarily the patient's satisfaction with the environment of care, satisfaction surveys were later expanded to tap into the patients' views on the technical competence, interpersonal skills, and patient care attitudes of key program staff members. More recent studies have elaborated on the relationship between treatment response and patient satisfaction. As an example, satisfaction was examined in 183 patients and revealed that only 1 patient of 82 high responders expressed dissatisfaction with treatment, whereas 21 of the 22 most dissatisfied respondents had showed a poor treatment response. The study concluded that treatment response tends to correlate with elevated patient satisfaction scores (Agency for Health Care Policy and Research 1999).

When selecting patient satisfaction instruments, clinicians need to keep in mind that many of the most widely used measures have been imported into psychiatry from the nonmedical service sector or from the general medical sector. Instruments with specific application to psychiatric patients are being developed and tested for reliability and validity (for more details, please refer to Chapter 18, in this volume).

Systems of care that are interested in comparing their patient satisfaction outcomes with a national sample may want to consider the consumer survey component of the Mental Health Statistics Improvement Program (MHSIP). A 21-item portion of the MHSIP consumer survey is being evaluated for inclusion in the Health Plan Employer Data and Information Set (HEDIS) of the NCQA.

At Bellevue, in 1998, patient satisfaction surveys were taken one step further by including in the 39-item patient satisfaction assessment instrument questions designed to assess patients' knowledge of general aspects of their treatment, such as goals, objectives, length of treatment, and time to improvement. Items that received lower-than-expected evaluations by the patients were fed back to outpatient clinicians in the context of weekly staff and monthly quality improvement meetings. At resurvey (12 months later), those items showed statistically significant differences from baseline (Table 19–9).

It is interesting to note that the therapist effectiveness rating (items such as demonstrable interest; clear explanations about the goals, means and timeline of therapy; and explanation of available after hours crisis resources) can go a long way toward improving patient satisfaction with treatment. It can also be easy to correct these scores when they are found to be suboptimal. Because patient satisfaction responses are very specific to patient populations and treatment settings, it behooves each facility to tap into its patient perceptions and to design continuous medical education and other quality improvement initiatives focused on their specific findings. To paraphrase a well-known political adage, patient satisfaction is always local.

Table 19–9. Comparison of 1998 and 1999 patient satisfaction survey results

Survey item	1998 (%)	1999 (%)	Changes reaching statistical significance
Program efficacy			
Treatment right for you	94	93	
Reaching personal goals	90	90	
Like program	91	93	
Would recommend program	89	87	
Helping with a better life	90	92	
Therapist effectiveness			
Therapist interested	93	96	$\chi^2 (1, n=1,245)=4.24, P<0.05$
Therapist on time	93	94	
Therapist knowledgeable	92	93	
Therapist explains clearly	94	97	$\chi^2 (1, n=1,245)=5.89, P<0.05$
Comfortable disclosing	90	92	
Therapist noncoercive	91	90	
Can get help after hours	77	83	$\chi^2 (1, n=1,245)=7.81, P<0.01$
Environment of care			
Area attractive	73	75	
Area clean	82	88	$\chi^2 (1, n=1,203)=8.80, P<0.01$
Clerical staff helpful	92	95	$\chi^2 (1, n=1,203)=5.33, P<0.05$
Area safe	92	95	$\chi^2 (1, n=1,203)=6.20, P<0.05$
Bathrooms clean	64	74	$\chi^2 (1, n=1,203)=15.29, P<0.001$
Composite ratings			
Program efficacy	91	91	
Therapist effectiveness	90	92	$\chi^2 (1, n=8,715)=7.67, P<0.01$
Environment of care	80	86	$\chi^2 (1, n=6,015)=28.12, P<0.001$

As the consumer movement in the United States (and other countries) continues to mature and consumers achieve a greater voice in health care, patient satisfaction questionnaires designed to survey beyond environment-of-care items to clinically relevant domains can help clinical systems modify policies, programs, and clinical practices toward an optimum fit between stated program goals and actual program performance, as assessed by the recipients of such programs. It is possible for individual patient goals and expectations to be incorporated into treatment plans, thereby fulfilling in practice the often theoretical commitment of many treatment programs to individually tailor the treatment to the needs of each patient.

Lessons Learned During Implementation of an Outcome Measurement Program

The introduction of an outcome measurement program into a system of care is a delicate management process. If successful, the program can yield significant gains in clinical benefit to patients, knowledge and mastery to clinicians, and demonstrable performance to clinical managers and third parties. It can also provide evidence of quality care to regulators and value to health care plans and other care buyers.

If unsuccessful, the program can get mired in expensive and mindless data collection. It can alienate overburdened clinicians and support personnel as unproductive lines of inquiry are pursued or abandoned, one after another. Key steps to success include the following:

- Careful delineation of expected deliverables with the agency or group that originates the demand for outcome measurement.
- Designing the outcome measurement plan as a part of the existing continuous quality improvement plan to ensure strategic alignment with existing quality goals and objectives and the selection of outcomes that address the care system's core mission. Optimally, the outcomes to be measured should reflect significant community problems and assess high-volume, high-risk, or problem-prone interventions.
- Early participation (and buy-in) of clinicians in the design of the program, the selection of instruments, and the working through of technical issues such as validity, reliability, and generalizability of findings.
- Considerations of time and hidden costs, including clinician time (administration, scoring, and interpretation of results), patient time, and any effects on clinician-patient interaction. As a general rule, outcome measurement represents a significant time commitment for systems that already face huge administrative burdens. Clinicians thus react with considerable resistance to additional paperwork or erosions of their much-valued clinical autonomy. Clinicians' views need to be taken seriously and worked through by a process that demonstrates value to the clinician by better outcomes and/or meaningful gains in clinical knowledge. If outcome measurement is part of a provider-profiling plan, with a potential adverse effect on a clinician's evaluations and compensation, due process safeguards must be established up front. These may include the opportunity to review findings for possible correction of false-positive and false-negative results.
- Considerations of the applicability of outcome measurements across different linguistic and cultural groups. It is well known that social, economic, educational, and cultural factors affect the measurement of

psychiatric disorders. Test score thresholds, boundaries between normal and pathological phenomena, and symptom content and themes vary widely from one culture to another. Translation and adaptations of diagnostic instruments present additional problems that may adversely affect the reliability and validity of findings.

For an implementation example, the reader is referred to Appendix A, which includes a depression treatment and outcome pathway.

CONCLUSION

At the dawn of the new millennium, health care in general, and psychiatric care in particular, are the target of many revolutionary forces. Research continues to transform the understanding of mental disorders and provide more and better means for their treatment. At the same time, payers demand evidence of efficiency and effectiveness; the public demands easy service access and affordable care; and consumers (both patients and families) seek a larger voice in mental health policies, programs, and practices. In short, the public and our patients want results. Emphasis on results (outcomes) is becoming a necessary feature in organized systems of care and for individual practitioners.

In this chapter, through theory and a case study covering the different levels of care (inpatient, partial hospital, and outpatient), a framework was provided for large systems of care to participate in the exciting development of outcome assessment. In addition, suggestions were offered regarding ways by which the systematic assessment of outcomes can contribute to better programs that are tailored to the individual needs of the patients we are called on to serve.

REFERENCES

Agency for Health Care Policy and Research: Treatment of Depression—Newer Pharmacotherapies (Evidence Report/Technology Assessment No 7) (Publ No 99-E014). Rockville, MD, Agency for Health Care Policy and Research, 1999

American Psychiatric Association: Diagnostic and Statistical Manual of Mental Disorders, 4th Edition, Text Revision. Washington, DC, American Psychiatric Association, 2000

Andrews G: Efficacy, effectiveness and efficiency in mental health service delivery. Aust N Z J Psychiatry 33:316–322, 1999

Bluestone H, Vela RM: Transcultural aspects in the psychotherapy of the Puerto Rican poor in New York City. J Am Acad Psychoanal 10:269–283, 1982

Carpinello S, Felton CJ, Pease EA, et al: Designing a system for managing the performance of mental health managed care: an example from New York State's prepaid mental health plan. J Behav Health Serv Res 25:269–278, 1998

Conte G, Ferrari R, Guarneri L, et al: Reducing the "revolving door" phenomenon. Am J Psychiatry 153:1512, 1996

Eisen SV, Grob MC: Patient outcome after transfer within a psychiatric hospital. Hospital and Community Psychiatry 43:803–806, 1992

Falloon IH, Kydd RR, Coverdale JH, et al: Early detection and intervention for initial episodes of schizophrenia, in Schizophrenia. Edited by Moscarelli M, Rupp A, Sartorius N (Handbook of Mental Health Economics and Health Policy, Vol 1). New York, Wiley, 1996, pp 167–178

Jones SH, Thornicroft G, Coffey M, et al: A brief mental health outcome scale: reliability and validity of the Global Assessment of Functioning (GAF). Br J Psychiatry 166:654–659, 1995

Juran JM: Juran on Leadership for Quality. New York, Free Press, 1989

Klein DN, Schwartz JE, Rose S, et al: Five-year course and outcome of dysthymic disorder: a prospective, naturalistic follow-up study. Am J Psychiatry 157:931–939, 2000

Leff JP, Kuipers L, Burkowitz R, et al: A controlled trial of social intervention in the families of schizophrenic patients: two year follow-up. Br J Psychiatry 146:594–600, 1985

Lehman AF, Steinwachs DM, Dixon LB, et al: Translating research into practice: the Schizophrenia Patient Outcomes Research Team (PORT) Treatment Recommendations. Schizophr Bull 24:1–20, 1998

Lyons JS, O'Mahoney MT, Miller SI, et al: Predicting readmission to the psychiatric hospital in a managed care environment: implications for quality indicators. Am J Psychiatry 154:337–340, 1997

McFarlane WR: FACT: integrating family psychoeducation and assertive community treatment. Adm Policy Ment Health 25:191–198, 1997

McFarlane WR, Lukens E, Link B, et al: Multiple-family groups and psychoeducation in the treatment of schizophrenia. Arch Gen Psychiatry 52:679–687, 1995

Patterson DA, Lee M: Intensive case management and rehospitalization: a survival analysis. Research on Social Work Practice 8:152–171, 1998

Regier DA, Narrow WE, Rae DS, et al: The de facto U.S. mental and addictive disorders service system: Epidemiologic Catchment Area prospective 1-year prevalence rates of disorders and services. Arch Gen Psychiatry 50:85–94, 1993

Swett C: Symptom severity and number of previous psychiatric admissions as predictors of readmission. Psychiatr Serv 46:482–485, 1995

Thomas MR, Rosenberg SA, Giese AA, et al: Shortening length of stay without increasing recidivism on a university-affiliated inpatient unit. Psychiatr Serv 47:996–998, 1996

Trujillo M: Cultural psychiatry, in Comprehensive Textbook of Psychiatry, 7th Edition. Edited by Sadock B, Sadock V. Baltimore, MD, Williams & Wilkins, 2000, pp 492–499

Waxman HM: Using outcomes assessment for quality improvement, in Outcomes Assessment in Clinical Practice. Edited by Sederer LI, Dickey B. Baltimore, MD, Williams & Wilkins, 1996, pp 25–99

Resistance to the Implementation of Outcome Measures

John M. Oldham, M.D.
Lloyd I. Sederer, M.D.

Concerns about quality are finally emerging from the persistent shadow of cost that has preoccupied health care for over a decade. In a recent policy article, Bodenheimer (1999a) described a national trend among health care leaders to establish a "culture of quality" within their institutions. A report of the Institute of Medicine (Kohn et al. 2000) on medical errors received widespread attention and reinforced the need for a focus on quality and improved health care outcomes. This chapter presents the current state of the art of outcome measures in psychiatry—measures that are increasingly being utilized by mental health provider organizations to meet the quality mandate.

But all is not smooth sailing in the world of performance measurement, and a number of sources of resistance—some overt and some covert—to the implementation of outcome measures exist. In this chapter, we comment on the following categories of resistance: 1) time and money, 2) mistrust of the system, 3) loss of control, and 4) fear of the consequences. We believe that a better understanding of the reasons for resistance to the adoption of performance measurement will better inform health care providers and will diminish that resistance, encouraging greater utilization of performance measurement programs.

TIME AND FINANCIAL ISSUES

In a project to develop a system for primary care physicians to screen for psychiatric illness, Spitzer and colleagues (1994) developed the PRIME-MD, a mental health screening tool estimated to take an average of 6 minutes to administer. In field trials of this new instrument, however, these researchers determined that primary care physicians did not have 6 minutes to spare in their evaluations of patients. Any added requirement for systematic, standardized evaluation within a health care system consumes more time; that time, in short supply, can come only from other activities (including patient care) and costs money.

In a survey on attitudes of mental health personnel about outcome measurement, Walter et al. (1998) reported that the majority of respondents were disinclined to do outcome measures in the future even if it meant providing a better service to patients. These researchers noted that the only predictor of a willingness to routinely measure outcome was if it was perceived as not being too time consuming. The authors concluded, "Instruments will need to be short and the battery of instruments kept to a minimum." However, as Ware (1999) pointed out, "short-form surveys are not up to the next generation of assessment. The very thing that makes them popular, their brevity, limits them in terms of another important requirement: score precision." On the other hand, Schade and associates (1998) reported on the validity and clinical utility of depression screening instruments and concluded that less is more. Their findings were that brief screening instruments performed as well as longer instruments in detecting the presence of depression.

As a rule, brief screening instruments are high on sensitivity but low on specificity (i.e., they tend to be overinclusive). Brief screening instruments can be efficient first steps that require further specific diagnostic precision to differentiate patients with true disorders from those with false-positive scores. Because it is well known that depression is underdetected (and undertreated) in the general population (Wells 1999), better case finding is needed, although this does not necessarily lead to appropriate treatment. A common time saver utilized in quality measurement is to employ self-report inventories of patients, which can save staff time and lessen their burden. However, even data produced by self-report questionnaires are limited by the level of enthusiasm and understanding that patients have of the information requested. In effect, professional and support staff need to prime the pump of inquiry for patients to effectively use screening instruments.

In a large study of Partners in Care, a system designed to improve the treatment of depression in primary care settings, Wells (1999) reported that quality improvement systems may increase direct costs, with uncertainty about future benefits or long-term savings. The use of any instrument—screening or follow-through specific assessment tool—has to cost money. Tools in the public domain (i.e., wherein no royalty payments are charged) still require expenditures for printing, data collection and analysis, and reporting. Some may require training. Although these costs can be kept low, they still strain mental health budgets that are already operating on little or no margin.

Busch and Sederer (in press) urge specificity in decision making before beginning a program of outcomes assessment; they describe examples of common problems in setting up a quality measurement system. They emphasize the importance of ensuring the reliability and validity of the measures chosen; the crucial need to choose measures that best fit the population or problem under study; the need to focus the study questions and avoid overly broad and complex inquiry; and not asking more of the clinical or information systems staff than they can deliver. Poorly designed outcomes programs backfire when they require additional time from usually already overburdened staffs or are excessively complex and do not provide meaningful and swift feedback that is useful to the clinical staff and patients.

MISTRUST OF MEASUREMENT SYSTEMS AND "GAMING"

In 1998 and 1999, we were members of an American Psychiatric Association Task Force on Quality Indicators, charged to create a conceptual framework and developing a process for the development of clinically based quality indicators in psychiatry. One of the principles articulated by the task force was that indicators should be as impervious as possible to "gaming" by health care organizations. Although many systems of care genuinely welcome performance measurement as a way of improving patient care and enhancing cost-effectiveness, others generate positive data in response to imposed external requirements from payers and accreditors, which may not substantively represent the actual quality of care provided. The Joint Commission on Accreditation of Healthcare Organizations (JCAHO) sought to establish an ambitious outcomes-based performance measurement program but encountered great resistance by hospital organizations (Bodenheimer 1999b). Instead, JCAHO introduced a system called ORYX, in which hospitals must initially select and report two measures relevant to at least 20% of their patient populations. In subsequent years, the hospitals will be required to increase the number of measures reported. Many JCAHO-accredited hospitals in large networks or systems selected measures that were already in use (and hence inexpensive and with low burden) and that already showed favorable profiles (e.g., length of stay). As the number of required measures increases, organizations are apt to play the game rather than seriously attempt to assess and improve outcomes. The collapse of the Charter proprietary hospital system, for example, illustrates a large-scale system in which profit goals obliterated appropriate health care values. It took a long time for the systemic problems in Charter's delivery of clinical care to surface, during which report after report contended that quality care was being provided.

Another process that can engender mistrust of measurement systems is the notorious inaccuracy of data. Bodenheimer (1999a) made the following observation:

> Each intervention requires its own particular measurement of quality; some elucidate the processes of care, and some focus on outcomes.... Even when considering only one health care intervention—for example, coronary-artery bypass surgery—it is treacherous to compare the outcomes of one surgical team with those of another without adjusting for the age of the patients and the severity of their illness. (p. 488)

Case-mix adjustment for psychiatric care is only at the beginning of its development, and it can be complicated, time consuming, and costly. But proper case-mix adjustment is the only way to ensure that meaningful data can be compared across systems. Frequently, data are far more imprecise than they appear to be. For example, in large public databases, even ostensibly simple information such as diagnoses can be quite muddled and inaccurate and yet be presented as definitive DSM-IV-TR statistics. This occurs, for example, when admission diagnoses are recorded rather than discharge diagnoses, because the former are easier to collect, although they are ultimately less accurate. In addition, although assessment may specify *primary* diagnoses, those entering the data from the medical records may result in various interpretations of *primary* as initial, Axis I, main, or first-listed diagnoses.

Clinicians, administrators, consumers, and payers all seek reliable and valid outcome data. Obtaining the data is another matter. Until trust improves about data measurement and reporting, resistance to its implementation will continue.

LOSS OF CONTROL

The practice patterns of experienced clinicians are not easy to change (Ellrodt et al. 1997). In part, this may derive from strongly held assumptions by practitioners that they are providing quality treatment based on sound training. In today's managed care world, however, other factors have aggressively intruded into the practitioner's world. For example, disease management programs have been developed, with explicit goals of prevention and early identification of problems.

Care paths, or decision trees, have been developed for the treatment of almost all the major psychiatric disorders. However, as Bodenheimer (1999b) pointed out, these programs often "place little value in the role of a trusted personal physician." The doctor-patient relationship is surprisingly absent from these algorithms. Nor does their introduction seem to attend to the difficulties of changing physicians' practice patterns. These omissions serve to impede the effectiveness of management programs designed to improve health and enhance treatment. Moreover, practitioners enrolled in managed care organizations (MCOs) frequently become embittered and disenchanted by the constant review and micromanagement of their medical decision making. As a result, it can become very difficult for clinicians to see quality management systems introduced by health management organizations (HMOs) or MCOs as anything more than efforts to control cost.

FEAR OF THE CONSEQUENCES

Variations in the provision of clinical services in different geographic localities have been attributed to many factors, including ease of access to health care, differing severities of illness, and differential practice patterns. Physician profiling has been undertaken in an attempt to study differences in decision making and care delivery. This concept is being incorporated into report cards for health care systems and individual practitioners. Hofer and associates (1999) sounded an alarm about such practices, citing the risk that for fear of being deselected from HMOs, physicians in turn deselect patients from their caseloads. By avoiding high-cost, complex, or severely ill patients, physicians may attempt to shape their performance reports to demonstrate a pleasing set of cost-effectiveness statistics.

Similarly, as pointed out by Bindman (1999):

> While the health care community awaits clarification on the benefits of reliable physician profiling, investigators should carefully scrutinize the costs of establishing physician profiles. Not only are there financial costs

associated with collecting these data, but also there are risks that these tools, which have been used to limit physicians' admitting privileges and contracting opportunities with managed care organizations, may likely contribute to physicians' increasing dissatisfaction with the health care system. (p. 2143)

The ambitious American Medical Accreditation Program (AMAP), developed by the American Medical Association as a program to accredit the practices of its individual physician members, was launched with great fanfare. However, resistance to this program led to its dismantlement.

CONCLUSION

Resistance to change is a normative process. When it appears not to be there, one should look harder, because it is probably just hidden. For the new and demanding enterprise of outcomes assessment, there are many reasons for clinicians and clinical administrators to resist its adoption. In this chapter, we have offered four categories of resistance to performance measurement, attempting to highlight some of the principal barriers to change. Improving patient care is fundamental to the covenant that clinicians have with patients. Using data to understand and improve patient care is the essence of empirical medicine. We hope that an understanding of the barriers to the use of data will lead to improved methods and enhanced trust of performance measurement systems, and that the result will be better patient outcomes and clinicians taking greater pride in their work.

REFERENCES

Bindman AB: Can physician profiles be trusted? JAMA 281:2142–2143, 1999

Bodenheimer T: The American health care system: the movement for improved quality in health care. N Engl J Med 340:488–492, 1999a

Bodenheimer T: Disease management—promises and pitfalls. N Engl J Med 340: 1202–1205, 1999b

Busch A, Sederer LI: Problems and solutions in implementing outcomes assessment. Harv Rev Psychiatry 8:323–327, 2000

Ellrodt G, Cook DJ, Lee J, et al: Evidence-based disease management. JAMA 278: 1687–1692, 1997

Hofer TP, Hayward RA, Greenfield S, et al: The unreliability of individual physician "report cards" for assessing the costs and quality of care of a chronic disease. JAMA 281:2098–2105, 1999

Kohn LT, Corrigan JM, Donaldson MS (eds): To Err Is Human: Building a Safer Health System. Committee on Quality Health Care in America, Institute of Medicine. Washington, DC, National Academy Press, 2000

Schade CP, Jones ER, Wittlin BJ: A ten-year review of the validity and clinical utility of depression screening. Psychiatr Serv 49:55–61, 1998

Spitzer RL, Williams JB, Kroenke K, et al: Utility of a new procedure for diagnosing mental disorders in primary care. The PRIME-MD 1000 study. JAMA 272:1749–1756, 1994

Walter G, Cleary M, Rey JM: Attitudes of mental health personnel towards rating outcome. J Qual Clin Pract 18:109–115, 1998

Ware JE: Future directions in health status assessment. Journal of Clinical Outcomes Management 6:34–37, 1999

Wells KB: The design of Partners in Care: evaluating the cost-effectiveness of improving care for depression in primary care. Soc Psychiatry Psychiatr Epidemiol 34:20–29, 1999

21

Efforts of Regulatory, Professional, and Accreditation Authorities

Russell F. Lim, M.D.

Outcome measures in mental health have been used for many years in the academic sector, but in recent years they have also been increasingly used by managed care organizations (MCOs). Within the last decade, there has been increasing attention paid to the utilization of medical services by the United States government and by MCOs themselves. This chapter describes outcome measurements in managed care environments, as well as the evolution of outcome assessments for MCOs, as influenced by the government, patient advocacy groups, and professional organizations. The chapter concludes with a discussion of the future of outcome measurement in MCOs.

A BRIEF HISTORY

The first effort at outcome measurement among MCOs consisted of report cards for consumers with the goal of increasing enrollment by self-promotion. The belief was that the consumer's level of satisfaction with services was a good marketing device. Information was easy to obtain through surveys either mailed or given to clients or gathered by telephone. What was measured was patient satisfaction—how much patients liked the services—rather than a quantitative measure of how much clinical improvement was received. Thus, measures such as reduction in depressive symptoms or relapse rate would not be used, in favor of time spent waiting for an appointment, thoroughness of the physician, and degree of comfort felt in the waiting room. These measures are a mixture of quantitative measures and qualitative measures; they do not include measures of quality, or how much clinical improvement consumers receive from their treatment. These outcome measurements have been more of a marketing tool to increase revenues, not necessarily to improve the quality of care as measured by clinically relevant parameters. MCOs tend not to use clinical performance measures, which help to determine if the proper care was given at the right time. For example, PacifiCare Behavioral Health offers only credentialing information for its providers.

INFLUENCES ON THE EVOLUTION OF THE USE OF OUTCOME MEASUREMENTS IN MANAGED CARE ORGANIZATIONS

Some MCOs, such as Kaiser Permanente of northern California (which published the first report card by a health plan) and United Behavioral Healthcare of Minneapolis (which published the first behavioral health plan report card), have published their own report cards since the early 1990s. These report cards contained the results of simple patient satisfaction measures that could be given when the service was completed. The MCO could then report a level of satisfaction with reception, length of waiting time, how much patients liked their doctor, and whether or not patients would refer their friends to that doctor. General Motors and other companies produce report cards for their employees, prompting the U.S. General Accounting Office (GAO) to report on the usefulness (or lack thereof) of report cards. "Individual consumers have had minimal input into selecting report card indicators, and little is known about their needs or interests," the GAO reported. "As a result, their needs may not be met" (U.S. General Accounting Office 1994). The report cautioned against a noncritical reading of these report cards, because the MCOs may have chosen nonrepresentative quality measures, such as the number of board-certified doctors, and because the databases used may not be representative of the patient population. The GAO recommended that there be a standard measure and database structure, so that all data would be comparable (U.S. General Accounting Office 1994).

In the past 5 years there has been a trend toward the use of more specific information. This trend was begun by consumer activist groups, such as the Pacific Business Group on Health (PBGH) and the National Alliance for the Mentally Ill (NAMI). The PBGH, formed in 1990, is a coalition of 32 large purchasers of health care and more than 8,000 small businesses. It was a pioneer in patient satisfaction surveys. Its report card (available on its Web site at The California Consumer Healthscope at http://www.healthscope.org) allows consumers to compare physician groups on items such as preventive care, member satisfaction, and accreditation, and to compare hospitals and complication rates of selected procedures at hospitals. PBGH also manages the California Information Exchange (CALINX), which hopes to create a universal data structure that would allow MCOs to share data by agreeing on which characteristics to be collected, such as ethnicity or diagnoses, and then to come to an agreement on outcome measurements for particular diagnoses. NAMI also produced a report card in 1997 that detailed what its 168,000 members thought was needed in health plans. They surveyed nine MCOs (including Green Spring, Merit, and PacifiCare) and asked if they had treatment guidelines, had adequate access to newer medications, used patient outcomes to determine policy, offered rehabilitation and housing services, or involved family members in treatment. All nine companies were unable to successfully pass these categories and received failing grades from NAMI.

Two newer organizations have also developed clinical outcome performance measures: the American Managed Behavioral Healthcare Association (AMBHA)—which has developed the Performance Measurement System (PERMS)—and the Foundation for Accountability (FACCT)—which has developed a module to measure depression outcomes. FACCT, founded in 1995 as a nonprofit foundation, has a mission to develop quality measures that meet the needs of buyers and users of health care. Its depression outcome module is comprehensive but not widely used, probably because of its complexity of administration.

The AMBHA is a coalition of 11 major behavioral health organizations, representing almost 80% of the 142 million Americans who have managed behavioral health care benefits. Formed in 1994, its goal is the promotion of accountability of health plans, managed behavioral health care organizations, and providers through performance measurement. PERMS is based on three classifications of indicators, access to care, consumer satisfaction, and quality of care, and includes expenditure rates by treatment settings, measures of telephone responsiveness, medication management visits for persons with the diagnosis of schizophrenia, and family visits for children under age 12, as well as a consumer satisfaction measure testing set.

SELF-REGULATION OF MANAGED CARE ORGANIZATIONS

MCOs have also regulated themselves, forming the National Committee for Quality Assurance (NCQA) in 1991, which is a private, not-for-profit organization whose mission is to evaluate and report on the quality of the nation's MCOs. The primary methods used by the NCQA are assessing and reporting on the quality of managed care plans by accreditation and performance measurement. During an NCQA accreditation survey, health plans are reviewed with regard to how they meet more than 60 different standards. Unions such as the United Auto Workers, which have determined that only health plans accepted by the NCQA will be offered to their members, take these surveys very seriously. According to the NCQA, these standards fall into five broad categories:

> *Access and service*—Do health plan members have access to the care and service they need? For example: are doctors in the health plan free to discuss all treatment options available? Do patients report problems getting needed care? How well does the health plan follow up on grievances?

> *Qualified providers*—Does the health plan assess each doctor's qualifications and what health plan members say about their providers? For example: does the health plan regularly check the licenses and training of physicians? How do health plan members rate their personal doctor or nurse?

> *Staying healthy*—Does the health plan help people maintain good health and avoid illness? Does it give its doctors guidelines about how to provide appropriate preventive health services? Are members receiving tests and screenings as appropriate?

> *Getting better*—How well does the health plan care for people when they become sick? How does the health plan evaluate new medical procedures, drugs and devices to ensure that patients have access to safe and effective care?

> *Living with illness*—How well does the health plan care for people with chronic conditions? Does the plan have programs in place to assist patients in managing chronic conditions like asthma? Do diabetics, who are at risk for blindness, receive eye exams as needed? (National Committee for Quality Assurance 2001)

The principal performance measurement tool used by the NCQA for managed care is the Health Plan Employer Data and Information Set (HEDIS), which was first developed by the HMO Group, and then taken over by the NCQA and released in 1993 as HEDIS 2.0. HEDIS is a set of standardized measures used to compare health plans, now in its fifth revision, known as HEDIS 2000. HEDIS was quickly adopted as a standard in the health care industry for performance measures. Using HEDIS, the NCQA can evaluate the results a health plan actually achieves in many key areas of care and service such as effectiveness, access and availability, satisfaction, cost, stability of the health plan, presence of informed health care choices, use of services, and health plan descriptive information. Specific examples of services for diseases evaluated are cancer, heart disease, smoking, asthma, and diabetes. The strengths of HEDIS are that it contains broad focused performance measures, can be used on both private and public patients, has testing standards for future inclusion in the measures set, and is specifically designed to be used for comparisons.

HEDIS 3.0 has been criticized by the Substance Abuse and Mental Health Services Administration (SAMHSA) for not having behavioral health measures, including screening for substance abuse; continuity of care for substance abuse patients; failure of substance abuse treatment; availability of treatment for schizophrenic patients; family visits for children; and penetration rate by setting, age, and diagnostic category. Other criticisms of HEDIS include that its functional outcomes are used only on patients who are over age 65, that there is no representation of mental health professionals on committees, that there are no measures for consumer involvement, that cultural competence standards are not addressed, and that the emphasis on the credentialing of individuals instead of programs inappropriately deemphasizes the use of multidisciplinary teams. In response to these criticisms, the NCQA created a Behavioral Health Measurement Advisory Panel (MAP) in July 1997 to develop better measures related to behavioral health. The MAP made several recommendations—including adding family visits for children, using more outcome measures from the Mental Health Statistics Improvement Program (MHSIP), and tracking initial substance abuse disorder—but the only ones that were implemented in 1999 were the management of antidepressant medications and the addition of MHSIP measures to the testing set.

Another tool used by the NCQA is the Consumer Assessment of Health Plans Study 2.0H (CAHPS 2.0H) survey, developed with the help of the Agency for Health Care Policy and Research (ACHPR), which combines the best features of the 1998 HEDIS Member Satisfaction Survey with the current CAHPS instrument. Data collected by the NCQA using HEDIS and CAHPS 2.0H constitute the data set known as Quality Compass, containing comparative data on more than 400 participating health plans. The plan's specific data are tabulated, including clinical, access, financial, utilization, and member satisfaction. Then, interested companies can order copies of the report to help them choose health plans. HEDIS data collected by the NCQA are also used to create HMO report cards and health plan report cards, as reported by HealthGrades. com. These report cards, however, measure only certain satisfaction attributes. HealthGrades.com also lists physician information, but this is limited to mostly demographic information, such as medical school graduated from, specialty, address, and telephone number. The AMBHA's most recent version of PERMS, 2.0, released in September 1998, has been designed to address specific shortcomings of HEDIS 3.0 with regard to behavioral health measures. A limitation of both PERMS and HEDIS is that they do not require the modification of existing data sets and concentrate mostly on access to care and appropriateness of care, and not on outcomes. Thus, the classification *quality of care* refers to outpatient follow-up and utilization of services by adults with adjustment disorder, but it does not assess symptom reduction, return to work, etc. In addition, FACCT is critical of the use of HEDIS and CAHPS measures to assess health plans, stating that they only assess "The Basics," that is, doctor care, rules for getting care, information and service satisfaction, and do not address issues of preventive care, reduction of health risks, early detection of illness, education ("Staying Healthy"); recovery from illness and follow-up ("Getting Better"); chronic conditions management ("Living With Illness"); or disability and/or terminal illness, comprehensive services, caregiver support, and hospice care ("Changing Needs") (Skolnick 1997).

The Joint Commission on Accreditation of Healthcare Organizations (JCAHO)—founded in 1951 by a coalition of the American College of Physicians, the American Hospital Association, the American Medical Association, the Canadian Medical Association, and the American College of Surgeons—is another example of a privately run regulatory agency. The JCAHO has created the ORYX performance system, which combines both accreditation and performance measures. Accredited hospitals and long-term care organizations are required to select at least 1 of more than 200 performance measurement systems (or 70 companies, if behavioral health care measures are required) that have signed a contract with the JCAHO to perform the ORYX evaluation (Joint Commission on Accreditation of Healthcare Organizations 2001).

Other professional organizations have become involved in the standardization of performance measures, such as the American College of Mental Health Administrators (ACMHA), which adopted a core set of values and indicators in March 1997. The ACMHA has formed a coalition to standardize performance measure usage. As of November 1998, the coalition members included the JCAHO, the Council on the Accreditation of

Rehabilitation Facilities (CARF), the Council on Quality and Leadership in Supports for People with Disabilities, the AMBHA, NAMI, the NCQA, the SAMHSA, and the National Mental Health Association (NMHA), along with ACMHA members.

Their organizational framework includes outcome indicators and recommended measures for outcomes, process, access, and structure. The intent was to identify measures that were already in use and to specify where additional measures could be used. It should be noted that the best-represented measures were the structural measures administered by the NCQA. These structural measures were only a quarter of the ACMHA recommended set.

Outcome indicators endorsed by the ACMHA include housing, work status, safety, legal difficulties, self-management, and quality of life; the corresponding measures were taken from the Lehman's Quality of Life Scale, the Behavior and Symptom Identification Scale (BASIS-32), MHSIP, and PERMS. Process indicators include that consumers participate in their care decisions, time to follow-up appointment is reasonable, and treatment is continuous—all measured by items in the MHSIP. Access indicators include service denials and access to a full range of services. Structure indicators include secure data, appropriate staffing, and follow-up on adverse events.

ROLE OF PROFESSIONAL ORGANIZATIONS

The American Psychiatric Association (APA) has played a meaningful role in the evolution of outcome measurements. The production of the Diagnostic and Statistical Manual, now in its fourth edition, by the APA has made psychiatric diagnosis more systematic. The APA has produced practice guidelines for the treatment of mental illnesses as a step toward unifying standards of care, but it has not yet published any position statements on the use of outcome measurements. The APA has also started to collect demographic data on its psychiatrists to describe their practices, with its Practice Research Network (PRN) project (Zarin et al. 1998), but has not collected outcome data in any systematic way on the treatment of psychiatric disorders. The American Psychological Association has a working group on outcome assessment but also does not have a position statement on outcome measurement. It is unclear why the two largest organizations of mental health professionals have not come to some consensus about outcome measurement, but it is most likely due to the complexity of outcome measurement, as well as the wide variety of practice settings represented by the two organizations.

ROLE OF THE FEDERAL GOVERNMENT IN OUTCOME MEASUREMENT

The federal government has also responded to the need for standardization through the AHCPR, founded in 1989, now renamed the Agency for Healthcare Research and Quality (AHRQ, pronounced "arc"), which has produced Computerized Needs Oriented Quality Measurement Evaluation System 2.0 (CONQUEST). CONQUEST is a database of 1,197 specific measures and 53 sets of clinical performance measures. The AHCPR has also developed CAHPS, a standardized, more in-depth patient satisfaction report. More recently, it has collaborated with the NCQA to produce CAHPS 2.0, which is a convergence of CAHPS 1.0 and the NCQA Member Satisfaction Survey. The AHCPR sponsors research on the development and evaluation of performance measures, and in so doing promotes scientific rigor in performance measurement. The agency has also released two reports on measure development and evaluation (Agency for Health Care Policy and Research 1995a, 1995b).

CAHPS was developed by a consortium of Harvard Medical School, RAND, and the Research Triangle Institute and was sponsored by the AHCPR. CAHPS 2.0 is designed to go beyond simple patient satisfaction and to do the following:

- Focus on information that consumers want when choosing a plan and present this information in easily understood formats.
- Address consumers' need for more detailed information by covering specific plan features such as access to care and quality of patient/physician interaction.
- Include questions that are targeted to persons with chronic conditions or disabilities, children, and Medicaid and Medicare beneficiaries.
- Provide standardized questionnaires for assessing experience across different populations and care delivery systems.
- Improve the utility and value of the survey questions through a combination of cognitive and psychometric testing that enhances the reliability and thus the comparability of results across different plans and population groups (Agency for Health Care Policy and Research 1998a, 1998c).

The benefits of CAHPS are that it is easy to use, accurate and clear, useful for comparison because it is universal, flexible, personalizable, free of charge, relevant, decision oriented, understandable, and instructive.

CONQUEST was developed by The Harvard School of Public Health, The MEDSTAT Group, Mikalix and Company, and the Center for Health Policy Studies and is designed to collect and evaluate health care quality measures to help users find those suited to or adaptable to their needs. CONQUEST contains measures that can be searched by specific conditions; age groups; primary and secondary prevention, managed care, and particular health care settings; process, outcome, and proxy outcome measurement; and administrative, medical records, and patient survey data. Users can limit their search to measures with reliability and validity testing or to measures currently in use. Each measure in the database has a short description of the measure's numerator, denominator, and clinical rationale. The clinical rationale includes a description of the condition the measure is intended to assess, the importance of measuring performance for that condition, and how the instrument measures an aspect of quality of clinical performance. CONQUEST also contains recommended services and the complications that may occur in different time frames for each condition, allowing users to compare actual services versus recommended services. Finally, CONQUEST helps users to create performance measure sets by walking them through the necessary components by means of a checklist.

In addition, in March of 1998, the President's Advisory Commission on Consumer Protection and Quality in the Health Care Industry proposed that the Forum for Health Care Quality Measurement and Reporting "serve as a vehicle to develop a comprehensive national plan for quality measurement, data collection, and reporting standards" (U.S. Department of Health and Human Services 1998). The Forum could periodically endorse core sets of measures for standardized reporting of health care quality. Specifically, its aims are the following:

- Identify core sets of quality measures for standardized reporting by all sectors of the health care industry.
- Establish a framework and capacity for quality measurement and reporting.
- Support the focused development of quality measures that enhance and improve the ability to evaluate and improve care.
- Make recommendations regarding an agenda for research and development needed to advance quality measurement and reporting.
- Ensure that comparative information on health care quality is valid, reliable, comprehensible, and widely available in the public domain (U.S. Department of Health and Human Services 1998).

Another instrument—the Consumer Assessment of Behavioral Health Services (CABHS), which is being developed by the AHCPR—is also under consideration by the NCQA as a behavioral health version of the

CAHPS 2.0H. Both instruments are being tested through the Human Services Research Institute (HSRI) so that one of the instruments—or some combination—can be recommended for use by the NCQA. Eisen and her colleagues (1999) reported on the development process of CABHS, which included a review of current satisfaction studies (Eisen et al. 1999). The intent was to design a survey that could compare mental health plans between different service settings, which focused on three quality domains believed by consumers to be useful, such as respect for consumer patient rights, consumer patient participation in the treatment process, and information about the benefits and risks of psychotropic medications. Consumer focus groups were also used to further develop the survey measures. Finally, there is the Integrated Mental Health, Substance Abuse, and Medicaid Data Project, sponsored by SAMHSA's Center for Substance Abuse Treatment (CSAT) and the Center for Mental Health Services (CMHS), known as the Integrated Database and Spending Estimate (IDBSE). The IDBSE is designed to help states prepare accurate estimates of the health care costs of clients with mental health and substance abuse disorders, as well as the benefits of mental health and substance abuse treatment and help states understand how best to integrate such data.

MHSIP

The Mental Health Statistics Improvement Program (MHSIP) was established in 1976 by the CMHS "to continue and expand the collaborative relationship with the states and to evolve data standards that reflected current developments in mental health services." In 1989, the National Institute of Mental Health (NIMH) published a report, which came to be known as "F-10," which summarized the key ideas the MHSIP Ad Hoc Group had been developing for several years. The report was called "Data Standards for Mental Health Decision Support," and it outlined a framework for the analysis of mental health client data that included standards for minimum data sets (Leginski 1989). F-10 has been the reference document for much of the public mental health data system development since then. Also in 1989, NIMH, and later CMHS, began awarding grants to help states and treatment agencies develop mental health data systems and use the data collected in those systems. In 1993, the MHSIP convened a task force to create a consumer-oriented report card to assess the quality and cost of substance abuse and mental health services. The critical domains included in the report card included access, appropriateness, outcomes, consumer satisfaction, and prevention. A report was released in April 1996, and a grant program was set up by CMHS to allow states to implement the guidelines and produce a report card of their own following the guidelines. Five states piloted the report card, and a 40-item survey was developed, with a 21-item survey developed for use in managed care settings. The grants are issued annually to states that are willing to develop outcome projects using the report card on different populations. The MHSIP report card is different from other report cards in that it includes a consumer focus, an emphasis on outcomes, and relevance to a range of mental health conditions; it is grounded in research but tempered with a consideration of practical issues. For example, it includes items on decreased level of psychological distress, involvement in self-help activities, increased activities with families and friends, etc. In contrast to HEDIS and PERMS, it does not focus on fiscal issues like utilization.

Many states have their own outcome measurement strategies. The Texas Mental Health Outcomes Project Workgroup used the Brief Psychiatric Rating Scale (BPRS), the Multnomah Community Ability Scale, the Clinical Alcohol and Drug Use Scale, a systems outcomes instrument, a consumer survey, and a family member survey. The state of California uses the BPRS and Kennedy subscales, as well as the Global Assessment of Functioning (GAF), BASIS-32, the Zung Self-Rating Scale for depressed patients, the MHSIP consumer satisfaction survey, and Lehman's Quality of Life Scale. Finally, the state of Utah uses the General Well-Being Plus (GWB), the Mental Health Corporation of America: Customer Satisfaction Survey (MHCA), the Managed Care Plan (MCP), BPRS, and the Youth Consumer Satisfaction (YCS) scale. It seems clear from these examples that there is little consensus on what constitutes an adequate outcomes measure set.

CURRENT STATUS OF PERFORMANCE MEASURES

Assessing how performance measures are currently being used is difficult for many reasons. Methods change quickly, and they are not always published in the literature. A literature search found two articles describing data found by CentraLink, in cooperation with the Institute for Behavioral Healthcare, during a national survey of MCOs in 1994, assessing the state of the art in mental health performance outcomes. In 1995 Kurland, using a framework developed by the AHCPR, found that a variety of instruments were being used by the 73 mental health care organizations that answered the survey. These organizations ranged in size from single-site facilities to multisite managed health care corporations, and were government and nongovernment agencies and profit and nonprofit organizations. A total of 10 measures were found, and none were designed as guides for individual consumers of care. The primary condition assessed was major depression, and there were no measures for child and adolescent or geriatric disorders, nor any measures for psychosocial stressors, such as violence, suicidality, or family disorders. In addition, no measures were included that measured mental health promotion, outreach, or prevention. There were no home, emergency room, or non–medical setting measures, reflecting an emphasis on medical settings. Outcome measures were limited to only the effects on the identified patient, and not on the family. The best systems were noted to be disease specific, had process and outcome measures, included measures for psychotherapy and pharmacotherapy, detection and treatment, allowance for patient variables, and consideration for timing. Kurland's (1995) recommendations were that there needed to be more attention paid to the settings in which the treatment occurs, as well as the systems affected, and there needs to be more emphasis on prevention and detection of illness. In 1994 Pallak, using the same data, reported that most of the organizations (71%) used patient satisfaction surveys, whereas 65% used symptom severity, and 58% used level of functioning. The majority of the respondents (82%) used self-reporting for their data source. The most predominant method was pretreatment/posttreatment/follow-up (61%), followed by retrospective (29%), prospective (21%), and randomized (18%), whereas matched control groups were the least used (7%). Finally, the survey revealed that only 11% of the projects followed up with patients 3–12 months after the treatment episode. The results of the survey and the two articles suggested that more MCOs were using outcome measures, but also that more needed to be done to improve the quality of their results.

An informal telephone survey and interview revealed that at least two of the behavioral health MCOs have both a research division and a quality demonstration division. The two divisions do parallel work, but their work is not duplicated. One division's charge is to perform naturalistic observations, whereas the other's is to test PERMS measures.

CONCLUSION

The process of choosing and implementing outcome measures is a difficult and complex task that has been taken on by consumer organizations, such as NAMI and FAACT; by MCOs and large business coalitions, such as the ACMHA's core indicators project, PBGH (CALINX), and AMBHA (PERMS); and by private accreditation organizations such as NCQA (HEDIS) and JCAHO (ORYX); and by the federal government, through AHCPR (CONQUEST, CAHPS, and CABHS) and CMHS (MHSIP). By agreeing on a set of standard measures and procedures, many health care organizations can compare their outcome data to those of other organizations in a more meaningful way. It has been difficult to come to a consensus, because different organizations have different priorities. For example, consumer groups are more interested in quality and prevention, whereas MCOs are more interested in satisfaction and utilization. The evolution of these systems is continuing, and if the current experience of CAHPS, MHSIP, and ACMHA can be used as an example, we can expect some agreement as time passes and new research is done. Any public or privately owned health care organization can be expected to undergo scrutiny by some outcome measure, whether it be dictated by an outside regulatory agency or used internally for justification of funding. Outcome measures can be very helpful to mental health care organizations if chosen critically and implemented carefully and conscientiously to assess outcomes, process, access, and structure.

REFERENCES

Agency for Health Care Policy and Research: Understanding and Choosing Clinical Performance Measures for Quality Improvement: Development of a Typology (AHCPR Publ No 95-N001 and 95-N002). Rockville, MD, Agency for Health Care Policy and Research, 1995a

Agency for Health Care Policy and Research: Using Clinical Practice Guidelines to Evaluate Quality of Care: Issues and Methods (AHCPR Publ No 95-0045 and 95-0046). Rockville, MD, Agency for Health Care Policy and Research, 1995b

Agency for Health Care Policy and Research: CAHPS 2.0 Questionnaires. Rockville, MD, Agency for Health Care Policy and Research, 1998a (available at http://www.ahcpr.gov/qual/cahps/cahpques.htm)

Agency for Health Care Policy and Research: Consumer Assessment of Health Plans (CAHPS): Fact Sheet (AHCPR Publ No 97-R079). Rockville, MD, Agency for Health Care Policy and Research, 1998c (available at http://www.ahcpr.gov/qual/cahpfact.htm)

Eisen SV, Shaul JA, Clarridge B, et al: Development of a consumer survey for behavioral health services. Psychiatr Serv 50:793–798, 1999

Kurland D: A review of quality evaluation systems for mental health services. Am J Med Qual 10:141–148, 1995

Leginski WA, Croze C, Driggers J, et al: Data Standards for Mental Health Decision Support Systems (Series FN No 10) (DHHS Publ No ADM 89–1589). Washington, DC, U.S. Government Printing Office, 1989

National Committee for Quality Assurance: NCQA Overview: Measuring the Quality of America's Health Care. Washington, DC, National Committee for Quality Assurance, 2001 (available at http://www.ncqa.org/Communications/Publications/overviewncqa.pdf)

Pallak MS: National Outcomes Management Survey: Summary Report. Behavioral Healthcare Tomorrow, September/October, 1994, pp 63–69

Skolnick AA: A FACCT-filled agenda for public information. JAMA 278:1558, 1997

U.S. Department of Health and Human Services: The Challenge and Potential for Assuring Quality Health Care for the 21st Century (Publ No OM 98–0009). Washington, DC, U.S. Department of Health and Human Services for the Domestic Policy Council, 1998 (available at http://www.ahcpr.gov/qual/21stcena.htm)

U.S. General Accounting Office: Health Care Reform: Report Cards Are Useful, but Significant Issues Need to Be Addressed (GAO/HEHS-94–219), Washington, DC, U.S. General Accounting Office, 1994

Zarin DA, Pincus HA, Peterson BD, et al: Characterizing psychiatry with findings from the 1996 National Survey of Psychiatric Practice. Am J Psychiatry 155:397–404, 1998

CHAPTER 22

Confidentiality and Outcome

Zebulon Taintor, M.D.

To judge an outcome well, one must know all the variables: what went into the process and what happened thereafter. In addition to the cost of the intervention, outcome measures evaluate how well the patient functions at various times after the intervention. Those who provide treatment have come to recognize that data can be retrieved about them; service data are available from clinical and administrative information systems. It is generally considered that the best way to follow what happens to the recipient of care is to retrieve data by use of a personal identifier. A law requiring a National Patient Identifier was passed in 1996 (Health Insurance Portability and Accountability Act of 1996, P.L. 104-191), but public outcry on proposed regulations to implement the identifier led to a consensus not to proceed (Peel 2000). The battle has now moved to issues of access to personal health records stored electronically.

Although outcome studies seek to share the high status of medical research, patients may not want to have their diagnoses or other facts about them known, especially with diagnoses and symptoms that can be stigmatizing (e.g., human immunodeficiency virus infection, alcohol or drug abuse, schizophrenia, suicide attempts). Some treatments carry their own stigma (e.g., electroconvulsive therapy, antipsychotic medications). Some outcomes may be stigmatizing, such as disability or incarceration. In this chapter, current laws and practices are examined, and ways to conduct specific assessment programs without compromising privacy are proposed.

CURRENT STATUS

Laws Governing Confidentiality

Written Records

Laws governing access to written records are well established at the state level. These are generally held to be tough. Even when a patient has access to his or her own record, this access is still limited (Aswad 1999). Twenty-five states have specific legislative wording in their laws allowing the provider to decide if patients should be given access to their own medical records. Case law provides additional precedents for medical record protection. For example, Dr. Robert Newman maintained photographs to identify his methadone maintenance patients, one of whom was suspected of murder (Pear 1999). Dr. Newman defied a court order to release the photographs to the police, arguing that he had taken the pictures with the promise that their purpose was only identification for methadone distribution. The court order was withdrawn, establishing an important precedent.

Electronic Records

Three forms of electronic records currently exist: computer-based patient records (CPRs), electronic patient records (EPRs), and the more comprehensive electronic medical records (EMRs). CPRs usually capture data at the point of care and allow for data manipulation, trending, and outcomes analysis. EPRs are the historical, archival copies of all the documents generated in the course of treatment and may include scanned images of handwritten progress notes and other documents that were originally in paper form (Smallwood 1999). It is rare for an EPR to be the sole data source for a patient.

Among the various issues on which there is disagreement are the desirability of EMRs versus CPRs; what constitutes a legally acceptable signature; and technology for protection against tampering. Generally, electronic data are regarded as secondary sources of information. The federal government's regulations for the Health Care Financing Administration (HCFA) (Health Care Financing Administration 1998) allow no identifiable patient data (as defined in the Privacy Act of 1974 on federal information systems) to be transmitted on the Internet. Despite general agreement that legislation for EMRs is required, disagreements over many specific aspects of proposed legislation persist. As a result, no standardized EMR legislation yet exists.

Confidentiality in Current Practice

Confidentiality varies by type of practice. A self-pay, purely private practice can be completely confidential, especially if there is an agreement with a patient that no written record is to be kept. But records must be kept when receiving third-party payment. To meet criteria for payment (or when the clinician is part of a hospital, clinical, or other institutional practice), some disclosure outside the doctor-patient relationship is required. In addition to third-party payment, information must be retained on prescriptions, which once never left the pharmacy where they were filled but now are computerized and available throughout very broad pharmacy databases.

Although it can be argued that written records are not secure, confidentiality breaches require actual contact with the written record, which is usually protected as property and by confidentiality laws. To obtain a written record, one must have access to its location. Certain licensing authorities, federal and state program audits, and judicial orders (e.g., medical record subpoenas) can authorize such access. A solo practitioner may use a billing service that retains some treatment and financial data even if no third-party payment is involved. Within group practices and institutions, record systems contain individual patient, treatment, and response-to-treatment data, all of which are potentially retrievable, with or without permission of the patient. However, until recently all such records were written and could be retrieved only by direct physical contact with the record. Although there may have been occasional abuses and some record rooms seemed to have lax security, a recent literature search yielded no cases of violation of confidentiality in which data on a patient had left the office or institution in which the patient was treated.

Despite many potential benefits and despite evidence of the lack of abuse, computerization of the medical record has been slow (Taintor 1997). This is partly due to confidentiality concerns that date back to the mid-1970s (Laska and Bank 1975). Records now contain a lot of data, especially in text form, which are increasingly easy to retrieve and can be transmitted widely. The amount of data and the ease with which they can move electronically make risks exponentially higher. For example, in 1999 sensitive information about thousands of patients was inadvertently placed on the Internet by a Midwestern university (Stout 1999). Fraudulent data about patients have been entered into computerized insurance records, adding the risk that the violation of confidentiality may involve "facts" that are untrue as well as detrimental (Raab 1996). It is not clear that there has been significant improvement since the 1996 Computer Crime and Security Survey (Industry Watch 1996), in which 41% of information systems surveyed had had their security systems compromised by unauthorized access. Of these, 50% were traced to current employees; many others were also traced to remote dial-in sources and Internet connections, with 36.8% of site attacks involving the unauthorized alteration of data.

Of note, it is legal for insurance companies to sell data about patients, including name, diagnosis, and other facts. The purchasers of the data can also make it public. Also, it is estimated that $15 billion is spent yearly on the acquisition and exchange of medical information (Scarf 1999).

Ironically, physicians may encounter unrealistic patient expectations that somehow the doctor can control data reported to third parties. Physicians are increasingly informing patients that they cannot ensure their privacy. Because of the lack of technical safeguards, legislation is required to protect the confidentiality of computerized patient records.

Types and Uses of Medical Data Available

There is a wide variety of medical data available: patient demographics, clinical diagnoses and severity of illness, providers, treatment services and medications, costs, and quality indicators.

Although the use of medical data is often seen as an intrusion on patients' privacy, its positive uses by health services researchers was cited in testimony by the Association of American Medical Colleges on proposed federal confidentiality legislation. Findings offered included that "pediatric patients treated for [attention-deficit/hyperactivity] disorder (ADHD) were less likely to use and become dependent upon illegal drugs during adolescence and young adulthood than patients with ADHD who had not received appropriate treatment" (McCabe 1999). Studies of this type focusing on the outcome of psychiatric interventions or their adverse effects are extremely useful for patients, clinicians, and researchers, but they require access to relevant data over time that may compromise confidentiality.

ACCESS TO OUTCOME DATA

Technological Advances and Access

While laws have languished unpassed, the technology of retrieval and access is outpacing that of encryption and privacy. Computerized data, even data thought to reside only on a single computer, can be retrieved whenever that computer is connected to another. No computer data system is absolutely secure from technical breaches. Computerized data reported to third parties are typically stored in a large computer and can be retrieved from other computers on the network, exponentially increasing the risk of a breach of confidentiality. Any applicant for health, life, or disability insurance is typically asked for permission to confirm what was said in the medical history and to enter that history into the data bank of the Medical Information Bureau (Grugle 1998).

A survey of 21 health-related Web sites that found 1) visitors are not anonymous, even though they think they are; 2) privacy policies have been established, but these do not provide complete consumer protection; 3) actual practice falls short of policy; 4) consumer personal data are not adequately protected; 5) third parties can gain access to data with neither the site nor the third party being liable; and 6) protection does not follow the data when they leave the site (Goldman et al. 2000).

Who Should Have Access?

It is in everyone's interest for people to know what information on them is available, because it may be false or violate their privacy. Existing legislation (e.g., the Privacy Act of 1974) requires that a person identified in federal files can know what information is contained therein. Patients can check what is on file about them through the Medical Information Bureau (Crowley 2000).

One answer to the access question is "no one besides the patient and doctor." Complete confidentiality requires the clinician not to disclose any information or data to anyone without the patient's expressed permission. Data outside the purely private doctor-patient relationship could then be shared at various levels on a need-to-know basis. Insurers have objected to being required to ask a patient's permission every time data need to be released, because it is too time consuming and costly.

FUTURE DIRECTIONS: WHAT NEEDS TO BE DONE?

Legislation, rather than the present regulation process, will be needed to deal with patient privacy concerns. Many comments on the proposed regulations have asked for criminal penalties (Peel 2000). This is recommended for serious breaches of confidentiality, with penalties scaled according to the damage done.

At a technical level, patient identifiers can be easily eliminated when using the data to measure the outcome of treatment by facility and/or population. For example, data on cost can be studied without identifiers.

Difficulties may be encountered with impersonal identifiers (e.g., patients involved in events extensively covered by the media) that can reveal the identity of the patient. The Health Plan Employer Data and Information Set (HEDIS) is an example of the ability to look at certain outcomes (e.g., immunization rates) without compromising confidentiality. However, HEDIS mental health measures are few and have been criticized for being limited to major affective disorder and not dealing with outcome (Robinson 1996).

CONCLUSION

There must be a universal acceptance that data belong first to the patient, second to clinicians, third to researchers, fourth to those who must be involved in paying the bills, and probably to no one else.

It is not costly and need not be time consuming to get a patient's permission every time data need to be released. Current legislation does not make it clear that the record belongs to the patient. Every patient should have a copy of his or her record and own it, just as should every physician have his or her copy and own it. But the issue is who has a greater right to the patient's identifying data. That should be the person most concerned and with the most to lose—the patient.

REFERENCES

Aswad C: Privacy issue: highest New York court gives patient access to own records (EVPgram). Lake Success, NY, Medical Society of the State of New York, 1999

Crowley S: Snoops finding new ways to breach medical files. AARP Bulletin, March 3, 2000

Grugle TA: Medical Information Bureau. CyberCouch Library, March 27, 1998. Accessed March 12, 2002 <http://www.cybercouch.com/library/medi.tag.html>

Goldman J, Hudson Z, Smith RM: Report on the Privacy Policies and Practices of Health Web Sites. Oakland, CA, California HealthCare Foundation, 2000

Health Care Financing Administration: HCFA Internet Security Policy. Health Care Financing Administration, November 24, 1998. Accessed March 12, 2002 <http://www.hcfa.gov/security/isecplcy.htm>

Health Insurance Portability and Accountability Act of 1996, Pub. L. No. 104-191

Industry Watch: 1996 computer crime and security survey. HealthManagement Technology 17(8):10, 1996

Laska EM, Bank R: Safeguarding Psychiatric Privacy. New York, Wiley Biomedical, 1975

McCabe C: AAMC presents confidentiality testimony before Ways and Means Subcommittee. Washington Highlights, Association of American Medical Colleges, July 23, 1999

Pear R: Future bleak for bill to keep health records confidential. New York Times, June 21, 1999, p. 12

Peel L: Washington update—the latest on privacy. APA Member-to-Member listserv, March 22, 2000

Raab S: New Jersey officials say Mafia infiltrated health-care industry. New York Times, August 21, 1966, p A1

Robinson G: Mental health measures in Medicaid HEDIS (CMHS Knowledge Exchange Network). Rockville, MD, Center for Mental Health Services, Substance Abuse and Mental Health Administration, 1996

Scarf M: The privacy threat that didn't go away. The New Republic, July 12, 1999, pp 16–18

Smallwood R: Healthcare, trends in patient record technologies. Inform Magazine (Association for Information and Image Management International), February 1999

Stout D: GOP sees privacy threat in Democrats' bid for documents, New York Times, June 10, 1999, p. 24

Taintor Z (ed): Computers and the Psychiatric Patient. Washington, DC, American Psychiatric Press, 1997, p. 87

CHAPTER 23

Training Psychiatry Residents in Outcome Measurement

Carol A. Bernstein, M.D.
Waguih William IsHak, M.D.

IMPORTANCE OF OUTCOME MEASUREMENT TRAINING

Teaching residents to measure the outcome of psychiatric treatments has tremendous educational value. Residents today frequently treat patients in a wide variety of settings without receiving systematic feedback about which interventions work and which do not. With the exception of those in some research-oriented settings, trainees in psychiatry are rarely taught how to scientifically evaluate the effect of their interventions. In addition, research on treatment is generally quite selective and hence cannot represent the patient populations customarily treated by residents. Therefore, it is particularly important that residents be provided the opportunity to experience firsthand the effects of their interventions during the course of their training.

During the past decade, there have been many changes in the way patients are treated and the way residents are trained (Kaplan 1997). The requirements of managed behavioral health programs and of regulatory and accrediting agencies and the expectations of consumer groups, patients, and families have resulted in increasing emphasis on accountability and cost-effectiveness. Training programs cannot be sheltered from these pressures, nor should they be. Demonstrating results and value for medical services is an important new dimension of health care that trainees need to understand. Moreover, to the extent that reimbursement will be tied to treatment outcome, training residents in the use of outcome measures will be important for the survival of psychiatric departments and graduate training programs.

There are few psychiatry training curricula or service programs that include systematic outcome assessment. In addition, residents do not always have the opportunity to follow patients through different levels of care and hence cannot evaluate the outcome of their care. Inpatient rotations in acute care are now relatively short (as are lengths of stay) and do not allow the time needed to see patients recompensate or to observe the courses of most major psychiatric illnesses. Residents generally do not have the opportunity to witness the long-term outcome of patients they see in the emergency room, acute care units, and walk-in clinics (O'Reilly and Parker 1990). Fragmented care systems with little continuity and the lack of accessible comprehensive medical record systems make it logistically difficult for residents to obtain outcome information that may be educational for them. (For more details on technological solutions for clinical care and training problems see Chapter 24, in this volume.)

Notably, many activities compete for resident training time today. Service demands, supervision sessions, and didactic teaching schedules fill up trainees' schedules. In larger academic centers, especially those with public hospital affiliations, the necessity for numerous in-house training sessions and administrative and program meetings has contributed to the competition for residents' time. In addition, charting requirements are more complex and time consuming, with demands for more detailed treatment plans, elaborate progress notes, and a variety of assessments. Outcome assessment may be perceived as another administrative burden due to the time it takes to complete clinician-based measures. In addition, residents are frequently reluctant to collect outcome information, because of resistance to completing new forms and concerns about reducing the patient to "a number."

EDUCATIONAL VALUE OF TRAINING RESIDENTS TO USE OUTCOME MEASURES

Modern psychiatric methodology trains residents to rely on empirical evidence rather than anecdotal reports. Yet clinical improvement or deterioration too often remains a subjective report by the resident, who draws on a mix of observations and clinical intuition. Teaching systematic outcome assessment adds a more precise dimension to the assessment of change in clinical conditions. The notion that outcome measurement is relevant only to psychopharmacologic treatments is continually being challenged by research findings (e.g., Barber et al. 1996). Whether the treatment modality used is psychotherapy or pharmacotherapy, monitoring outcome during residency training enables residents to understand more about clinician factors associated with positive and negative outcomes. In psychotherapy training, learning about clinician factors in outcome is generally accomplished by surveying the resident's psychotherapy supervisors (Buckley et al. 1979). Adding periodic outcome measures to assess the therapeutic alliance, defensive operations, and severity of symptoms could enhance training in clinician factors and the doctor-patient relationship. (For more details see Chapter 8, in this volume.)

The integration of the previously mentioned measures into the supervisory process should enrich the learning experience for residents, advance their training, and enhance patient outcome. Where possible, residents should be exposed to outcome measurement methodology during the initial evaluation of patients and as part of ongoing patient management. In the United States, the Residency Review Committee is now requiring that training programs demonstrate that residents are competent to provide different psychiatric treatments as a requirement of successful completion of residency training. However, measuring competence is a difficult and challenging task and remains a debatable issue. The use of outcome measures to facilitate the evaluation of resident competencies may be a useful adjunct to the process, if cases can be adjusted for demographic, clinical, and other factors that influence treatment. An attempt to address some of those factors is through the use of scales that quantify clinical complexity. (For more information see the Clinical Complexity Scale in Appendix A, in this volume.)

IMPLEMENTATION OF OUTCOME MEASUREMENT TRAINING FOR RESIDENTS

An educational program for outcome assessment should be composed of hands-on training and didactic teaching. Outcome measures customarily focus on four areas: symptoms, functioning, quality of life, and patient (or family) satisfaction with treatment (Sederer et al. 1995). If it is presented as part of an overall educational program, outcome measurements can help residents learn more about the initial status of their patients as well as their progress and experience of care (i.e., satisfaction) over time.

The following example shows how outcome assessments are used to monitor a depressed patient during the training of fourth-year residents in intensive short-term dynamic psychotherapy at Bellevue Hospital Center and New York University School of Medicine.

At intake:
1. The patient completes the Beck Depression Inventory
2. The resident administers the Hamilton Rating Scale for Depression
3. The resident scores the Global Assessment of Functioning (GAF: Axis V of the DSM-IV-TR)
4. The patient completes the Quality of Life Inventory
5. The patient completes the Client Satisfaction Questionnaire (CSQ-8) at the end of the intake.

During continued care:
These measures are repeated at 3, 6, 9 and 12 months. Ideally, the resident and the supervisor would review the results at every data point to determine whether treatment is effective and to assess the patient's perception of the care received. Using this information, decisions would be made whether to alter treatment strategies and/or modalities or to identify limitations in resident skills. The inclusion of these data may also help residents (and patients) see progress or deterioration that may not be overtly apparent. In either scenario, residents should benefit from the periodic evaluation of treatment outcomes.

If outcome measures are to be incorporated into the educational program, the didactic curriculum must include lectures on the appropriate use of outcome measures (Tasman and Minkoff 1997). Instruction and periodic training in the application of various rating scales as well as clinical opportunities to implement these measures will be equally important. Academic and departmental leaders need to ensure that this clinical training is regularly provided in their institutions.

CONCLUSION

Outcome measurement needs to become an important aspect of the educational and training experience in psychiatry. It not only should be a response to cost-effectiveness pressures but should also be a means to monitor the application of psychiatric knowledge attained during the years of training and to help residents measure cause-and-effect aspects of their evaluation and treatment. Outcome measurements also need to be implemented as new and complex treatment interventions are developed and introduced into practice. The next century will witness increasing sophistication and accountability in medical and psychiatric practice. Training future psychiatrists in outcome assessment will become a necessity to achieve the results that patients, families, and clinicians all desire.

REFERENCES

Barber JP, Crits-Christoph P, Luborsky L: Effects of therapist adherence and competence on patient outcome in brief dynamic therapy. J Consult Clin Psychol 64:619–622, 1996

Buckley P, Karasu TB, Charles E: Common mistakes in psychotherapy. Am J Psychiatry 136:1578–1580, 1979

Kaplan M: Creating the new psychiatric residency, in Training Behavioral Healthcare Professionals: Higher Learning in the Era of Managed Care. Edited by Schuster JM, Lovell MR, Trachta AM. San Francisco, CA, Jossey-Bass, 1997

O'Reilly RL, Parker Z: Resolving the conflict of training and therapy in psychiatry. Psychiatric Journal of the University of Ottawa 15:28–31, 1990

Sederer LI, Hermann R, Dickey B: The imperative of outcome assessment in psychiatry. Am J Med Qual 10:127–132, 1995

Tasman A, Minkoff K: Educational and training issues in public sector managed mental health care, in Managed Mental Health Care in the Public Sector: A Survival Manual. Edited by Minkoff K, Pollack Dl. Singapore, Harwood, 1997

CHAPTER 24

Use of Technology in Outcome Measurement

Tal Burt, M.D.
Waguih William IsHak, M.D.

Attempts at incorporating computerized technology into outcome assessment in psychiatry can be traced back to the 1960s (Hargreaves and Blacker 1966). Since then, the mental health field has been faced with an increasing amount and complexity of data retrieved from patients. It has also been faced with pressures from regulatory agencies and third-party payers to process the data and implement the results in the immediate management of the patients. Both collection and processing of data require significant resources in personnel time, hardware, and software. The time spent on processing of the collected data often prevents their implementation in the immediate management of individual patients and therefore provides little reward and incentive to clinicians and patients alike. Data collected in the process of outcome measurement can be of limited use unless it is processed in the context of the continuous evaluation of the patient or groups of patients. There is also a need to compare these data to current standards of care and guidelines of treatment. Moreover, there is a growing need to keep clinicians abreast of improvement, deterioration, or absence of either, in the condition of their patients. Clinicians should also be aware of the adverse effects of the treatment provided.

During the process of outcome measurement, a large amount of information is collected. Since outcome measurement detects change in the patient's condition and/or response to therapeutic interventions, it is imperative to relate outcome assessment chronologically to all factors affecting the patient's condition. Biological factors, psychosocial stressors, and treatment interventions have to be considered in relation to outcome measurement. For example, in the treatment of an acute manic episode with lithium, at least four separate categories of data are involved: manic symptoms, lithium dose, lithium level, and lithium side effects. The clinician has to process this information and also remember information gathered from previous encounters with the patient (or recheck the medical record). Computer processing of those four items could assist the clinician in making the appropriate decisions regarding lithium dosing. Using computerized graphic representation of data, as shown in Figure 24–1, the clinician will be able to continuously monitor and choose the optimal dose sufficient to resolve manic symptoms without causing undue side effects. The practice of considering all these factors can be referred to as data processing.

NECESSITY OF USING COMPUTER TECHNOLOGY IN OUTCOME MEASUREMENT

Computer technology has gained tremendous ground in the field of data processing. Data processing can be conceptualized as the conversion of raw data into usable information. Computer technology offers the advantages of speed, reliability of storage and retrieval, and data processing, which can yield significant savings in time, effort, and cost. The incorporation of technological advances into the provision of care can enable a wealth of information on treatment effectiveness and can offer great opportunities for quality improvement. Randomized controlled trials are routinely criticized for their lack of relevance to everyday clinical practice. The use of standard computerized medical records can help clinicians organize large databases of clinical experience and can assist in analyzing illness characteristics, the epidemiology of diseases, treatment response, and management practices and costs across varied treatment centers and countries.

Certain characteristics of outcome data make them ideally suited for use in electronic systems. Outcome data are usually numerical and categorical and can be followed over time. Electronic information systems provide reliability and legibility of retrieved data, as well as ease of access that

■ Young Mania Rating Scale   ▨ Lithium level
■ Side effects   ▢ Daily dose

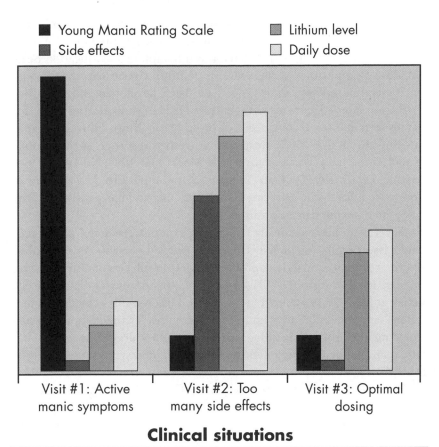

Clinical situations

Figure 24–1. Computerized graphing of multiple factors in the treatment of mania.

eludes paper-and-pencil retrieval systems. These systems also can increase the speed by which clinicians are given feedback regarding the patient's condition and allow comparisons among practitioners and systems of care.

COMPUTER TECHNOLOGY APPLICATION IN OUTCOME MEASUREMENT

Computer technology in measuring outcome in psychiatric care includes the applications described below.

Computerized Outcome Tools

Computerized outcome measurement tools are now becoming increasingly available. These instruments are easy to computerize and can be made friendly to use by patients and clinicians. Results are calculated and tabulated automatically. Global outcome measures such as the Global Assessment of Functioning (GAF), Behavior and Symptom Identification Scale (BASIS-32), and other scales exist in computerized form. Diagnosis-specific computerized rating scales have been developed and tested for depression (Beck Depression Inventory-II, Hamilton Rating Scale for Depression), obsessive-compulsive disorder (Yale-Brown Obsessive-Compulsive Scale, BT STEPS), posttraumatic stress disorder, social phobia, alcohol abuse, and personality disorders (Marks et al. 1998; Neal et al. 1994; Rosenfeld et al. 1992). Results indicate that computerized assessment of these varied diagnostic categories can be reliable and inexpensive and can yield instantaneous data acquisition.

Several studies specifically comparing computerized and paper-and-pencil assessments concluded that computerized versions have equal or superior reliability and did not produce anxiety in subjects of different sexes or educational backgrounds (Baer et al. 1993; Bendtsen and Timpka 1999; Kobak et al. 1999; Rosenfeld et al. 1992). Other studies concluded that patients are generally more honest and often prefer the computer when providing information regarding suicide, alcohol or drug abuse, sexual behavior, and human immunodeficiency virus–related symptoms (Kobak et al. 1996).

The use of interactive voice response (IVR), whereby patients record their symptoms using a Touch-Tone telephone, is also gaining popularity. The results are calculated and posted automatically for the clinician to inspect. Direct patient-computer interviews offer several advantages for collecting data from subjects in clinical trials. Perfect standardization and reliability are achieved in the interviewing process because each subject responds to exactly the same information and questions. Computer interviews are also adaptive and personalize each interview, pursuing positive lines of inquiry but branching away from topics irrelevant to the subject. Respondents are more candid about socially sensitive subject matter when interviewed by a computer; error checking occurs as the interview progresses; and data are stored in relational databases, permitting immediate analyses.

IVR uses ubiquitous Touch-Tone telephones as computer terminals, which helps overcome the functional illiteracy that is present in more than 20% of the United States population (Koback et al. 1997). Accessibility of phones makes frequent interviewing possible, to assess rapid onset of effect and to obtain daily or more frequent ratings. Patients like computer interviews at least as well as they do human interviews, and clinicians are relieved at not having to do repetitive assessments. Patient perspective is critical in clinical trials. Ultimately, patients are subject experts on the effects of disorders they experience and treatments they receive to reduce symptoms and improve quality of life. The technology is available in a variety of languages and has been used in countries other than the United States.

There is still a need to link clinical outcomes to treatment plans to make timely clinical use of the information. Greist et al. (1998) demonstrated feasibility and good outcomes when a self-assessment/self-treatment computerized IVR system was incorporated into a treatment program for obsessive-compulsive disorder. It is also important to link outcome measures to the medical record, to graph the results, and to consider the other factors influencing improvement or deterioration of the patient's condition. More work is needed in developing these types of linkages. Other tools use the Internet as a medium to reach patients in the privacy of their own home, school, or work environments (e.g., the Online Depression Screening Test [ODST], available at http://www.med.nyu.edu/Psych/screens/depres.html).

Computerized Performance and Outcome Measurement Systems

The Joint Commission on Accreditation of Healthcare Organizations (JCAHO) has listed 68 performance and outcome measurement systems in its ORYX initiative. Many of these systems are now computerized (for an up-to-date listing, please visit the JCAHO Web site at http://www.jcaho.org/perfmeas/steps/systems.html).

Computerized Medical Records

A comprehensive computerized medical record (CMR) could provide a reliable and standardized means for measuring outcome of psychiatric interventions. Attempts to create the ideal system are under way in the United States, United Kingdom, and other parts of the world (Powsner et al. 1998). Characteristics of an ideal system include ease of use, versatility, powerful graphical capabilities, and easy accessibility and retrieval capabilities by multiple users (simultaneously). It should have the ability to compare data with those of other centers, should have the ability to maintain data integrity and confidentiality, and should possess powerful data processing capabilities. It should provide regular feedback to clinicians regarding significant deviations in the conditions of patients and should provide feedback to clinical administrators about significant deviations from standard management.

Cannon and Allen (2000) compared the effects of computer and manual reminders on compliance with mental health clinical practice guidelines. They found that computer reminders are superior to manual ones in improving adherence to depression practice guidelines in an outpatient mental health clinic. The system also should be able to provide powerful graphic feedback to its users, and that interface should be tailored to maximize relevant data for rapid interpretation and implementation. The system should be designed to receive direct input from patients through the use of self-rated electronic instruments and should be able to have a limited automatic first-pass evaluation of such data to immediately identify any alarming deviations in a patient's condition.

An important value of a CMR system lies in the ability to keep track of almost all events of psychiatric significance in the patient's life, including biological and psychosocial precipitating and predisposing factors as well as psychiatric interventions. Various authors have shown the importance and usefulness to the treating clinician of graphic representations of severity of symptoms over time (Harding et al. 1989; Kraepelin 1921; Marks 1998; Post et al. 1988; Powsner and Tufte 1997). We suggest an expansion of this concept by using computer technology to graph not only the severity of symptoms, but, as previously mentioned, all events of psychiatric significance according to a biopsychosocial model. The hexagraph shown in Figure 24–2 is an example of the use of computer technology in providing the clinician with a concise, comprehensive view of the patient's condition that is linked to outcome measurement.

OBSTACLES IN IMPLEMENTATION OF COMPUTER TECHNOLOGY IN PSYCHIATRIC OUTCOME ASSESSMENT

Any discussion of implementing technological advances in outcome measurement cannot be complete without discussing the obstacles. For many consumers and professionals in the mental health field, confidentiality is a major concern regarding the implementation of electronic record systems (Wedding et al. 1995). Technological advances in data encryption, firewalls, and password/key-protected access are providing some solutions to the problem, but concern appropriately persists. Financial institutions and government agencies have implemented some of these technologies to protect confidential and classified information. These technologies show high levels of security but are not infallible.

One major obstacle to broad implementation remains clinician resistance to computers. Many clinicians believe that the nature of the human psychological experience evades being captured in numerical or analog systems. In one assessment of the self-reporting of alcohol habits, subjects reported concerns about confidentiality and loss of personal contact (Bendtsen and Timpka 1999). Concerns exist regarding the replacement of

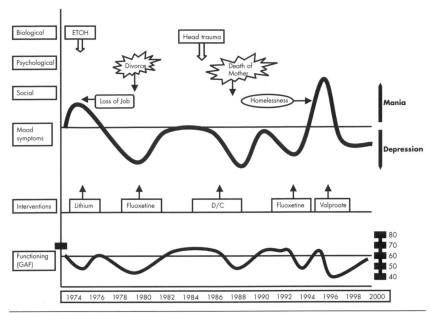

Figure 24–2. Example of a computer-generated biopsychological hexagraph that presents a graphical representation of numerous patient factors of psychiatric significance over time.

Note. D/C=discontinued; ETOH=alcohol abuse; GAF=Global Assessment of Functioning score.

the traditional clinical judgment with automated decisions based on the processing of only a limited number of clinical parameters. There are also real-time and cost limitations to computer technology. Other obstacles include the cost of infrastructure, training, maintenance, and data entry itself. There is debate over the amount of training required of data entry persons and how to avoid or minimize errors in the collection and recording of data. Time spent on data entry continues to be an important concern in most systems. Advances in voice recognition, touch-screen, and other means may be a promising alternative. Other difficulties are inherent in the nature of computerized systems and include their propensity to fail, to become infected by electronic viruses, and to be violated by remote users over wide area networks.

CONCLUSION

The field of psychiatric outcome measurement has witnessed the introduction of computerized technology in the last few decades of the twentieth century. Driven by demand for reliable data processing, and made possible by a growing industry of both software and hardware utilities, computerized technology appears to hold a potential for a significant contribution to the filed of outcome assessment in psychiatry. On the way to realizing its beneficial potential, the new technology will have to answer to concerns regarding confidentiality and regarding the appropriateness of the electronic medium to convey psychiatric data.

REFERENCES

Baer L, Brown-Beasley MW, Sorce J, et al: Computer-assisted telephone administration of a structured interview for obsessive-compulsive disorder. Am J Psychiatry 150:1737–1738, 1993

Bendtsen P, Timpka T: Acceptability of computerized self-report of alcohol habits: a patient perspective. Alcohol Alcohol 34:575–580, 1999

Cannon DS, Allen SN: A comparison of the effects of computer and manual reminders on compliance with a mental health clinical practice guideline. J Am Med Inform Assoc 7:196–203, 2000

Greist JH, Marks IM, Baer L, et al: Self-treatment for obsessive compulsive disorder using a manual and a computerized telephone interview: a U.S.-U.K. study. MD Comput 15:149–157, 1998

Harding CM, McCormick RV, Strauss JS, et al: Computerized life chart methods to map domains of function and illustrate patterns of interactions in the long-term course trajectories of patients who once met the criteria for DSM-III schizophrenia. Br J Psychiatry Suppl 5:100–106, 1989

Hargreaves WH, Blacker KH: The computer: a new tool for psychiatry. Charting changes in patients' daily behavior. Hospital and Community Psychiatry 17:70–73, 1966

Kobak KA, Greist JH, Jefferson JW, et al: Computer-administered clinical rating scales. A review. Psychopharmacology (Berl) 127:291–301, 1996

Kobak KA, Taylor LH, Dottl SL, et al: A computer-administered telephone interview to identify mental disorders. JAMA 278:905–910, 1997

Kobak KA, Greist JH, Jefferson JW, et al: Computerized assessment of depression and anxiety over the telephone using interactive voice response. MD Comput 16:64–68, 1999

Kraepelin E: Manic-Depressive Insanity and Paranoia. Edinburgh, Livingstone, 1921

Marks I: Overcoming obstacles to routine outcome measurement: the nuts and bolts of implementing clinical audit (editorial) (see comments). Br J Psychiatry 173:281–286, 1998

Marks IM, Baer L, Greist JH: Home self-assessment of obsessive-compulsive disorder. Use of a manual and a computer-conducted telephone interview: two UK-US studies. Br J Psychiatry 172:406–412, 1998

Neal LA, Busuttil W, Herapath R, et al: Development and validation of the computerized clinician administered Post-Traumatic Stress Disorder Scale-1-Revised. Psychol Med 24:701–706, 1994

Post RM, Roy-Byrne PP, Uhde TW: Graphic representation of the life course of illness in patients with affective disorder. Am J Psychiatry 145:844–848, 1988

Powsner SM, Tufte ER: Summarizing clinical psychiatric data. Psychiatr Serv 48:1458–1461, 1997

Powsner SM, Wyatt JC, Wright P: Opportunities for and challenges of computerization. Lancet 352:1617–1622, 1998

Rosenfeld R, Dar R, Anderson D, et al: A computer-administered version of the Yale-Brown Obsessive-Compulsive Scale. Psychol Assess 4:329–332, 1992

Wedding D, Topolski J, McGaha A: Maintaining the confidentiality of computerized mental health outcome data. Journal of Mental Health Administration 22:237–244, 1995

CHAPTER 25

Innovative Approaches in Outcome Measurement

A Futuristic View

Waguih William IsHak, M.D.
Antonio Almoguera-Abad, M.D.
Murray Alpert, Ph.D.

The future holds a significant amount of innovation for the accurate measurement of outcomes of psychiatric treatments. In this regard, the history of medicine is inspiring. Hundreds of years ago, detecting that a patient had a fever was dependent on two means: the patient's subjective reporting of heat and the physician's impression from feeling the patient's forehand using the back of the hand. Determining the severity of the fever was more difficult and was determined by the presence of fever-associated symptoms and signs such as headache and obtundation. The invention of the thermometer brought an end to dependence on these subjective means. In 1615, Santorio Santorio, an Italian physician, added a numerical scale to Galileo's 1603 thermoscope, thereby creating the first thermometer (Figure 25–1). In

1866, British physician Sir Thomas Allbutt invented the modern mercury clinical thermometer, which became a useful medical tool, replacing a foot-long model that required 20 minutes to operate (Middleton 1966).

At that point, a new era began for the assessment of fever. In addition to the patient's report and the physician's impression, a new method was introduced: the ability to assign a quantitative numerical value to the fever symptom, defining it as body temperature of more than 98.6 F. This new method also allowed for the differentiation between a low-grade fever and a high-grade fever (above 100.7°F). Incidentally, data from recent research suggest that normal body temperature should be revised from 98.6°F to 98.2°F based on statistical analysis of temperature readings in large samples (Mackowiak et al. 1992).

This numerical value (the temperature) permitted measurement of symptoms and assessment of progress or deterioration over time. More importantly, it was independent of what the patient feels or what the clinician thinks—that is, an objective measure for fever. The reader is invited to draw a parallel between fever in this example and a psychiatric symptom such as depressed mood.

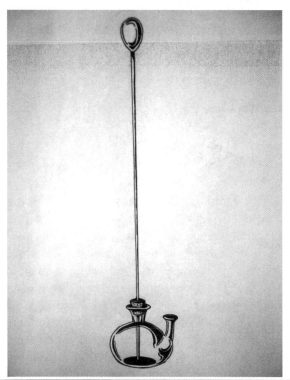

Figure 25–1.   Galileo's thermoscope.

This chapter is an attempt to highlight some of the objective potential measures of outcome, notwithstanding the fact that many of these measures may be experimental (as in Galileo's thermoscope), expensive, or difficult to use (as with early thermometers) or will bring revision or modification of the definitions of pathology (as in possibly changing the definition of fever to a temperature above 98.2°F). Brain imaging, laboratory investigations, and technological tests are all part of this promising growth of objective outcome measurement in psychiatric disorders.

OUTCOME MEASUREMENT USING BRAIN IMAGING

Structural and functional changes in many psychiatric illnesses have been detected using brain imaging techniques. Some of these changes normalize after treatment, giving rise to the possibility of measuring the change for purposes of outcome assessment. However, the reliability and validity of imaging methods and recorded changes are still being determined. This section focuses on the use of imaging techniques in measuring symptom change in pretreatment and posttreatment stages as opposed to the prediction of treatment outcome.

Positron Emission Tomography

Positron emission tomography (PET) is an imaging method that enables the visualization of organ physiology by detection of positrons emitted from radioactively tagged compounds such as glucose, oxygen, or pharmacologic agents. PET quantitatively measures metabolic, biochemical, and functional activity in vivo.

A critical review of PET studies (from 1966 to 1999) showed evidence that patients with major depression have reduced blood flow and metabolism in the prefrontal cortex as well as abnormalities in the anterior cingulate gyrus and the basal ganglia (Videbech 2000). Baxter et al. (1989) showed reductions of glucose concentration in the dorsal anterolateral prefrontal cortex in major depression, which resolved with remission of depressive episodes and were significantly correlated with rating scales of depression severity (Figure 25–2). Buchsbaum et al. (1997) showed that depressed patients had relatively increased metabolic activity bilaterally in the middle frontal gyrus (an area with decreased metabolic activity in depression) after sertraline treatment. Brody et al. (1999) used PET to examine outpatients with major depressive disorder (MDD) before and after treatment with paroxetine. Patients who responded to treatment had significantly greater decreases in normalized metabolism in the ventrolateral prefrontal cortex and the orbitofrontal cortex. This study showed a positive correlation between change in scores on the Hamilton Rating Scale for Depression and change in normalized ventrolateral prefrontal cortex metabolism.

Similarly, studies of patients with obsessive-compulsive disorder (OCD) before and after treatment revealed a significant decrease in normalized right caudate nucleus metabolism correlating with scores on the Yale-Brown Obsessive Compulsive Scale (Y-BOCS) in those who responded to treatment with fluoxetine or cognitive-behavioral therapy (CBT) (Baxter 1992). Schwartz et al. (1996) replicated these findings, showing significant decreases in glucose metabolism in the caudate nucleus in those who responded to treatment compared with nonresponders. Furthermore, percentage change in the Y-BOCS score was positively correlated with percentage change in metabolism in the left orbital cortex. Saxena et al. (1995, 1998) replicated the findings of decreasing metabolism in the right caudate nucleus and orbitofrontal cortex in patients with OCD who responded to treatment with paroxetine.

The findings described earlier suggest that during remission after using medications or psychotherapy, changes in specific brain areas as visualized by PET correspond with changes in symptoms as measured by rating scales. These findings suggest that PET could be used as a method to measure clinical changes and ultimately outcome of treatment interventions.

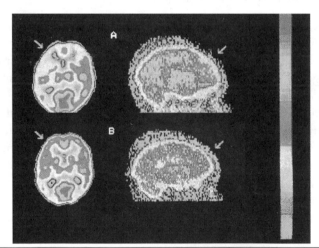

Figure 25–2.   Positron emission tomographic scans of a patient with obsessive-compulsive disorder and secondary major depression. *Arrows* indicate the dorsolateral prefrontal cortex. *A:* Before treatment. *B:* After treatment with antidepressants.

Source.   Reprinted from Baxter LR, Schwartz JM, Phelps ME, et al.: "Reduction of Prefrontal Cortex Glucose Metabolism Common to Three Types of Depression." *Archives of General Psychiatry* 46:243–250, 1989. Used with permission. Copyright 1989 American Medical Association. Figure printed in color in original publication.

Single Photon Emission Computed Tomography

Single photon emission computed tomography (SPECT) is another technique that uses the detection of emitted photons from compounds containing small amounts of short-lived radioactive isotopes (such as technetium 99m) to visualize organ blood flow and ligand binding.

In several case reports in which SPECT was used before and after treatment, significant changes in regional cerebral blood flow (rCBF) were demonstrated. However, these findings need to be replicated in controlled studies. Wada et al. (1999) reported marked improvement in rCBF after treatment and resolution of hypochondriacal delusions. Similarly, Laatsch et al. (1997) reported significant improvements on measures of neuropsychological functioning and improvements in rCBF in three patients with known brain injury after cognitive rehabilitation therapy. Rodriguez and Andree (1996) used SPECT to examine perfusion in different brain regions before and after clozapine administration to 24 patients with treatment-resistant schizophrenia. Patients who responded to treatment with clozapine showed higher thalamic, left basal ganglia, and right prefrontal perfusion in addition to decreased subcortical perfusion, whereas nonresponders had lower prefrontal perfusion. In patients with major depression, Klimke et al. (1999) showed that age-corrected baseline binding of the dopamine type 2 (D_2) receptor antagonist [^{123}I] iodobenzamide (IBZM) in the striatum was significantly lower in patients who responded to treatment than in nonresponders.

Magnetic Resonance Imaging and Functional Magnetic Resonance Imaging

Magnetic resonance imaging (MRI) was originally used to visualize soft tissue abnormalities associated with particular disease processes. Nevertheless, current studies suggest that it could be a useful outcome measurement tool in psychiatric disorders. MRI was used to test volume changes in cortical areas in connection with clinical improvement after treatment. Lauriello et al. (1998) showed that in patients with schizophrenia who were treated with clozapine, improvement in scores on the Brief Psychiatric Rating Scale (BPRS) correlated with MRI values. Patients with larger anterior superior temporal lobe cerebrospinal fluid volumes showed greater reduction in BPRS scores and improvement of withdrawal and retardation symptoms.

Functional MRI (fMRI) provides a high-resolution reporting of neural activity as detected by signals dependent on blood oxygen level. Use of fMRI as a method of detecting treatment change in schizophrenia and mood disorders is still in the experimental phase. fMRI is the most promising brain imaging method for clinical measurement based on its noninvasive nature, its favorable cost, and the availability of equipment in medical centers.

Summary: Application of Imaging in Outcome Measurement

Many studies have shown the value of imaging in detecting changes in different areas of the brain before and after treatment. However, the use of brain imaging as an outcome tool is still in its early stages and will remain bound by the ability to increase its specificity to the disorders being assessed. In addition, studies are needed to establish more reliable correlations with clinical changes.

OUTCOME MEASUREMENT USING LABORATORY TESTS

The clinical laboratory provides psychiatry with promising outcome assessment tools developed over the last few decades and enhanced by recent technological advances. However, because there is insufficient evidence-based knowledge on the neurochemical changes involved in the etiopathogenic and therapeutic processes, it is still not possible to attribute with certainty a predictive or outcome assessment value to changes in laboratory values. Cyclic and compensatory physiologic changes, the effect of drugs and other therapeutic interventions, and many other contributors to "noise" all decrease the signal-to-noise ratio in measurements. Described below are laboratory markers that may contribute to outcome assessment in the future as technology and specificity improve.

Homovanillic Acid

Poor outcome of patients with schizophrenia and depression, as evidenced by their suicide, is correlated with low levels of homovanillic acid (HVA) and 5-hydroxyindoleacetic acid (5-HIAA) in cerebrospinal fluid (CSF) in postmortem studies (Engstroem et al. 1999). Other studies have suggested that good treatment outcome in depression and aggressive behavior is associated with increased 5-hydroxytryptamine (5-HT) levels in CSF. Successful outcome in the treatment of refractory schizophrenia with clozapine has also been associated with an increased ratio of HVA to 5-HIAA in the CSF (Szymansky et al. 1993). However, the detection of these substances or their metabolites in plasma and urine (to avoid the risks and discomfort of lumbar puncture) is complicated by the filter effect created by the blood-brain barrier and other causes of "noise." These causes include the contribution of metabolites by the peripheral neurovegetative system, circadian rhythms, diet, and differences in interindividual elimination rates.

The study of changes in plasma HVA in response to neuroleptic treatment in schizophrenia has also provided encouraging correlations of this marker to outcome. During treatment with haloperidol, plasma HVA initially increases, reflecting an increment of dopamine release in an attempt by the system to overcome postsynaptic dopamine blockade. This is followed, after approximately 2 weeks, by a significant reduction due to down-regulation (by depolarization inactivation of the dopaminergic system) at the presynaptic level. Multiple reports have confirmed that patients who had the greatest changes in plasma HVA in response to neuroleptic blockade showed the greatest clinical improvement as measured by clinical assessment scales (Davila et al. 1997). The study of these metabolites during treatment in schizophrenia has supported their value as pathophysiologic and pharmacologic outcome indicators. Further evidence supporting the outcome assessment value of drug metabolites includes reports on platelet serotonin content in various treatment options (Lestra et al. 1998).

Immunologic Tests, G Protein, and Plasma Prolactin

Immunologic investigation of patients with mental disorders is a novel laboratory aspect of outcome assessment in psychiatry. Although they are still in the research phase, various outcome prediction candidates have been proposed. For instance, G protein acts as a messenger for transducing signals for a variety of hormones that cause cellular responses such as activating the production of cyclic adenosine monophosphate. There are reports indicating that the low levels of G protein functioning and immunoreactivity found in depression might be reliable and accurate indicators (as well as predictors) of change due to treatment. In one study, repeated assays performed after successive electroconvulsive therapy sessions showed that the normalization of G protein measures preceded, and thus predicted, clinical improvement (Avissar et al. 1998).

Interestingly, similar effects on measurements of G protein have been positively correlated with good outcome in seasonal affective disorder. In this illness, normalization of G protein was significantly correlated both with successful therapy and with season change (Avissar et al. 1999). In parallel lines of immunologic research, interleukin-2 receptor–mediated blastoformation (Kanba et al. 1998) and changes in interleukin-1β (Anisman et al. 1999) and CD4 and CD8 lymphocyte counts have also been proposed as indicators in the interface between the central nervous system and the immune system in depression, stress-related disorders (Scanlan et al. 1998), and schizophrenia (Zorrilla et al. 1998). Plasma prolactin response to fenfluramine treatment in OCD has also been significantly correlated with outcome (Monteleone et al. 1997).

Hypothalamic-Pituitary-Adrenal Axis

Another category of laboratory tests in psychopharmacologic outcome assessment includes a variety of hormones, metabolites, and drug challenges to the hypothalamic-pituitary-adrenal (HPA) axis. HPA axis studies, particularly the dexamethasone suppression test (DST), have been performed for many years in treatment studies using a variety of polycyclic antidepressants and selective serotonin reuptake inhibitors. However, these tests have not proved useful because only a fraction of depressed patients have abnormal responses. Currently, tests involving challenges with corticotropin-releasing factor (CRF), metyrapone, and other drugs are being performed as a potential alternative to the DST. Although the tests are relatively inexpensive, the use of DST and other HPA studies remain controversial and are not recommended for outcome assessment at this time.

Other Laboratory Measures

The laboratory detection of substances of abuse is the most reliable indicator of outcome for patients with substance abuse with or without coexisting mental illness. Random or scheduled toxicologic examination of urine and other body elements is relatively inexpensive and constitutes the main tool to ascertain the overall success of treatment. Also highly reliable are the assays of whole blood–associated acetaldehyde and carbohydrate-deficient transferrin in serum for the outcome assessment of alcohol dependence. These two assays show better reliability and specificity than γ-glutamyl transpeptidase (GGT) or red blood cell volume assays, at a similar cost (Schmidt et al. 1997). Quantitative electroencephalography (QEEG) also showed promising data that is similar to brain imaging studies and may be of use in the future.

Summary and Future Directions

The cost of advanced laboratory technologies has so far limited their use and investigation. The cost-effectiveness ratio of these and other novel outcome indicators, such as those derived from recently developed genetic, spectrographic, and other technologies, may soon reach levels acceptable for clinical use and empirical investigation.

Although there are still very few tests available to measure the outcome of psychiatric interventions, there are preliminary data regarding the effects of psychiatric interventions on the metabolites of serotonin, norepinephrine, dopamine, and other catecholamines, as well as of peptides, amino acids, and other molecules. The future will bring more developments in this area, especially progress in the correlation between laboratory measures and changes in the clinical picture.

OUTCOME MEASUREMENT USING TECHNOLOGICAL TESTS

Vocal Acoustic Measures of the Patient's Voice: The "Flat Affect" Example

Although clinical ratings of flat affect and alogia achieve acceptable reliability, they lack precision. Subscales overlap with each other, with ratings of depression, and with neuroleptic motor side effects. A study to compare ratings of flat affect and alogia with acoustic measures of the patient's prosody and fluency included patients with schizophrenia who were evaluated using the Scale for the Assessment of Negative Symptoms (SANS) and the St. Hans Extrapyramidal Rating Scale. Fifteen-minute free-speech samples were recorded and analyzed acoustically. Data analysis was based on the VoxCom system (Alpert et al. 1986), a hybrid analog-digital speech analysis program. Correlations between pairs of SANS items and acoustic measures (e.g., vocal inflection and fundamental frequency variance; response latency and duration of switching pauses; and poverty of speech and the percentage of time talking) were weak. For example, response latency, an acoustic measure, is defined as the space following the end of the question and the beginning of the response. In the SANS, the interviewer must estimate the patient's response latency, a rather difficult task. Clinical ratings are unable to achieve precise assessments of small latency differences. In a randomized clinical trial comparing an atypical with a typical neuroleptic as well as a placebo, it was possible to show that the use of acoustic analysis to measure the increased latency of response was more effective in distinguishing outcome than was clinical rating. (Alpert et al. 1995).

Summary

Acoustic analysis shows promise as a precise method of assessing patients before and after treatment. The development of acoustic and other technological measures may enhance outcome assessment in psychiatric disorders.

CONCLUSION

The innovative imaging, laboratory, and technical approaches to outcome measurement described in this chapter are still in early phases of development. More research is needed to develop tests with better validity, reliability, sensitivity, and specificity. Research in the area of brain imaging (especially fMRI) may show the greatest potential for practical applications in outcome assessment. The future is promising for a comprehensive outcome measurement system that could encompass the patient's subjective report and the clinician's impression in addition to the "temperature" of each psychiatric symptom.

REFERENCES

Alpert M, Merewether F, Homel P, et al: Voxcom: a system for analyzing natural speech in real time. Behav Res Methods Instrum Comput 18:267–272, 1986

Alpert M, Pouget ER, Sison C, et al: Clinical and acoustic measures of the negative syndrome. Psychopharmacology Bulletin 31:321–326, 1995

Anisman H, Ravindram AV, Griffiths J, et al: Interleukin-1-beta production in dysthymia before and after pharmacotherapy. Biol Psychiatry 46:1649–1655, 1999

Avissar S, Nechamkin Y, Roitman G, et al: Dynamics of ECT normalization of low G protein function and immunoreactivity in mononuclear leukocytes of patients with major depression. Am J Psychiatry 155:666–671, 1998

Avissar S, Schreiber G, Nechamkin Y, et al: The effects of seasons and light therapy on G protein levels in mononuclear leukocytes of patients with seasonal affective disorder. Arch Gen Psychiatry 56:178–183, 1999

Baxter LR, Schwartz JM, Phelps ME, et al: Reduction of prefrontal cortex glucose metabolism common to three types of depression. Arch Gen Psychiatry 46: 243–250, 1989

Baxter LR Jr, Schwartz JM, Bergman KS, et al: Caudate glucose metabolic rate changes with both drug and behavior therapy for obsessive-compulsive disorder. Arch Gen Psychiatry 49(9):681–689, 1992

Brody AL, Saxena S, Silverman DHS, et al: Brain metabolic changes in major depressive disorder from pre- to post-treatment with paroxetine. Psychiatry Res 91:127–139, 1999

Buchsbaum MS, Wu J, Siegel BV, et al: Effect of sertraline on regional metabolic rate in patients with affective disorder. Biol Psychiatry 41:15–22, 1997

Davila R, Zumarzraga M, Andia I, et al: Early increase in plasma HVA during neuroleptic treatment: a tool for outcome prediction in schizophrenia, in Plasma Homovanillic Acid in Schizophrenia: Implications for Presynaptic Dopamine Dysfunction. Edited by Friedhoff AJ, Amin F. Washington DC, American Psychiatric Press, 1997

Engstroem G, Alling C, Blennow K, et al: Reduced cerebrospinal HVA concentrations and HVA/5-HIAA ratios in suicide attempters: monoamine metabolites in 120 suicide attempters and 47 controls. Eur Neuropsychopharmacol 9:399–405, 1999

Kanba S, Manki H, Shintani F, et al: Aberrant interleukin-2-receptor-mediated blastoformation of peripheral blood lymphocytes in a severe major depressive episode. Psychol Med 28:481–484, 1998

Klimke A, Larisch R, Janz A, et al: Dopamine D2 receptor binding before and after treatment of major depression measured by [^{123}I]IBZM SPECT. Psychiatry Res 90:91–101, 1999

Laatsch L, Jobe T, Sychra J, et al: Impact of cognitive rehabilitation therapy on neuropsychological impairments as measured by brain perfusion SPECT: a longitudinal study. Brain Injury 11:851–863, 1997

Lauriello J, Mathalon DH, Rosenbloom M, et al: Association between regional brain volumes and clozapine response in schizophrenia. Biol Psychiatry 43:879–886, 1998

Lestra C, D'Amatto T, Ghaemmaghami C, et al: Biological parameters in major depression: effects of paroxetine, viloxacine, moclobemide, and electroconvulsive therapy. Relation to early clinical outcome. Biol Psychiatry 44:274–289, 1998

Mackowiak PA, Wasserman SS, Levine MM: A critical appraisal of 98.6 degrees F, the upper limit of the normal body temperature, and other legacies of Carl Reinhold August Wunderlich. JAMA 268:1578–1580, 1992

Middleton WEK: The History of the Thermometer and its Use in Meteorology Baltimore, MD, Johns Hopkins University Press, 1966

Monteleone P, Catapano F, Di Martino S, et al: Prolactin response to d-fenfluramine in obsessive compulsive patients, and outcome of fluvoxamine treatment. Br J Psychiatry 170:554–557, 1997

Rodriguez VM, Andree RM: SPECT study of regional cerebral perfusion in neuroleptic-resistant schizophrenic patients who responded or did not respond to clozapine. Am J Psychiatry 153:1343–1346, 1996

Saxena S, Brody AL, Schwartz JM, et al: Neuroimaging and frontal-subcortical circuitry in obsessive-compulsive disorder. Br J Psychiatry 173:26–37, 1998

Scanlan JM, Vitaliano PP, Ochs H, et al: CD4 and CD8 counts are associated with interactions of gender and psychosocial stress. Psychosom Med 60:644–653, 1998

Schmidt LG, Schmidt K, Dufeu P, et al: Superiority of carbohydrase-deficient transferrin to gamma-glutamyltranspeptidase in detecting relapse in alcoholism. Am J Psychiatry 154:75–80, 1997

Szymansky S, Liebman J, Pollack S: The dopamine-serotonin relationship in clozapine response. Psychopharmacology 112:585–589, 1993

Videbech P: PET measurements of brain glucose metabolism and blood flow in major depressive disorder: a critical review. Acta Psychiatr Scand 101:11–20, 2000

Wada T, Kawakatsu S, Komatani A: Possible association between delusional disorder, somatic type and reduced regional cerebral blood flow. Prog Neuropsychopharmacol Biol Psychiatry 23:353–357, 1999

Zorrilla EP, Cannon TD, Kessler J, et al: Leukocyte differentials predicts short-term clinical outcome following antipsychotic treatment in schizophrenia. Biol Psychiatry 43:887–896, 1998

Example of a Depression Treatment and Outcome Monitoring Pathway

Waguih William IsHak, M.D.
Joseph P. Merlino, M.D., M.P.A.
Manuel Trujillo, M.D.

The Depression Treatment and Outcome-Monitoring Pathway (NYU/ Bellevue-DTP) was developed at the Bellevue Hospital Center Division of Outpatient and Community Psychiatry and New York University School

We thank Carlos Ortiz, M.D., for his active participation and continuous feedback during the process of development; Hector Varas, M.D., for providing the original direction; David Nardacci, M.D., for inspiring the process through the first outcome initiative; A. John Rush, M.D., for giving permission to use the Inventory of Depressive Symptomatology and its quick version; and the Bellevue Outpatient attending psychiatrists for all their tremendous efforts in implementation of the pathway, valuable teaching of residents, and advanced clinical work with patients.

Do not use this material without written permission from Waguih William IsHak, M.D.

of Medicine. To develop the pathway, the authors utilized the Expert Consensus Guidelines (Frances et al. 1998), the American Psychiatric Association Practice Guidelines for depression (American Psychiatric Association 2000b), and a comprehensive review of depression outcome measures as highlighted in Chapter 10, in this volume. These reviews, together with numerous critiques of the literature, revealed that the most commonly used instruments in diagnosing or rating depression—that is, the Beck Depression Inventory (BDI) and the Hamilton Rating Scale for Depression (Ham-D or HRSD)—do not correspond with the current definitions of depression as defined by DSM-IV-TR or ICD-10 (American Psychiatric Association 2000a; World Health Organization 1992).

Utilizing a best practices approach, it was decided for the purposes of this pathway to use a DSM-IV-TR–based tool that had both a patient self-report and clinician-rated instrument. The Inventory for Depressive Symptomatology (IDS) (Rush et al. 1986) was selected for this pathway, adopting the shorter form, the Quick Inventory for Depressive Symptomatology (QIDS), in both its self-report (QIDS-SR) and clinician-rated (QIDS-C) versions (see the instruments in Appendix B).

The pathway involves measuring the outcome of treatment interventions in a timely manner. Those interventions include psychotherapy, the use of medication(s), medication augmentation, and the use of antidepressant classes that have been shown to be effective in the treatment of refractory depression. The pathway incorporates significant flexibility, allowing the clinician numerous choices in selection and dosage of medication.

Patients are enrolled in this program at the time they are assigned to clinicians for treatment. Participating patients are treated by psychiatry residents (supervised by pathway attending MDs) or by attending psychiatrists participating in the pathway. Through their involvement, the clinicians are taught more scientific and cost-effective ways to treat depressive disorders. This is achieved through regularly scheduled group supervision and reviews of the latest literature on the topic. Administrative support for data entry and analysis is also provided.

The pathway calls for the administration of the QIDS-SR at the time the patient begins the triage or intake evaluation. This evaluation establishes a preliminary diagnosis. After the score is noted and the biopsychosocial assessment is reviewed for exclusion criteria, the clinician follows the pathway as outlined below.

I. At Points of Entry (e.g., Triage or Intake Assessment) Administer QIDS-SR to Every Patient

IF score is ≤ 9:	Patient excluded (not depressed)
IF score is ≥ 10–17:	Mild to moderate depression
IF score is ≥ 18:	Severe depression

II. A Biopsychosocial Evaluation Is Conducted (see Section VIII), a Working Diagnosis Is Determined (Using the DSM-IV-TR), the Clinical Complexity Scale Is Administered (See Section X), and the Following Diagnoses Are to Be Excluded:

- Mood disorder due to general medical conditions
- Substance-induced mood disorders
- Mood disorders with psychotic features

III. Using the Severity of Depression as Determined by the QIDS-SR Score, Follow the Treatment Guidelines Below:

Disorder	Mild to moderate (QIDS-SR≥10–17)	Severe (QIDS-SR≥18)
Major depression	Psychotherapy and/or medications (see A)	Medications mandatory (see A) ±psychotherapy
Dysthymic disorder	Psychotherapy and/or medications (see A)	Medications mandatory (see A) ±psychotherapy
Bipolar disorder, depressed	Psychotherapy and/or medications (see B)	Medications mandatory (see C) ±psychotherapy

A. Medications for Dysthymic Disorder and Major Depression (With No Psychotic Features):

Step 1.

Start with the clinician's choice of selective serotonin reuptake inhibitor (SSRI), norepinephrine serotonin reuptake inhibitor (NSRI), tricyclic antidepressant (TCA), or atypical antidepressant **for 6 full weeks on an adequate dose** (see discussion of adequate dose in Sections V and VI below).

At the end of the sixth week, **reapply QIDS-SR**. If there is no response, or partial response (for definitions of response, see Section IV below), go to Step 2.

Step 2.

Switch class of antidepressant at this point and give new medication **for 6 weeks on an adequate dose.**

At the end of this sixth week period (twelfth week of the pathway), reapply QIDS-SR. Also administer the QIDS-C and the Ham-D (because the Ham-D is still the most commonly used clinician-administered measure).

If there is no response, or partial response, go to Step 3.

Step 3.

The patient should now have a biopsychosocial reevaluation to reassess diagnosis and to identify comorbidities or stresses requiring other interventions. If the diagnosis remains the same, then start augmentation with lithium or thyroxin **for 12 more weeks.**

After the twelfth week, reapply QIDS-SR, QIDS-C, and the Ham-D. If there is no response, or partial response, go to Step 4.

Step 4.

Repeat biopsychosocial reevaluation. If the diagnosis remains the same, then use a monoamine oxidase inhibitor (MAOI) **for 12 weeks on an adequate dose.** After the twelfth week, reapply QIDS-SR, QIDS-C, and the Ham-D. If there is no response, the patient is considered treatment refractory, and other assessment and treatment alternatives should be pursued to address predisposing and precipitating factors.

B. Medications for MILD TO MODERATE Bipolar Disorder Depressed (Without Psychotic Features):

Step 1.

Start with the clinician's choice of lithium, valproate (Depakote), or lamotrigine (Lamictal) **for 6 weeks on an adequate dose** (see discussion of adequate dose in Sections V and VII below). Reapply QIDS-SR. If there is no response, or partial response, go to Step 2.

Step 2.

Switch to a different mood stabilizer **for 6 weeks on an adequate dose.** Again administer the QIDS-SR and apply QIDS-C and the Ham-D (because the Ham-D is still the most commonly used clinician-administered measure).

   If there is no response, or partial response, go to Step 3.

Step 3.

The patient should now have a biopsychosocial reevaluation. If the diagnosis remains the same, then use a combination of two mood stabilizers **for 12 weeks on an adequate dose.**

   After the twelfth week, reapply QIDS-SR, QIDS-C, and the Ham-D. If there is no response, then proceed to C. Step 4.

C. Medications for SEVERE Bipolar Disorder Depressed (With No Psychotic Features):

Step 1.

Start with the clinician's choice of lithium, valproate (Depakote), or lamotrigine (Lamictal) **combined with** bupropion (Wellbutrin) or SSRI **for 6 weeks on an adequate dose.** Reapply QIDS-SR. If there is no response, or partial response, go to Step 2.

Step 2.

Use the clinician's choice of lithium, valproate (Depakote), or lamotrigine (Lamictal) **combined with** venlafaxine (Effexor) or MAOI **for 6 weeks on an adequate dose.**

   Reapply QIDS-SR and apply QIDS-C and the Ham-D (because the Ham-D is still the most commonly used clinician-administered measure). If there is no response, or partial response, go to Step 3.

Step 3.

The patient should now have a biopsychosocial reevaluation. If the diagnosis remains the same, then switch the mood stabilizer and **combine with** venlafaxine (Effexor) or MAOI **for 6 weeks on an adequate dose.**

   After the sixth week, reapply QIDS-SR, QIDS-C, and the Ham-D. If there is no response, or partial response, go to Step 4.

Step 4.

Use a combination of two mood stabilizers **with** venlafaxine (Effexor), or MAOI **for 6 weeks on an adequate dose.**

After the sixth week, reapply QIDS-SR, QIDS-C, and the Ham-D. If there is no response, or partial response, go to Step 5.

Step 5.

The patient should now have a biopsychosocial reevaluation. If the diagnosis remains the same, then augment the above treatment regiment **with** thyroxin **for 12 weeks on an adequate dose.**

After the twelfth week, reapply QIDS-SR, QIDS-C, and the Ham-D. If there is no response, the patient is considered treatment refractory, and other assessment and treatment alternatives should be pursued to address predisposing and precipitating factors.

Note. Antidepressants should be tapered 2 to 6 months after remission to prevent antidepressant-induced manic episodes.

IV. Response and Partial Response Definitions

- *RESPONSE* is defined as a decrease in the QIDS-SR/QIDS-C score to ≤9 or a 50% reduction in the score.
- *PARTIAL RESPONSE* is defined as a decrease in the QIDS-SR/QIDS-C score from SEVERE to MILD-MODERATE or a 25% reduction in the score.

V. Adequate Dose General Guidelines

The adequate dose guidelines below were derived from literature reviews and U.S. Food and Drug Administration (FDA)–approved labeling information. Common practice strategies of increasing the medications to maximum doses had proven to be inferior to adequate trials of a different class or the use of augmenting agents. This pathway offers the clinician the flexibility of increasing the dosage as long as it meets the minimum requirement for ADEQUATE DOSE.

VI. Guidelines for Adequate Dose of Recommended Antidepressants

Medication	Initial	ADEQUATE DOSE is at least	Notes
1. SSRIs			
Prozac	20 mg qam	20 mg daily	Max. dose=80 mg daily
Zoloft	50 mg qd	50 mg daily	Dose changes should not occur at intervals of less than 1 week. Max. dose=200 mg daily
Paxil	20 mg qd	40 mg daily	Dose changes should occur at intervals of at least 1 week in 10-mg/day increments. Max. dose=50 mg daily
Luvox	50 mg qhs	200 mg daily	Dose should be increased in 50-mg increments every 4 to 7 days, as tolerated. Max. dose=200 mg daily
Celexa	20 mg qd	40 mg daily	Dose increases should usually occur in increments of 20 mg at intervals of no less than 1 week. Max. dose=60 mg daily
2. NSRIs			
Effexor XR	75 mg qd	225 mg daily	When increasing the dose, increments of up to 75 mg/day should be made at intervals of no less than 4 days. Max. dose=375 mg daily
3. Wellbutrin SR	100 mg bid	300 mg daily	No single dose of Wellbutrin should exceed 200 mg. Max. dose=400 mg daily
4. Serzone	100 mg bid	600 mg daily	Dose increases should occur in increments of 100 mg/day at intervals of no less than 1 week. Dose-response relationship is undetermined; the use of the maximum dose of 600 mg daily is preferred.
5. Remeron	15 mg qd	45 mg daily	Dose changes should not be made at intervals of less than 1–2 weeks. Dose-response relationship is undetermined; the use of the maximum dose of 45 mg daily is preferred.

VI. Guidelines for Adequate Dose of Recommended Antidepressants *(continued)*

Medication	Initial	ADEQUATE DOSE is at least	Notes
6. TCAs			
Pamelor	25 mg qhs	100 mg daily to maintain a blood level of at least 100 μg.	Max. dose=150 mg daily
Tofranil	50 mg qhs	200 mg daily to maintain a blood level of at least 150 μg.	Max. dose=300 mg daily
Elavil	50 mg qhs	200 mg daily to maintain a blood level of at least 150 μg.	Max. dose=300 mg daily
7. Parnate	30 mg qd	30 mg daily	Diet precautions. Max. dose=60 mg daily

Note.   bid=twice a day; qam=every morning; qd=every day; qhs=every night.

VII. Guidelines for Adequate Dose of Recommended Mood Stabilizers

Medication	Initial	ADEQUATE DOSE	Notes
Lithium	300 mg tid	Doses maintaining a blood level between 1.0 and 1.4 mEq/L	Dose changes should occur at intervals of at least 1 week. Blood level should not be exceed 1.4 mEq/L
Valproate (Depakote)	250 mg tid	Doses maintaining a blood level between 50 μg/mL and 125 μg/mL	The dose should be increased as rapidly as possible to achieve the lowest therapeutic dose that produces the desired clinical effect or the desired range of plasma concentrations. Dose should not exceed 60 mg/kg per day.

VII. Guidelines for Adequate Dose of Recommended Mood Stabilizers *(continued)*

Medication	Initial	ADEQUATE DOSE	Notes
Lamotrigine (Lamictal)	25 mg qd	At least 200 mg qd	Off-label use. Titrate very gradually (by 25 mg–100 mg/week). Stop if rash develops for potential danger of Stevens-Johnson syndrome (0.3%)

Note. Carbamazepine (Tegretol) is not used in this project due to partial evidence in depression. qd=every day; tid=three times a day.

VIII. Guidelines for Biopsychosocial Evaluation

1. Identify biological factors related to the etiology of depressive symptoms.
   a. Medical causes of depression
   b. Substance abuse, including intoxication and withdrawal
   c. Medications/dietary supplements implicated in depression
2. Identify psychological factors related to the etiology of depressive symptoms.
   a. Significant psychological traumas
   b. Significant psychological losses
   c. Unresolved grief
   d. Interpersonal conflicts (family, work)
3. Identify social factors related to the etiology of depressive symptoms.
   a. Residential problems
   b. Employment problems
   c. Financial problems
4. Rule out malingering, factitious disorders, and somatoform disorders.
5. Review the working diagnosis and consider alternative diagnoses.
6. Implement treatment interventions to address the identified etiological factors above.

IX. Guidelines for Psychotherapy

1. Individual psychotherapy
   a. Frequency: weekly
   b. Duration: 30- to 45-minute sessions
   c. Type: identify the type of psychotherapy used:

      (1) Eclectic (most common, ongoing)
      (2) Supportive (ongoing)
      (3) Psychodynamic (ongoing)
      (4) Cognitive-behavioral therapy (CBT) (12–16 sessions)
      (5) Brief dynamic (12 sessions)
      (6) Intensive short-term dynamic (up to 40 sessions)
      (7) Interpersonal (12–16 sessions)

2. Group psychotherapy
  a. Frequency: weekly
  b. Duration: 60- to 90-minute sessions
  c. Type: identify the type of group psychotherapy used
      (1) Eclectic (most common, ongoing)
      (2) Supportive (ongoing)
      (3) Psychodynamic (ongoing)
      (4) CBT (12–16 sessions)
      (5) Interpersonal (12–16 sessions)

3. Family psychotherapy is used only as an adjunct treatment.
4. FREQUENCY OF OUTCOME EVALUATIONS DURING PSY-
    CHOTHERAPY

Step 1.

Before the first scheduled session, apply QIDS-SR.

    After 12 weeks, reapply QIDS-SR. If there is no response, or partial response, go to Step 2.

Step 2.

The patient should now have a biopsychosocial reevaluation. If the diagnosis remains the same, then consider medications and continue psychotherapy for 12 weeks. After the twelfth week, reapply QIDS-SR, QIDS-C, and the Ham-D (because the Ham-D is still the most commonly used clinician-administered measure). If there is no response, or partial response, go to Step 3.

Step 3.

The patient should now have a biopsychosocial reevaluation. If the diagnosis remains the same, then antidepressant medications are mandatory; follow medication guidelines in addition to ongoing psychotherapy.

    Note. Reapply QIDS-SR, QIDS-C, and the Ham-D at the end of briefer therapies.

X. Guidelines for Clinical Complexity Determination

Use the Clinical Complexity Scale (CCS) at the time of case assignment (triages, disposition, or team conference) to measure the level of clinical complexity. This determination will assist the clinician in addressing all the prognostic factors, which might affect the expected outcome of treatment.

Clinical Complexity Scale (CCS)

Item	0 (none)	1 (mild)	2 (moderate)	3 (severe)
1. Family history of mental illness		3rd-degree relative(s)	2nd-degree relative(s)	1st-degree relative(s)
2. Perinatal events Medications, infections, anoxia, etc.		Mild	Moderate	Severe
3. Psychological traumas/loss in childhood Abuse, neglect, abandonment, overgratification, or overprotection.		Mild	Moderate	Severe
4. Substance abuse		Abstinent for >1 year	Abstinent for >3 months	Active
5. Medical problems DM, HTN, TBI, CP, etc.		Mild	Moderate	Severe
6. Axis II diagnosis Cluster A, B, or C		Mild	Moderate	Severe
7. Duration of illness		>6 months	>1 year	>5 years
8. Residential problems		Conflict at residence	Impending homelessness	Homelessness
9. Financial problems		Barely making it (living from check to check)	Significant debt	Bankruptcy (actual or impending)
10. Vocational problems		Conflict at work	Impending unemployment	Unemployment

Clinical Complexity Scale (CCS) *(continued)*

Item	Score			
	0 (none)	1 (mild)	2 (moderate)	3 (severe)
11. Relationship problems		Conflict in close relationships	Impending loss of relationships	No close relationships
12. Psychological traumas/losses in adulthood				
Death of loved ones, exposure to violence, etc.		Mild	Moderate	Severe
13. Noncompliance with appointments		25% of the time	50% of the time	Near 100% of the time
14. Noncompliance with treatment plan				
Refusal of treatment recommendations such as tests, medications, and treatment modalities.		Mild	Moderate	Severe
15. Functioning level as measured using the GAF score		≥75	<75 and >30	≤30

Note. 1–15=mild complexity; 16–30=moderate complexity; 30–45=severe complexity; CP=cardiopulmonary; DM=diabetes mellitus; HTN=hypertension; TBI=traumatic brain injury. © 2001 Waguih William IsHak, M.D.

References

American Psychiatric Association: Diagnostic and Statistical Manual of Mental Disorders, 4th Edition, Text Revision. Washington, DC, American Psychiatric Association, 2000a

American Psychiatric Association: Practice Guidelines for the Treatment of Psychiatric Disorders, Compendium 2000, Washington, DC, American Psychiatric Press, 2000b

Frances AJ, Kahn DA, Carpenter D, et al: The Expert Consensus Guidelines for treating depression in bipolar disorder. J Clin Psychiatry 59 (suppl 4):73–79, 1998

Rush AJ, Giles DE, Schlesser MA, et al: The Inventory for Depressive Symptomatology (IDS): Preliminary findings. Psychiatry Res 18(1):65–87, 1986

World Health Organization: International Statistical Classification of Diseases and Related Health Problems, 10th Revision. Geneva, World Health Organization, 1992

Suggested Readings

Compton MT, Nemeroff CB: The treatment of bipolar depression. J Clin Psychiatry 61 (suppl 9):57–67, 2000

Crismon ML, Trivedi M, Pigott TA, et al: The Texas Medication Algorithm Project: report of the Texas Consensus Conference Panel on Medication Treatment of Major Depressive Disorder. J Clin Psychiatry 60(3):142–156, 1999

Persons JB, Thase ME, Crits-Christoph P: The role of psychotherapy in the treatment of depression: review of two practice guidelines. Arch Gen Psychiatry 53(4):283–290, 1996

Post RM, Leverich GS, Denicoff KD, et al: Alternative approaches to refractory depression in bipolar illness. Depress Anxiety 5(4):175–189, 1997

Rush AJ, Crismon ML, Toprac MG, et al: Consensus guidelines in the treatment of major depressive disorder. J Clin Psychiatry 59 (suppl 20):73–84, 1998

Sachs GS, Printz DJ, Kahn DA, et al: The Expert Consensus Guidelines Series: Medication Treatment of Bipolar Disorder 2000. Postgrad Med Spec No:1–104, 2000

Thase ME, Sachs GS: Bipolar depression: pharmacotherapy and related therapeutic strategies. Biol Psychiatry 48(6):558–572, 2000

Trivedi MH, Shon S, Crismon ML, et al: Texas Implementation of Medication Algorithms (TIMA) Guidelines for Treating Major Depressive Disorder: TIMA Physician Procedural Manual. Austin, TX, Texas Department of Mental Health and Mental Retardation, 2000 (available at http://www.mhmr.state.tx.us/centraloffice/medicaldirector/timaMDDman.pdf)

B

Selected Outcome Measures

ABNORMAL INVOLUNTARY MOVEMENT SCALE (AIMS)

Examination Procedure

Either before or after completing the examination procedure, observe the patient unobtrusively at rest (e.g., in the waiting room).

The chair to be used in this examination should be a hard, firm one without arms.

1. Ask the patient whether there is anything in his or her mouth (such as gum or candy) and, if so, to remove it.
2. Ask about the *current* condition of the patient's teeth. Ask if he or she wears dentures. Ask whether teeth or dentures bother the patient *now*.
3. Ask whether the patient notices any movements in his or her mouth, face, hands, or feet. If yes, ask the patient to describe them and to indicate to what extent they *currently* bother the patient or interfere with activities.
4. Have the patient sit in chair with hands on knees, legs slightly apart, and feet flat on floor. (Look at the entire body for movements while the patient is in this position.)
5. Ask the patient to sit with hands hanging unsupported—if male, between his legs, if female and wearing a dress, hanging over her knees. (Observe hands and other body areas).
6. Ask the patient to open his or her mouth. (Observe the tongue at rest within the mouth.) Do this twice.
7. Ask the patient to protrude his or her tongue. (Observe abnormalities of tongue movement.) Do this twice.
8. Ask the patient to tap his or her thumb with each finger as rapidly as possible for 10–15 seconds, first with right hand, then with left hand. (Observe facial and leg movements.) [activated movement]
9. Flex and extend the patient's left and right arms, one at a time.
10. Ask the patient to stand up. (Observe the patient in profile. Observe all body areas again, hips included.)
11. Ask the patient to extend both arms out in front, palms down. (Observe trunk, legs, and mouth.) [activated movement]
12. Have the patient walk a few paces, turn, and walk back to the chair. (Observe hands and gait.) Do this twice. [activated movement]

Scoring Procedure

Complete the examination procedure before making ratings.

For the movement ratings (the first three categories below), rate the highest severity observed. 0=none, 1=minimal (may be extreme normal), 2=mild, 3=moderate, and 4=severe. According to the original AIMS instructions, one point is subtracted if movements are seen only on activation, but not all investigators follow that convention.

Abnormal Involuntary Movement Scale (AIMS)

	None	Minimal	Mild	Moderate	Severe
Facial and oral movements					
1. Muscles of facial expression (e.g., movements of forehead, eyebrows, periorbital area, cheeks; include frowning, blinking, smiling, grimacing)	0	1	2	3	4
2. Lips and perioral area (e.g., puckering, pouting, smacking)	0	1	2	3	4
3. Jaw (e.g., biting, clenching, chewing, mouth opening, lateral movement)	0	1	2	3	4
4. Tongue Rate only increase in movement both in and out of mouth, NOT inability to sustain movement	0	1	2	3	4
Extremity movements					
5. Upper (arms, wrists, hands, fingers) Include choreic movements (i.e., rapid, objectively purposeless, irregular, spontaneous), athetoid movements (i.e., slow, irregular, complex, serpentine). Do NOT include tremor (i.e., repetitive, regular, rhythmic)	0	1	2	3	4
6. Lower (legs, knees, ankles, toes) (e.g., lateral knee movement, foot tapping, heel dropping, foot squirming, inversion and eversion of foot)	0	1	2	3	4
Trunk movements					
7. Neck, shoulders, hips (e.g., rocking, twisting, squirming, pelvic gyrations)	0	1	2	3	4
Global judgments					
8. Severity of abnormal movements	0	1	2	3	4
9. Incapacitation due to abnormal movements	0	1	2	3	4

10. Patient's awareness of abnormal movements Rate only patient's report	No awareness	0
	Aware, no distress	1
	Aware, mild distress	2
	Aware, moderate distress	3
	Aware, severe distress	4
11. Current problems with teeth and/or dentures	No	0
	Yes	1
12. Does patient usually wear dentures?	No	0
	Yes	1

Source. Reprinted from Guy W: *ECDEU Assessment Manual for Psychopharmacology, Revised* (DHEW Publ. No. ADM 76-338). Rockville, MD, U.S. Department of Health, Education, and Welfare, Public Health Service, Alcohol, Drug Abuse, and Mental Health Administration, NIMH Psychopharmacology Research Branch, Division of Extramural Research Programs, 1976.

Addiction Severity Index (ASI)

INSTRUCTIONS

1. Leave No Blanks - Where appropriate code:
   X = question not answered
   N = questions not applicable
   Use only one character per item.

2. Item numbers circled are to be asked at follow-up. Items with an asterisk are cumulative and should be rephrased at follow-up (see Manual).

3. Space is provided after sections for additional comments.

ADDICTION SEVERITY INDEX
SEVERITY RATINGS

The severity ratings are interviewer estimates of the patient's need for additional treatment in each area. The scales range from 0 (no treatment necessary) to 9 (treatment needed to intervene in life-threatening situation). Each ratings is based upon the patient's history of problem symptoms, present condition and subjective assessment of his treatment needs in a given area. For a detailed description of severity ratings' derivation procedures and conventions, see manual. **Note:** These severity ratings are optional.

Fifth Edition

SUMMARY OF PATIENTS RATING SCALE

0 - Not at all
1 - Slightly
2 - Moderately
3 - Considerably
4 - Extremely

G1. I.D. NUMBER

G2. LAST 4 DIGITS OF SSN

G3. PROGRAM NUMBER

G4. DATE OF ADMISSION

G5. DATE OF INTERVIEW

G6. TIME BEGUN

G7. TIME ENDED

G8. CLASS:
1 - Intake
2 - Follow-up

G9. CONTACT CODE:
1 - In Person
2 - Phone

G10. GENDER:
1 - Male
2 - Female

G11. INTERVIEWER CODE NUMBER

G12. SPECIAL:
1 - Patient terminated
2 - Patient refused
3 - Patient unable to respond

GENERAL INFORMATION

NAME _____

CURRENT ADDRESS _____

_____

G13. GEOGRAPHIC CODE

G14. How long have you lived at this address?

G15. Is this residence owned by your or your family?

G16. DATE OF BIRTH

G17. RACE
1 - White (Not of Hispanic Origin)
2 - Black (Not of Hispanic Origin)
3 - American Indian
4 - Alaskan Native
5 - Asian or Pacific Islander
6 - Hispanic - Mexican
7 - Hispanic - Puerto Rican
8 - Hispanic - Cuban
9 - Other Hispanic

G18. RELIGIOUS PREFERENCE
1 - Protestant
2 - Catholic
3 - Jewish
4 - Islamic
5 - Other
6 - None

G19. Have you been in a controlled environment in the past 30 days?
1 - No
2 - Jail
3 - Alcohol or Drug Treatment
4 - Medical Treatment
5 - Psychiatric Treatment
6 - Other

G20. How many days?

ADDITIONAL TEST RESULTS

G21. Shipley C.Q.

G22. Shipley I.Q.

G23. Beck Total Score

G24. SCL-90 Total

G25. MAST

G26.

G27.

G28.

SEVERITY PROFILE

9
8
7
6
5
4
3
2
1
0

PROBLEMS | MEDICAL | EMP/SUP | ALCOHOL | DRUG | LEGAL | FAM/SOC | PSYCH

Addiction Severity Index (ASI) *(continued)*

MEDICAL STATUS

M1. How many times in your life have you been hospitalized for medical problems? (Include o.d.'s, d.t.'s, exclude detox.)

M2. How long ago was your last hospitalization for a physical problem?
Years   Months

M3. Do you have any chronic medical problems which continue to interfere with your life?

M4. Are you taking any prescribed medication on a regular basis for a physical problem? 0 - No 1 - Yes

M5. Do you receive a pension for a physical disability? (Exclude psychiatric disability.)
0 - No
1 - Yes ____
Specify

M6. How many days have you experienced medical problems in the past 30 days?

FOR QUESTIONS M7 & M8 PLEASE ASK PATIENT TO USE THE PATIENT'S RATING SCALE

M7. How troubled or bothered have you been by these medical problems in the past 30 days?

COMMENTS

M8. How important to you now is treatment for these medical problems?

INTERVIEWER SEVERITY RATING

M9. How would you rate the patient's need for medical treatment?

CONFIDENCE RATINGS

Is the above information significantly distorted by:

M10. Patient's misrepresentation ?
0 - No 1 - Yes

M11. Patient's inability to understand ?
0 - No 1 - Yes

EMPLOYMENT/SUPPORT STATUS

E1. Education completed
Years   Months

E2. Training or technical education completed
Months

E3. Do you have a profession, trade or skill?
0 - No
1 - Yes ____
Specify

E4. Do you have a valid driver's license ?
0 - No 1 - Yes

E5. Do you have an automobile available for use? (Answer No if no valid driver's license.) 0 - No 1 - Yes

E6. How long was your longest full-time job?
Years   Months

E7. Usual (or last) occupation ?

Specify in detail

E8. Does someone contribute to your support in any way?

E9. (ONLY IF ITEM 8 IS YES)
Does this constitute the majority of your support?

E10. Usual employment pattern , past 3 years.

1 - full time (40 hrs/wk)
2 - part time (reg. hrs.)
3 - part time (irreg., daywork)
4 - student
5 - service
6 - retired/disability
7 - unemployed
8 - in controlled environment

E11. How many days were you paid for working in the past 30? (include "under the table" work.)

How much money did you receive from the following sources in the past 30 days?

E12. Employment (net income)

E13. Unemployment compensation

E14. DPA

E15. Pension, benefits or social security

E16. Mate, family or friends (Money for personal expenses)

E17. Illegal

COMMENTS

E18. How many people depend on you for the majority of their food, shelter, etc.?

E19. How many days have you experienced employment problems in the past 30?

FOR QUESTIONS E20&E21 PLEASE ASK THE PATIENT'S RATING SCALE

E20. How troubled or bothered have you been by these employment problems in the past 30 days?

E21. How important to you now is counseling for these employment problems?

INTERVIEWER SEVERITY RATING

E22. How would you rate the patient's need for employment counseling?

CONFIDENCE RATINGS

Is the above information significantly distorted by:

E23. Patient's misrepresentation ?
0 - No 1 - Yes

E24. Patient's inability to understand ?
0 - No 1 - Yes

Addiction Severity Index (ASI) *(continued)*

DRUG/ALCOHOL USE

	PAST 30 DAYS	LIFETIME YEARS	USE (Rt of admin)
D1. Alcohol - any use at all			
D2. Alcohol - to intoxication			
D3. Heroin			
D4. Methadone			
D5. Other opiates/ analgesics			
D6. Barbiturates			
D7. Other sed/ hyp/tranq.			
D8. Cocaine			
D9. Amphetamines			
D10. Cannabis			
D11. Hallucinogens			
D12. Inhalants			
D13. More than one substance per day (include alcohol)			

Note: See manual for representative examples for each drug class

*Route of Administration: 1 = Oral, 2 = Nasal, 3 = Smoking, 4 = Non IV inj., 5 = IV inj.

D14. Which substance is the major problem? Please code as above or 00-No problem; 15-Alcohol & Drug (Dual addiction); 16-Polydrug; when not clear, ask patient.

D15. How long was your last period of voluntary abstinence from this major substance? (00 - never abstinent)   Months

D16. How many months ago did this abstinence end? (00 - still abstinent)

How many times have you:

D17. Had alcohol d.t.'s ?

D18. Overdosed on drugs ?

How many time in your life have you been treated for:

D19. Alcohol Abuse :

D20. Drug Abuse :

How many of these were detox only?

D21. Alcohol :

D22. Drug :

How much would you say you spent during the past 30 days on:

D23. Alcohol ?

D24. Drugs ?

D25. How many days have you been treated in an outpatient setting for alcohol or drugs in the past 30 days? (Include NA, AA).

How many days in the past 30 have you experienced:

D26. Alcohol Problems?

D27. Drug Problems ?

FOR QUESTIONS D28-D31 PLEASE ASK PATIENT TO USE THE PATIENT'S RATING SCALE

How troubled or bothered have you been in the past 30 days by these:

D28. Alcohol Problems ?

D29. Drug Problems ?

How important to you now is treatment for these:

D30. Alcohol Problems ?

D31. Drug Problems ?

INTERVIEWER SEVERITY RATING

How would you rate the patient's need for treatment for:

D32. Alcohol Abuse ?

D33. Drug Abuse ?

CONFIDENCE RATINGS

Is the above information significantly distorted by:

D34. Patient's misrepresentation ?
0 - No 1 - Yes

D35. Patient's inability to understand?
0 - No 1 - Yes

COMMENTS

_____
_____
_____
_____
_____
_____
_____
_____
_____
_____
_____
_____
_____
_____
_____
_____
_____

Addiction Severity Index (ASI) *(continued)*

LEGAL STATUS

L1. Was this admission prompted or suggested by the criminal justice system (judge, probation/parole officer, etc.) 0 - No 1 - Yes

L2. Are you on probation or parole ? 0 - No 1 - Yes

How many times in your life have you been arrested and charged with the following:

L3. - shoplifting/vandalism

L4. - parole/probation violations

L5. - drug charges

L6. - forgery

L7. - weapons offense

L8. - burglary, larceny, B&E

L9. - robbery

L10. - assault

L11. - arson

L12. - rape

L13. - homicide, manslaughter

L14. - prostitution

L15. - contempt of court

L16. - other

L17. How many of these charges resulted in convictions?

How many time in your life have you been charged with the following:

L18. Disorderly conduct, vagrancy, public intoxication

L19. Driving while intoxicated

L20. Major driving violations (reckless driving, speeding, no license, etc.)

L21. How many months were you incarcerated in your life? Months

L22. How long was your last incarceration? Months

L23. What was it for? *(Use codes 3-16, 18-20. If multiple charges, code most severe)*

L24. Are you presently awaiting charges, trial or sentence? 0 - No 1 - Yes

L25. What for? (If multiple charges, use most severe).

L26. How many days in the past 30 were you detained or incarcerated?

L27. How many days in the past 30 have you engaged in illegal activities for profit?

FOR QUESTIONS L28 & L29 PLEASE ASK PATIENT TO USE THE PATIENT'S RATING SCALE

L28. How serious do you feel your present legal problems are? (Exclude civil problems)

L29. How important to you now is counseling or referral for these legal problems?

INTERVIEWER SEVERITY RATING

L30. How would you rate the patient's need for legal services or counseling?

CONFIDENCE RATINGS

Is the above information signficantly distorted by:

L31. Patient's misrepresentation ?

L32. Patient's inability to understand ?

COMMENTS

_____

_____

_____

_____

_____

_____

FAMILY HISTORY

Have any of your relatives had what you would call a significant drinking, drug use or psych problem - one that did or should have led to

Mother's Side	Alc	Drug	Psych	Father's Side	Alc	Drug	Psych	Siblings	Alc	Drug	Psych
H1. Grandmother				H6. Grandmother				H11. Brother			
H2. Grandfather				H7. Grandfather							
H3. Mother				H8. Father				H13. Sister			
H4. Aunt				H9. Aunt							
H5. Uncle				H10. Uncle							

Direction: Place "0" in relative category where the answer is clearly no for all relatives in the category; "1" where the answer is clearly yes for any relative within the category; "X" where the answer is uncertain or "I don't know" and "N" where there never was a relatives from that category. Code most problematic relative in cases of multiple members per category.

Addiction Severity Index (ASI) *(continued)*

FAMILY/SOCIAL RELATIONSHIPS

F1. Marital Status

1 - Married   4 - Separated
2 - Remarried   5 - Divorced
3 - Widowed   6 - Never Married

F2. How long have you been in this marital status? (If never married, since age 18).   Years   Months

F3. Are you satisfied with this situation ?
0 - No
1 - Indifferent
2 - Yes

F4. Usual living arrangements (past 3 yr.)
1 - With sexual partner and children
2 - With sexual partner alone
3 - With children alone
4 - With parents
5 - With family
6 - With friends
7 - Alone
8 - Controlled environment
9 - No stable arrangements

F5. How long have you lived in those arrangements? (If with parents or family, since age 18).   Years   Months

F6. Are you satisfied with these living arrangements?
0 - No
1 - Indifferent
2 - Yes

Do you live with anyone who: (0 - No 1 - Yes)

F7. Has a current alcohol problem ?

F8. Uses non-prescribed drugs ?

F9. With whom do you spend most of your free time:
1 - Family
2 - Friends
3 - Alone

F10. Are you satisfied with spending your free time this way?
0 - No
1 - Indifferent
2 - Yes

F11. How many close friends do you have?

Direction for F12-F26: Place "0" in relative category where the answer is clearly no for all relatives in the category; "1" where the answer is clearly yes for any relative within the category; "X" where the answer is uncertain or "I don't know" and "N" where there never was a relative from that category.

Would you say you have had close, long lasting, personal relationships with any of the following people in your life:

F12. Mother
F13. Father
F14. Brothers/Sisters
F16. Children
F17. Friends

Have you had significant periods in which you have experienced serious problems getting along with:

	PAST 30 DAYS	IN YOUR LIFE
F18. Mother		
F19. Father		
F20. Brothers/Sisters		
F21. Sexual partner/spouse		
F22. Children		
F23. Other signficant family		
F24. Close friends		
F25. Neighbors		
F26. Co-Workers		

Did any of these people (F18-F26) abuse you:

	PAST 30 DAYS	IN YOUR LIFE
F27. Emotionally (make you feel bad through harsh words)?		
F28. Physically (cause you physical harm)?		
F29. Sexually (force sexual advances or sexual acts)?		

How many days in the past 30 have you had serious conflicts:

F30. With your family ?

F31. With other people ? (excluding family)

FOR QUESTIONS F32-F35 PLEASE ASK PATIENT TO USE THE PATIENT'S RATING SCALE

How troubled or bothered have you been in the past 30 days by these:

F32. Family problems

F33. Social problems

How important to you now is treatment or counseling for these:

F34. Family problems

F35. Social problems

INTERVIEWER SEVERITY RATING

F36. How would you rate the patient's need for family and/or social counseling?

CONFIDENCE RATINGS

Is the above information significantly distorted by:

F37. Patient's misrepresentation ?
0 - No 1 - Yes

F38. Patient's inability to understand ?
0 - No 1 - Yes

COMMENTS

Addiction Severity Index (ASI) *(continued)*

PSYCHIATRIC STATUS

P1. How many times have you been treated for any psychological or emotional problems?

In a hospital

As an Outpatient or Private patient

P2. Do you receive a pension for a psychiatric disability? 0 - No 1 - Yes

Have you had a significant period, (that was not a direct result of drug/alcohol use), in which you have:

	PAST 30 DAYS	IN YOUR LIFE
P3. Experienced serious depression		
P4. Experienced serious anxiety or tension		
P5. Experienced hallucinations		
P6. Experienced trouble understanding, concentrating or remembering		
P7. Experienced trouble controlling violent behavior		
P8. Experienced serious thoughts of suicide		
P9. Attempted suicide		
P10. Been prescribed medication for any psychological emotional problem		

P11. How many days in the past 30 have you experienced these psychological or emotional problems?

FOR QUESTIONS P12 & P13 PLEASE ASK PATIENT TO USE THE PATIENT'S RATING SCALE

P12. How much have you been troubled or bothered by these psychological or emotional problems in the past 30 days?

P13. How important to you now is treatment for these psychological problems?

THE FOLLOWING ITEMS ARE TO BE COMPLETED BY THE INTERVIEWER
0 - No 1 - Yes

At the time of the interview, is patient:

P14. Obviously depressed/withdrawn

P15. Obviously hostile

P16. Obviously anxious/nervous

P17. Having trouble with reality testing , thought disorders, paranoid thinking

P18. Having trouble comprehending, concentrating, remembering

P19. Having suicidal thoughts

P20. How would you rate the patient's need for psychiatric/psychological treatment?

CONFIDENCE RATINGS

Is the above information significantly distorted by:

P21. Patient's misrepresentation ?
0 - No 1 - Yes

P22. Patient's inability to understand ?
0 - No 1 - Yes

COMMENTS

Source.   Reprinted from McLellan AT, Luborsky L, Woody GE, et al.: "An Improved Diagnostic Evaluation Instrument for Substance Abuse Patients: The Addiction Severity Index." *Journal of Nervous and Mental Disease* 168(1):26–33, 1980

Behavior and Symptom Identification Scale (BASIS-32)

FOR OFFICE USE ONLY   Site code ☐☐☐

INSTRUCTIONS TO STAFF: Please write the respondent's Identification Number and Visit Number, one digit in each box. Fill in the Visit Type and Level of Care using the code numbers below.

Identification Number .... ☐☐☐☐☐☐☐☐☐

Visit Number .... ☐☐☐☐☐☐

Visit Type...............................1 = Admission/Intake   3 = Discharge/Termination .... ☐
                            2 = Mid-Treatment   4 = Post-Treatment Follow-up

Level of Care...............................1 = Inpatient   3 = Partial Hospital/Day Treatment... ☐
                            2 = Outpatient

BASIS-32™
BEHAVIOR AND SYMPTOM IDENTIFICATION SCALE

INSTRUCTIONS TO RESPONDENT: Below is a list of problems and areas of life functioning in which some people experience difficulties. Using the scale below, fill in the box with the answer that best describes how much difficulty you have been having in each area during the **PAST WEEK.**

         0 = No difficulty
         1 = A little difficulty
         2 = Moderate difficulty
         3 = Quite a bit of difficulty
         4 = Extreme difficulty

Please respond to each item. Do not leave any blank. If there is an area that you consider to be inapplicable, indicate that it is *No Difficulty.*

IN THE PAST WEEK, how much difficulty have you been having in the area of:

1. **Managing Day-to-Day Life.** (For example, getting places on time, handling money, making everyday decisions)..1 ☐

2. **Household Responsibilities.** (For example, shopping, cooking, laundry, cleaning, other chores).. 2 ☐

3. **Work.** (For example, completing tasks, performance level, finding/keeping a job). 3 ☐

4. **School.** (For example, academic performance, completing assignments, attendance).4 ☐

5. Leisure time or recreational activities.. 5 ☐

6. **Adjusting to major life stresses.** (For example, separation, divorce, moving, new job, new school, a death)... 6 ☐

7. Relationships with family members.. 7 ☐

8. Getting along with people outside of the family... 8 ☐

PLEASE TURN PAGE TO CONTINUE.

Behavior and Symptom Identification Scale (BASIS-32) *(continued)*

0 = No difficulty
1 = A little difficulty
2 = Moderate difficulty
3 = Quite a bit of difficulty
4 = Extreme difficulty

9. Isolation or feelings of loneliness.. 9 ☐

10. Being able to feel close to others.. 10 ☐

11. Being realistic about yourself or others... 11 ☐

12. Recognizing and expressing emotions appropriately.................................... 12 ☐

13. Developing independence, autonomy... 13 ☐

14. Goals or direction in life... 14 ☐

15. Lack of self-confidence, feeling bad about yourself...................................... 15 ☐

16. Apathy, lack of interest in things.. 16 ☐

17. Depression, hopelessness.. 17 ☐

18. Suicidal feelings or behavior.. 18 ☐

19. Physical symptoms (For example, headaches, aches and pains, sleep
disturbance, stomach aches, dizziness).. 19 ☐

20. Fear, anxiety or panic... 20 ☐

21. Confusion, concentration, memory... 21 ☐

22. Disturbing or unreal thoughts or beliefs... 22 ☐

23. Hearing voices, seeing things.. 23 ☐

24. Manic, bizarre behavior.. 24 ☐

25. Mood swings, unstable moods... 25 ☐

26. Uncontrollable, compulsive behavior (For example, eating disorder,
hand-washing, hurting yourself).. 26 ☐

27. Sexual activity or preoccupation... 27 ☐

28. Drinking alcoholic beverages.. 28 ☐

29. Taking illegal drugs, misusing drugs... 29 ☐

30. Controlling temper, outbursts of anger, violence... 30 ☐

31. Impulsive, illegal or reckless behavior.. 31 ☐

32. Feeling satisfaction with your life.. 32 ☐

Behavior and Symptom Identification Scale (BASIS-32) *(continued)*

For the following questions, please write the response code in the appropriate box.

33. How old were you on your last birthday?...33 ☐

34. What is your sex?..34 ☐
     1 = Male   2 = Female

35. What is your race?...35 ☐
     1 = Black/African-American   4 = American Indian/Alaskan
     2 = White/Caucasian   5 = Other
     3 = Asian/Pacific Islander

36. Are you Hispanic or Latino?..36 ☐
     1 = Yes   2 = No

37. What is your marital status?..37 ☐
     1 = Never married   4 = Divorced
     2 = Married   5 = Widowed
     3 = Separated

38. How much school have you completed?...38 ☐
     1 = 8th grade or less   4 = Some college
     2 = Some high school, but did not graduate   5 = 4-year college graduate
     3 = High school graduate or GED

39. In the past 30 days, what were your usual living arrangements?.............39 ☐
     1 = Alone   4 = With non-relative
     2 = Halfway house/group home/hospital   5 = Shelter/Street
     3 = With family   6 = Other

40. In the past 30 days, were you working at a paid job?............................40 ☐
     1 = Yes   2 = No

41. If yes, how many hours per week? (If no, leave blank)........................41 ☐
     1 = 1 - 10 hours   3 = 21 - 30 hours
     2 = 11 - 20 hours   4 = More than 30 hours

42. What was your total household income before taxes last year from all sources?
     (job, unemployment, disability, social security, child support etc.)...............42 ☐
     1 = Less than $20,000   3 =$40,000 - $59,000
     2 = $20,000 - $39,000   4 = $60,000 or more

43. In the past 30 days, were you a student attending a high school,
     vocational training program, college or graduate degree program?................43 ☐
     1 = Yes   2 =No

44. Today's Date.......................................44 ☐☐ ☐☐ ☐☐
                                                 MONTH   DAY   YEAR

THANK YOU VERY MUCH.

Behavior and Symptom Identification Scale (BASIS-32) *(continued)*

Instructions to staff: Please fill in the following information.

Site number: ___ ___ ___-___ ___

Patient ID number: ___ ___ ___ ___ ___ ___ ___ ___ ___

Admission/intake date: ___ ___/___ ___/___ ___ ___ ___
                       Day   Month   Year

Time point: **1**=Admission/intake   **3**=Discharge/termination
                 2=Mid-treatment   **4**=Post-treatment follow-up

Level of care: **1**=Inpatient   **3**=Partial/Day Hospital
                 2=Outpatient   **4**=Residential

Program type: **1**=General adult   **6**=Anxiety disorders/trauma
                 2=Child/adolescent   **7**=Substance abuse/chemical dependency
                 3=Geriatric   **8**=Dual diagnosis
                 4=Affective/mood disorders **9**=Other
                 5=Psychotic disorders

Brief Psychiatric Rating Scale (BPRS)

DIRECTIONS: Place an X in the appropriate box to represent level of severity of each symptom.

	Not present	Very mild	Mild	Moderate	Moderately severe	Severe	Extremely severe
SOMATIC CONCERN—preoccupation with physical health, fear of physical illness, hypochondriasis.	❑	❑	❑	❑	❑	❑	❑
ANXIETY—worry, fear, overconcern for present or future, uneasiness.	❑	❑	❑	❑	❑	❑	❑
EMOTIONAL WITHDRAWAL—lack of spontaneous interaction, isolation deficiency in relating to others.	❑	❑	❑	❑	❑	❑	❑
CONCEPTUAL DISORGANIZATION—thought processes confused, disconnected, disorganized, disrupted.	❑	❑	❑	❑	❑	❑	❑
GUILT FEELINGS—self-blame, shame, remorse for past behavior.	❑	❑	❑	❑	❑	❑	❑
TENSION—physical and motor manifestations of nervousness, overactivation.	❑	❑	❑	❑	❑	❑	❑
MANNERISMS AND POSTURING—peculiar, bizarre unnatural motor behavior (not including tic).	❑	❑	❑	❑	❑	❑	❑
GRANDIOSITY—exaggerated self-opinion, arrogance, conviction of unusual power or abilities.	❑	❑	❑	❑	❑	❑	❑
DEPRESSIVE MOOD—sorrow, sadness, despondency, pessimism.	❑	❑	❑	❑	❑	❑	❑
HOSTILITY—animosity, contempt, belligerence, disdain for others.	❑	❑	❑	❑	❑	❑	❑
SUSPICIOUSNESS—mistrust, belief others harbor malicious or discriminatory intent.	❑	❑	❑	❑	❑	❑	❑
HALLUCINATORY BEHAVIOR—perceptions without normal external stimulus correspondence.	❑	❑	❑	❑	❑	❑	❑
MOTOR RETARDATION—slowed, weakened movements or speech, reduced body tone.	❑	❑	❑	❑	❑	❑	❑
UNCOOPERATIVENESS—resistance, guardedness, rejection of authority.	❑	❑	❑	❑	❑	❑	❑
UNUSUAL THOUGHT CONTENT—unusual, odd, strange, bizarre thought content.	❑	❑	❑	❑	❑	❑	❑
BLUNTED AFFECT—reduced emotional tone, reduction in formal intensity of feelings, flatness.	❑	❑	❑	❑	❑	❑	❑
EXCITEMENT—heightened emotional tone, agitation, increased reactivity.	❑	❑	❑	❑	❑	❑	❑
DISORIENTATION—confusion or lack of proper association for person, place, or time.	❑	❑	❑	❑	❑	❑	❑

Global Assessment Scale (Range 1–100) _____

Source. Reprinted from Overall JE: "The Brief Psychiatric Rating Scale (BPRS): Recent Developments in Ascertainment and Scaling." *Psychopharmacology Bulletin* 24:97–99, 1988. Used with permission.

Inventory of Depressive Symptomatology (Self-Report) (IDS-SR)

INVENTORY OF DEPRESSIVE SYMPTOMATOLOGY (SELF-REPORT)
(IDS-SR)

NAME: _____   TODAY'S DATE _____

Please circle the one response to each item that best describes you for the past seven days.

1. Falling Asleep:

   0   I never take longer than 30 minutes to fall asleep.
   1   I take at least 30 minutes to fall asleep, less than half the time.
   2   I take at least 30 minutes to fall asleep, more than half the time.
   3   I take more than 60 minutes to fall asleep, more than half the time.

2. Sleep During the Night:

   0   I do not wake up at night.
   1   I have a restless, light sleep with a few brief awakenings each night.
   2   I wake up at least once a night, but I go back to sleep easily.
   3   I awaken more than once a night and stay awake for 20 minutes or more, more than half the time.

3. Waking Up Too Early:

   0   Most of the time, I awaken no more than 30 minutes before I need to get up.
   1   More than half the time, I awaken more than 30 minutes before I need to get up.
   2   I almost always awaken at least one hour or so before I need to, but I go back to sleep eventually.
   3   I awaken at least one hour before I need to, and can't go back to sleep.

4. Sleeping Too Much:

   0   I sleep no longer than 7-8 hours/night, without napping during the day.
   1   I sleep no longer than 10 hours in a 24-hour period including naps.
   2   I sleep no longer than 12 hours in a 24-hour period including naps.
   3   I sleep longer than 12 hours in a 24-hour period including naps.

5. Feeling Sad:

   0   I do not feel sad
   1   I feel sad less than half the time.
   2   I feel sad more than half the time.
   3   I feel sad nearly all of the time.

6. Feeling Irritable:

   0   I do not feel irritable.
   1   I feel irritable less than half the time.
   2   I feel irritable more than half the time.
   3   I feel extremely irritable nearly all of the time.

7. Feeling Anxious or Tense:

   0   I do not feel anxious or tense.
   1   I feel anxious (tense) less than half the time.
   2   I feel anxious (tense) more than half the time.
   3   I feel extremely anxious (tense) nearly all of the time.

8. Response of Your Mood to Good or Desired Events:

   0   My mood brightens to a normal level which lasts for several hours when good events occur.
   1   My mood brightens but I do not feel like my normal self when good events occur.
   2   My mood brightens only somewhat to a rather limited range of desired events.
   3   My mood does not brighten at all, even when very good or desired events occur in my life.

9. Mood in Relation to the Time of Day:

   0   There is no regular relationship between my mood and the time of day.
   1   My mood often relates to the time of day because of environmental events (e.g., being alone, working).
   2   In general, my mood is more related to the time of day than to environmental events.
   3   My mood is clearly and predictably better or worse at a particular time each day.

   9A. Is your mood typically worse in the morning, afternoon or night? (circle one)

   9B. Is your mood variation attributed to the environment? (yes or no) (circle one)

10. The Quality of Your Mood:

   0   The mood (internal feelings) that I experience is very much a normal mood.
   1   My mood is sad, but this sadness is pretty much like the sad mood I would feel if someone close to me died or left.
   2   My mood is sad, but this sadness has a rather different quality to it than the sadness I would feel if someone close to me died or left.
   3   My mood is sad, but this sadness is different from the type of sadness associated with grief or loss.

Reprinted by permission of the author, A. John Rush, Jr., M.D.

Inventory of Depressive Symptomatology (Self-Report) (IDS-SR) *(continued)*

Please complete either 11 or 12 (not both)

11. Decreased Appetite:

    0   There is no change in my usual appetite.
    1   I eat somewhat less often or lesser amounts of food than usual.
    2   I eat much less than usual and only with personal effort.
    3   I rarely eat within a 24-hour period, and only with extreme personal effort or when others persuade me to eat.

12. Increased Appetite:

    0   There is no change from my usual appetite.
    1   I feel a need to eat more frequently than usual.
    2   I regularly eat more often and/or greater amounts of food than usual.
    3   I feel driven to overeat both at mealtime and between meals.

Please complete either 13 or 14 (not both)

13. Within the Last Two Weeks:

    0   I have not had a change in my weight.
    1   I feel as if I've had a slight weight loss.
    2   I have lost 2 pounds or more.
    3   I have lost 5 pounds or more.

14. Within the Last Two Weeks:

    0   I have not had a change in my weight.
    1   I feel as if I've had a slight weight gain.
    2   I have gained 2 pounds or more.
    3   I have gained 5 pounds or more.

15. Concentration/Decision Making:

    0   There is no change in my usual capacity to concentrate or make decisions.
    1   I occasionally feel indecisive or find that my attention wanders.
    2   Most of the time, I struggle to focus my attention or to make decisions.
    3   I cannot concentrate well enough to read or cannot make even minor decisions.

16. View of Myself:

    0   I see myself as equally worthwhile and deserving as other people.
    1   I am more self-blaming than usual.
    2   I largely believe that I cause problems for others.
    3   I think almost constantly about major and minor defects in myself.

17. View of My Future:

    0   I have an optimistic view of my future.
    1   I am occasionally pessimistic about my future, but for the most part I believe things will get better.
    2   I'm pretty certain that my immediate future (1-2 months) does not hold much promise of good things for me.
    3   I see no hope of anything good happening to me anytime in the future.

18. Thoughts of Death or Suicide:

    0   I do not think of suicide or death.
    1   I feel that life is empty or wonder if it's worth living.
    2   I think of suicide or death several times a week for several minutes.
    3   I think of suicide or death several times a day in some detail, or I have made specific plans for suicide or have actually tried to take my life.

19. General Interest:

    0   There is no change from usual in how interested I am in other people or activities.
    1   I notice that I am less interested in people or activities.
    2   I find I have interest in only one or two of my formerly pursued activities.
    3   I have virtually no interest in formerly pursued activities.

20. Energy Level:

    0   There is no change in my usual level of energy.
    1   I get tired more easily than usual.
    2   I have to make a big effort to start or finish my usual daily activities (for example, shopping, homework, cooking or going to work).
    3   I really cannot carry out most of my usual daily activities because I just don't have the energy.

21. Capacity for Pleasure or Enjoyment (excluding sex):

    0   I enjoy pleasurable activities just as much as usual.
    1   I do not feel my usual sense of enjoyment from pleasurable activities.
    2   I rarely get a feeling of pleasure from any activity.
    3   I am unable to get any pleasure or enjoyment from anything.

Inventory of Depressive Symptomatology
(Self-Report) (IDS-SR) *(continued)*

22. Interest in Sex (Please Rate <u>Interest</u>, not Activity):

    0   I'm just as interested in sex as usual.
    1   My interest in sex is somewhat less than usual or I do not get the same pleasure from sex as I used to.
    2   I have little desire for or rarely derive pleasure from sex.
    3   I have absolutely no interest in or derive no pleasure from sex.

23. Feeling slowed down:

    0   I think, speak, and move at my usual rate of speed.
    1   I find that my thinking is slowed down or my voice sounds dull or flat.
    2   It takes me several seconds to respond to most questions and I'm sure my thinking is slowed.
    3   I am often unable to respond to questions without extreme effort.

24. Feeling restless:

    0   I do not feel restless.
    1   I'm often fidgety, wring my hands, or need to shift how I am sitting.
    2   I have impulses to move about and am quite restless.
    3   At times, I am unable to stay seated and need to pace around.

25. Aches and pains:

    0   I don't have any feeling of heaviness in my arms or legs and don't have any aches or pains.
    1   Sometimes I get headaches or pains in my stomach, back or joints but these pains are only sometime present and they don't stop me from doing what I need to do.
    2   I have these sorts of pains most of the time.
    3   These pains are so bad they force me to stop what I am doing.

26. Other bodily symptoms:

    0   I don't have any of these symptoms: heart pounding fast, blurred vision, sweating, hot and cold flashes, chest pain, heart turning over in my chest, ringing in my ears, or shaking.
    1   I have some of these symptoms but they are mild and are present only sometimes.
    2   I have several of these symptoms and they bother me quite a bit.
    3   I have several of these symptoms and when they occur I have to stop doing whatever I am doing.

27. Panic/Phobic symptoms:

    0   I have no spells of panic or specific fears (phobia) (such as animals or heights).
    1   I have mild panic episodes or fears that do not usually change my behavior or stop me from functioning.
    2   I have significant panic episodes or fears that force me to change my behavior but do <u>not</u> stop me from functioning.
    3   I have panic episodes at least once a week or severe fears that stop me from carrying on my daily activities.

28. Constipation/diarrhea:

    0   There is no change in my usual bowel habits.
    1   I have intermittent constipation or diarrhea which is mild.
    2   I have diarrhea or constipation most of the time but it does not interfere with my day-to-day functioning.
    3   I have constipation or diarrhea for which I take medicine or which interferes with my day-to-day activities.

29. Interpersonal Sensitivity:

    0   I have not felt easily rejected, slighted, criticized or hurt by others at all.
    1   I have occasionally felt rejected, slighted, criticized or hurt by others.
    2   I have often felt rejected, slighted, criticized or hurt by others, but these feelings have had only slight effects on my relationships or work.
    3   I have often felt rejected, slighted, criticized or hurt by others and these feelings have impaired my relationships and work.

30. Leaden Paralysis/Physical Energy:

    0   I have not experienced the physical sensation of feeling weighted down and without physical energy.
    1   I have occasionally experienced periods of feeling physically weighted down and without physical energy, but without a negative effect on work, school, or activity level.
    2   I feel physically weighted down (without physical energy) more than half the time.
    3   I feel physically weighted down (without physical energy) most of the time, several hours per day, several days per week.

Please review this test and write in this space _____ the numbers of the 3 items that were the most difficult to understand.
Which 3 items (questions) were the easiest to understand? _____

Thank you

Range 0-90   Score: _____

Source. Reprinted from Rush AJ, Carmody T, Reimitz P-E: "The Inventory of Depressive Symptomatology (IDS): Clinician (IDS-C) and Self-Report (IDS-SR) Ratings of Depressive Symptoms." *International Journal of Methods in Psychiatric Research* 9:45–59, 2000. Used with permission.

Inventory of Depressive Symptomatology (Clincian Related) (IDS-C)

INVENTORY OF DEPRESSIVE SYMPTOMATOLOGY (CLINICIAN-RATED)
(IDS-C)

NAME: _____   TODAY'S DATE: _____

Please circle one response to each item that best describes the patient for the last seven days.

1. Sleep Onset Insomnia:

   0   Never takes longer than 30 minutes to fall asleep.
   1   Takes at least 30 minutes to fall asleep, less than half the time.
   2   Takes at least 30 minutes to fall asleep, more than half the time.
   3   Takes more than 60 minutes to fall asleep, more than half the time.

2. Mid-Nocturnal Insomnia:

   0   Does not wake up at night.
   1   Restless, light sleep with few awakenings.
   2   Wakes up at least once a night, but goes back to sleep easily.
   3   Awakens more than once a night and stays awake for 20 minutes or more, more than half the time.

3. Early Morning Insomnia:

   0   Less than half the time, awakens no more than 30 minutes before necessary.
   1   More than half the time, awakens more than 30 minutes before need be.
   2   Awakens at least one hour before need be, more than half the time.
   3   Awakens at least two hours before need be, more than half the time.

4. Hypersomnia:

   0   Sleeps no longer than 7-8 hours/night, without naps.
   1   Sleeps no longer than 10 hours in a 24 hour period (include naps).
   2   Sleeps no longer than 12 hours in a 24 hour period (include naps).
   3   Sleeps longer than 12 hours in a 24 hour period (include naps).

5. Mood (Sad):

   0   Does not feel sad.
   1   Feels sad less than half the time.
   2   Feels sad more than half the time.
   3   Feels intensely sad virtually all of the time.

6. Mood (Irritable):

   0   Does not feel irritable.
   1   Feels irritable less than half the time.
   2   Feels irritable more than half the time.
   3   Feels extremely irritable virtually all of the time.

7. Mood (Anxious):

   0   Does not feel anxious or tense.
   1   Feels anxious/tense less than half the time.
   2   Feels anxious/tense more than half the time.
   3   Feels extremely anxious/tense virtually all of the time.

8. Reactivity of Mood:

   0   Mood brightens to normal level and lasts several hours when good events occur.
   1   Mood brightens but does not feel like normal self when good events occur.
   2   Mood brightens only somewhat with few selected, extremely desired events.
   3   Mood does not brighten at all, even when very good or desired events occur.

9. Mood Variation:

   0   Notes no regular relationship between mood and time of day.
   1   Mood often relates to time of day due to environmental circumstances.
   2   For most of week, mood appears more related to time of day than to events.
   3   Mood is clearly, predictably, better or worse at a fixed time each day.

9A. Is mood typically worse in morning, afternoon, or night (circle one).

9B. Is mood variation attributed to environment by the patient? (yes or no) (circle one).

10. Quality of Mood:

   0   Mood is virtually identical to feelings associated with bereavement or is undisturbed.
   1   Mood is largely like sadness in bereavement, although it may lack explanation, be associated with more anxiety, or be much more intense.
   2   Less than half the time, mood is qualitatively distinct from grief and therefore difficult to explain to others.
   3   Mood is qualitatively distinct from grief nearly all of the time.

Reprinted by permission of the author, A. John Rush, Jr., M.D.

Inventory of Depressive Symptomatology
(Clincian Related) (IDS-C) *(continued)*

Complete <u>either</u> 11 <u>or</u> 12 (not both)

11. Appetite (Decreased):

    0   No change from usual appetite.
    1   Eats somewhat less often and/or lesser amounts than usual.
    2   Eats much less than usual and only with personal effort.
    3   Eats rarely within a 24-hour period, and only with extreme personal effort or with persuasion by others.

12. Appetite (Increased):

    0   No change from usual appetite.
    1   More frequently feels a need to eat than usual.
    2   Regularly eats more often and/or greater amounts than usual.
    3   Feels driven to overeat at and between meals.

Complete <u>either</u> 13 <u>or</u> 14 (not both)

13. Weight (Decrease) Within The Last Two Weeks:

    0   Has experienced no weight change.
    1   Feels as if some slight weight loss occurred.
    2   Has lost 2 pounds or more.
    3   Has lost 5 pounds or more.

14. Weight (Increase) Within the Last Two Weeks:

    0   Has experienced no weight change.
    1   Feels as if some slight weight gain has occurred.
    2   Has gained 2 pounds or more.
    3   Has gained 5 pounds or more.

15. Concentration/Decision Making:

    0   No change in usual capacity to concentrate and decide.
    1   Occasionally feels indecisive or notes that attention often wanders.
    2   Most of the time struggles to focus attention or make decisions.
    3   Cannot concentrate well enough to read or cannot make even minor decisions.

16. Outlook (Self):

    0   Sees self as equally worthwhile and deserving as others.
    1   Is more self-blaming than usual.
    2   Largely believes that he/she causes problems for others.
    3   Ruminates over major and minor defects in self.

17. Outlook (Future):

    0   Views future with usual optimism.
    1   Occasionally has pessimistic outlook that can be dispelled by others or events.
    2   Largely pessimistic for the near future.
    3   Sees no hope for self/situation anytime in the future.

18. Suicidal Ideation:

    0   Does not think of suicide or death.
    1   Feels life is empty or is not worth living.
    2   Thinks of suicide/death several times a week for several minutes.
    3   Thinks of suicide/death several times a day in depth, or has made specific plans, or attempted suicide.

19. Involvement:

    0   No change from usual level of interest in other people and activities.
    1   Notices a reduction in former interests/activities.
    2   Finds only one or two former interests remain.
    3   Has virtually no interest in formerly pursued activities.

20. Energy/Fatiguability:

    0   No change in usual level of energy.
    1   Tires more easily than usual.
    2   Makes significant personal effort to initiate or maintain usual daily activities.
    3   Unable to carry out most of usual daily activities due to lack of energy.

21. Pleasure/Enjoyment (exclude sexual activities):

    0   Participates in and derives usual sense of enjoyment from pleasurable activities.
    1   Does not feel usual enjoyment from pleasurable activities.
    2   Rarely derives pleasure from any activities.
    3   Is unable to register any sense of pleasure/enjoyment from anything.

22. Sexual <u>Interest</u>:

    0   Has usual interest in or derives usual pleasure from sex.
    1   Has near usual interest in or derives some pleasure from sex.
    2   Has little desire for or rarely derives pleasure from sex.
    3   Has absolutely no interest in or derives no pleasure from sex.

Inventory of Depressive Symptomatology
(Clincian Related) (IDS-C) *(continued)*

23. Psychomotor Slowing:

    0   Normal speed of thinking, gesturing, and speaking.
    1   Patient notes slowed thinking, and voice modulation is reduced.
    2   Takes several seconds to respond to most questions; reports slowed thinking.
    3   Is largely unresponsive to most questions without strong encouragement.

24. Psychomotor Agitation:

    0   No increased speed or disorganization in thinking or gesturing.
    1   Fidgets, wrings hands and shifts positions often.
    2   Describes impulse to move about and displays motor restlessness.
    3   Unable to stay seated. Paces about with or without permission.

25. Somatic Complaints:

    0   States there is no feeling of limb heaviness or pains.
    1   Complains of headaches, abdominal, back or joint pains that are intermittent and not disabling.
    2   Complains that the above pains are present most of the time.
    3   Functional impairment results from the above pains.

26. Sympathetic Arousal:

    0   Reports no palpitations, tremors, blurred vision, tinnitus or increased sweating, dyspnea, hot and cold flashes, chest pain.
    1   The above are mild and only intermittently present.
    2   The above are moderate and present more than half the time.
    3   The above result in functional impairment.

27. Panic/Phobic Symptoms:

    0   Has neither panic episodes nor phobic symptoms.
    1   Has mild panic episodes or phobias that do not usually alter behavior or incapacitate.
    2   Has significant panic episodes or phobias that modify behavior but do not incapacitate.
    3   Has incapacitating panic episodes at least once a week or severe phobias that lead to complete and regular avoidance behavior.

28. Gastrointestinal:

    0   Has no change in usual bowel habits.
    1   Has intermittent constipation and/or diarrhea that is mild.
    2   Has diarrhea and/or constipation most of the time that does not impair functioning.
    3   Has intermittent presence of constipation and/or diarrhea that requires treatment or causes functional impairment.

29. Interpersonal Sensitivity:

    0   Has not felt easily rejected, slighted, criticized or hurt by others at all.
    1   Occasionally feels rejected, slighted, criticized or hurt by others.
    2   Often feels rejected, slighted, criticized or hurt by others, but with only slight effects on social/occupational functioning.
    3   Often feels rejected, slighted, criticized or hurt by others that results in impaired social/occupational functioning.

30. Leaden Paralysis/Physical Energy:

    0   Does not experience the physical sensation of feeling weighted down and without physical energy.
    1   Occasionally experiences periods of feeling physically weighted down and without physical energy, but without a negative effect on work, school, or activity level.
    2   Feels physically weighted down (without physical energy) more than half the time.
    3   Feels physically weighted down (without physical energy) most of the time, several hours per day, several days per week.

Source.   Reprinted from Rush AJ, Carmody T, Reimitz P-E: "The Inventory of Depressive Symptomatology (IDS): Clinician (IDS-C) and Self-Report (IDS-SR) Ratings of Depressive Symptoms." *International Journal of Methods in Psychiatric Research* 9:45–59, 2000. Used with permission.

Quick Inventory of Depressive Symptomatology (Self-Report) (QIDS-SR)

Name:_____   Today's date _____

Please circle the one response to each item that best describes you for the past 7 days.

1. Falling asleep:
   - 0   I never take longer than 30 minutes to fall asleep.
   - 1   I take at least 30 minutes to fall asleep, less than half the time.
   - 2   I take at least 30 minutes to fall asleep, more than half the time.
   - 3   I take more than 60 minutes to fall asleep, more than half the time.

2. Sleep during the night:
   - 0   I do not wake up at night.
   - 1   I have a restless, light sleep with a few brief awakenings each night.
   - 2   I wake up at least once a night, but I go back to sleep easily.
   - 3   I awaken more than once a night and stay awake for 20 minutes or more, more than half the time.

3. Waking up too early:
   - 0   Most of the time, I awaken no more than 30 minutes before I need to get up.
   - 1   More than half the time, I awaken more than 30 minutes before I need to get up.
   - 2   I almost always awaken at least one hour or so before I need to, but I go back to sleep eventually.
   - 3   I awaken at least one hour before I need to, and can't go back to sleep.

4. Sleeping too much:
   - 0   I sleep no longer than 7-8 hours/night, without napping during the day.
   - 1   I sleep no longer than 10 hours in a 24-hour period including naps.
   - 2   I sleep no longer than 12 hours in a 24-hour period including naps.
   - 3   I sleep longer than 12 hours in a 24-hour period including naps.

5. Feeling sad:
   - 0   I do not feel sad.
   - 1   I feel sad less than half the time.
   - 2   I feel sad more than half the time.
       I feel sad nearly all of the time.

6. Decreased appetite:
   - 0   There is no change in my usual appetite.
   - 1   I eat somewhat less often or lesser amounts of food than usual.
   - 2   I eat much less than usual and only with personal effort.
   - 3   I rarely eat within a 24-hour period, and only with extreme personal effort or when others persuade me to eat.

7. Increased appetite:
   - 0   There is no change from my usual appetite.
   - 1   I feel a need to eat more frequently than usual.
   - 2   I regularly eat more often and/or greater amounts of food than usual.
   - 3   I feel driven to overeat both at mealtime and between meals.

8. Decreased weight (within the last 2 weeks):
   - 0   I have not had a change in my weight.
   - 1   I feel as if I've had a slight weight loss.
   - 2   I have lost 2 pounds or more.
   - 3   I have lost 5 pounds or more.

9. Increased weight (within the last 2 weeks):
   - 0   I have not had a change in my weight.
   - 1   I feel as if I've had a slight weight gain.
   - 2   I have gained 2 pounds or more.
   - 3   I have gained 5 pounds or more.

Quick Inventory of Depressive Symptomatology
(Self-Report) (QIDS-SR) (continued)

10. Concentration/decision making:
  - 0   There is no change in my usual capacity to concentrate or make decisions.
  - 1   I occasionally feel indecisive or find that my attention wanders.
  - 2   Most of the time, I struggle to focus my attention or to make decisions.
  - 3   I cannot concentrate well enough to read or cannot make even minor decisions.

11. View of myself:
  - 0   I see myself as equally worthwhile and deserving as other people.
  - 1   I am more self-blaming than usual.
  - 2   I largely believe that I cause problems for others.
  - 3   I think almost constantly about major and minor defects in myself.

12. Thoughts of death or suicide:
  - 0   I do not think of suicide or death.
  - 1   I feel that life is empty or wonder if it's worth living.
  - 2   I think of suicide or death several times a week for several minutes.
  - 3   I think of suicide or death several times a day in some detail, or I have made specific plans for suicide or have actually tried to take my life.

13. General interest:
  - 0   There is no change from usual in how interested I am in other people or activities.
  - 1   I notice that I am less interested in people or activities.
  - 2   I find I have interest in only one or two of my formerly pursued activities.
  - 3   I have virtually no interest in formerly pursued activities.

14. Energy level:
  - 0   There is no change in my usual level of energy.
  - 1   I get tired more easily than usual.
  - 2   I have to make a big effort to start or finish my usual daily activities (for example, shopping, homework, cooking or going to work).
  - 3   I really cannot carry out most of my usual daily activities because I just don't have the energy.

15. Feeling slowed down:
  - 0   I think, speak, and move at my usual rate of speed.
  - 1   I find that my thinking is slowed down or my voice sounds dull or flat.
  - 2   It takes me several seconds to respond to most questions and I'm sure my thinking is slowed.
  - 3   I am often unable to respond to questions without extreme effort.

16. Feeling restless:
  - 0   I do not feel restless.
  - 1   I'm often fidgety, wringing my hands, or need to shift how I am sitting.
  - 2   I have impulses to move about and am quite restless.
  - 3   At times, I am unable to stay seated and need to pace around.

Quick Inventory of Depressive Symptomatology (Self-Report) (QIDS-SR) *(continued)*

To score:

1. Enter the highest score on any 1 of the 4 sleep items (1–4) ____
2. Item 5 ____
3. Enter the highest score on any 1 appetite/weight item (6–9) ____
4. Item 10 ____
5. Item 11 ____
6. Item 12 ____
7. Item 13 ____
8. Item 14 ____
9. Enter the highest score on either of the 2 psychomotor items (15 and 16) ____

TOTAL SCORE (Range 0–27) ____

Source. Reprinted from Rush AJ, Carmody T, Reimitz P-E: "The Inventory of Depressive Symptomatology (IDS): Clinician (IDS-C) and Self-Report (IDS-SR) Ratings of Depressive Symptoms." *International Journal of Methods in Psychiatric Research* 9:45-59, 2000. Used with permission. ©2000, A. John Rush, M.D.

Quick Inventory of Depressive Symptomatology–Clinician (QIDS-C)

Name:_____   Today's date: _____

Please circle one response to each item that best describes the patient for the last seven days.

1. Sleep onset insomnia:
   - 0 Never takes longer than 30 minutes to fall asleep.
   - 1 Takes at least 30 minutes to fall asleep, less than half the time.
   - 2 Takes at least 30 minutes to fall asleep, more than half the time.
   - 3 Takes more than 60 minutes to fall asleep, more than half the time.

2. Mid-nocturnal insomnia:
   - 0 Does not wake up at night.
   - 1 Restless, light sleep with few awakenings.
   - 2 Wakes up at least once a night, but goes back to sleep easily.
   - 3 Awakens more than once a night and stays awake for 20 minutes or more, more than half the time.

3. Early Morning Insomnia:
   - 0 Less than half the time, awakens no more than 30 minutes before necessary.
   - 1 More than half the time, awakens more than 30 minutes before need be.
   - 2 Awakens at least 1 hour before need be, more than half the time.
   - 3 Awakens at least 2 hours before need be, more than half the time.

4. Hypersomnia:
   - 0 Sleeps no longer than 7-8 hours/night, without naps.
   - 1 Sleeps no longer than 10 hours in a 24-hour period (include naps).
   - 2 Sleeps no longer than 12 hours in a 24-hour period (include naps).
   - 3 Sleeps longer than 12 hours in a 24-hour period (include naps).

Enter the highest score on any 1 of the 4 sleep items (1–4 above) ____

5. Mood (sad):
   - 0 Does not feel sad.
   - 1 Feels sad less than half the time.
   - 2 Feels sad more than half the time.
   - 3 Feels intensely sad virtually all of the time.

6. Appetite (decreased):
   - 0 No change from usual appetite.
   - 1 Eats somewhat less often and/or lesser amounts than usual.
   - 2 Eats much less than usual and only with personal effort.
   - 3 Eats rarely within a 24-hour period, and only with extreme personal effort or with persuasion by others.

7. Appetite (increased):
   - 0 No change from usual appetite.
   - 1 More frequently feels a need to eat than usual.
   - 2 Regularly eats more often and/or greater amounts than usual.
   - 3 Feels driven to overeat at and between meals.

8. Weight (decrease) within the last 2 weeks:
   - 0 Has experienced no weight change.
   - 1 Feels as if some slight weight loss occurred.
   - 2 Has lost 2 pounds or more.
   - 3 Has lost 5 pounds or more.

9. Weight (increase) within the last 2 weeks:
   - 0 Has experienced no weight change.
   - 1 Feels as if some slight weight gain has occurred.
   - 2 Has gained 2 pounds or more.
   - 3 Has gained 5 pounds or more.

Enter the highest score on any 1 of the 4 appetite/weight change items (6–9 above) ____

10. Concentration/decision making:
   - 0 No change in usual capacity to concentrate and decide.
   - 1 Occasionally feels indecisive or notes that attention often wanders.
   - 2 Most of the time struggles to focus attention or make decisions.
   - 3 Cannot concentrate well enough to read or cannot make even minor decisions.

Quick Inventory of Depressive Symptomatology—
Clinician (QIDS-C) *(continued)*

11. Outlook (self):
    0   Sees self as equally worthwhile and deserving as others.
    1   Is more self-blaming than usual.
    2   Largely believes that he/she causes problems for others.
    3   Ruminates over major and minor defects in self.

12. Suicidal ideation:
    0   Does not think of suicide or death.
    1   Feels life is empty or is not worth living.
    2   Thinks of suicide/death several times a week for several minutes.
    3   Thinks of suicide/death several times a day in depth, or has made specific plans, or attempted suicide.

13. Involvement:
    0   No change from usual level of interest in other people and activities.
    1   Notices a reduction in former interests/activities.
    2   Finds only one or two former interests remain.
    3   Has virtually no interest in formerly pursued activities.

14. Energy/fatigability:
    0   No change in usual level of energy.
    1   Tires more easily than usual.
    2   Makes significant personal effort to initiate or maintain usual daily activities.
    3   Unable to carry out most of usual daily activities due to lack of energy.

15. Psychomotor slowing:
    0   Normal speed of thinking, gesturing, and speaking.
    1   Patient notes slowed thinking, and voice modulation is reduced.
    2   Takes several seconds to respond to most questions; reports slowed thinking.
    3   Is largely unresponsive to most questions without strong encouragement.

16. Psychomotor agitation:
    0   No increased speed or disorganization in thinking or gesturing.
    1   Fidgets, wrings hands and shifts positions often.
    2   Describes impulse to move about and displays motor restlessness.
    3   Unable to stay seated. Paces about with or without permission.

Enter the highest score on either of the 2 psychomotor items (15 or 16 above) _____

Total Score: _____   (Range 0–27)

Source. Reprinted from Rush AJ, Carmody T, Reimitz P-E: "The Inventory of Depressive Symptomatology (IDS): Clinician (IDS-C) and Self-Report (IDS-SR) Ratings of Depressive Symptoms." *International Journal of Methods in Psychiatric Research* 9:45–59, 2000. Used with permission. ©2000, A. John Rush, M.D.

Perceptions of Care (PoC) (Inpatient/Residential Version)

INSTRUCTIONS TO STAFF: Please fill in the Site Code and respondent's Identification Number, one digit in each box. Fill in the Admission Date, Level of Care, Time Point, and Program type using the codes below.

Site code ☐☐☐ ☐☐

Identification Number ☐☐☐☐☐☐☐☐☐

Admission Date ☐☐ ☐☐ ☐☐☐☐
                  Month   Day   Year

Level of care	1=Inpatient	2=Partial/Day Hospital	3=Residential	☐
Time Point	1=Mid-Treatment	2=End of Treatment	3=Post-Discharge Follow-up	☐
Program Type	1=Genral Adult	2=Child/Adolescent	3=Geriatric Dependency	☐
	4=Affective/Mood Disorders	5=Psychotic Disorders	6=Anxiety Disorders/ Trauma	
	7=Substance Abuse/ Chemical Dependency	8=Dual Diagnosis	9=Other	

INSTRUCTIONS TO Respondent: We would like to know your views about the services you received during your stay at this facility. We will use this information to improve our quality of care. Please fill in the circle that corresponds to your answer to each of the questions below. Please answer every question.

1. Did the staff give you information about the rules and policies of the programs?	① Yes	② No	
2. Did the staff give you information about your rights as a patient?	① Yes	② No	
3. Did the staff tell you about the benefits and risks of the medication(s) you are taking?	① Yes	② No	⑨ I am not taking any medication
4. Did the staff explain things in a way you could understand?	① Never	② Sometimes	③ Usually	④ Always
5. Were you involved as much as you wanted in decisions about your treatment?	① Never	② Sometimes	③ Usually	④ Always
6. How much did the staff involve your family in your treatment?	① More than I wanted	② Less than I wanted	③ About the right amount	④ No involvement, which is what I wanted
7. Did the staff listen carefully to you?	① Never	② Sometimes	③ Usually	④ Always
8. Did the staff who treated you work well together as a team?	① Never	② Sometimes	③ Usually	④ Always

Perceptions of Care (PoC) (Inpatient/Residential Version) *(continued)*

	①	②	③	④
9. Did the staff spend enough time with you?	Never	Sometimes	Usually	Always

	①	②	③	④
10. Did the staff treat you with respect and dignity?	Never	Sometimes	Usually	Always

	①	②	③	④
11. Did the staff give you reassurance and support?	Never	Sometimes	Usually	Always

	①	②	③
12. Did the staff review with you the plans for your continued treatment after you leave the program?	Yes	Unsure	No

	①	②	③
13. Were you told whom to contact if you have a problem or crisis after you leave the program?	Yes	Unsure	No

	①	②
14. Did the staff tell you about self-help or support groups?	Yes	No

	①	②
15. Did the staff give you information about how to reduce the chances of a relapse?	Yes	No

	①	②	③	④
16. How much were you helped by the care you received?	Not at all	Somewhat	Quite a bit	A great deal

17. Using any number from 1 to 10, what is your overall rating of the care you received in the program?

① ② ③ ④ ① ⑤ ⑥ ⑦ ⑧ ⑨ ⑩
Worst possible care   Best possible care

	①	②	③
18. Would you recommend this facility to someone else who needed mental health or substance abuse treatment?	Yes	Unsure	No

Please fill in today's date.

☐☐ ☐☐ ☐☐☐☐
Month   Day   Year

20. Please identify staff whom you feel deserve special recognition.

21. Is there anything else you would like to tell us about your care?

YOUR OPINIONS ARE IMPORTANT TO US.

THANK YOU VERY MUCH.

Source. Reprinted from Eisen SV, Idiculla T, Wilcox M, et al.: The Perceptions of Care Survey: A Consumer-Based Measure of Mental Health Treatment Quality. Poster presented at the 15th International Conference on Mental Health Services Research, Washington, DC, April 1, 2002. Used with permission. Copyright McLean Hospital Department of Mental Health Services Research.

Index

*Page numbers printed in **boldface** type refer to tables or figures.*